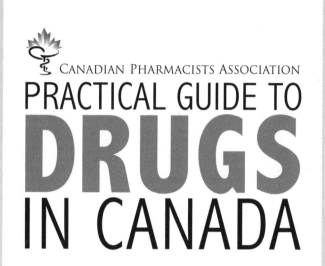

Canadian Pharmacists Association
PRACTICAL GUIDE TO
DRUGS
IN CANADA

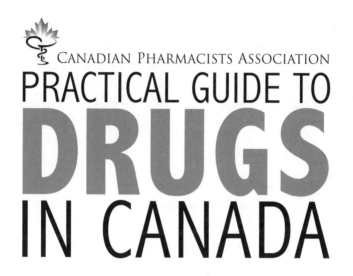

CANADIAN PHARMACISTS ASSOCIATION

PRACTICAL GUIDE TO
DRUGS
IN CANADA

EDITOR-IN-CHIEF
Lalitha Raman-Wilms
BScPHM, PharmD, FCSHP

CANADIAN PHARMACISTS ASSOCIATION

President Ruth Ackerman, BScPhm, MBA, RPh
Executive Director Jeff Poston, PhD, MRPharmS
Senior Director, Digital Publishing Solutions
James de Gaspé Bonar

Editor-in-Chief Carol Repchinsky
Editors Sonal Acharya, Jo-Anne Hutsul, Barbara Jovaisas, Geoff Lewis, Gustavo Paguaga, Hélène Perrier, Marc Riachi, Angela Ross, Louise Welbanks

DORLING KINDERSLEY LIMITED

Editor, Canada Barbara Campbell
Production Controller Erika Pepe
Jacket Designer Mark Cavanagh
Illustrations Karen Cochrane, Tony Graham, Mike Johnson, Kevin Marks, Coral Mula, Lynda Payne, Richard Tibbitts

DORLING KINDERSLEY INDIA

Design Manager Arunesh Talapatra
Senior Designer Mitun Banerjee
Designers Shreya Anand, Niyati Gosain, Zaurin Thoidingjam
Editorial Manager Rohan Sinha
Editors Aditi Ghosh, Ekta Sharma, Himanshi Sharma
DTP Manager Balwant Singh
DTP Designer Anita Yadav, Jaypal Chauhan, Vishal Bhatia

Front/back cover picture credit: © Nathan Griffith/Corbis

First Canadian edition 2011
Copyright © 2011 Dorling Kindersley Limited

Dorling Kindersley is represented in Canada by Tourmaline Editions Inc., 662 King Street West, Suite 304, Toronto, Ontario M5V 1M7

Some of the material in this book has been updated and adapted from the *Guide to Drugs in Canada*, published in Canada in 2009 by Dorling Kindersley Ltd.

The Canadian Pharmacists Association *Practical Guide to Drugs in Canada* provides information on a wide range of medications, drugs, and related subjects. The book is not a substitute for expert medical advice, however, and you are advised always to consult your physician or pharmacist for specific information on personal health matters. Never disregard expert medical advice or delay in seeking medical advice due to information obtained from this book. The naming of any product, treatment, or organization in this book does not imply endorsement by the Editor-in-Chief, the Canadian Pharmacists Association (CPhA), or the publisher, nor does the omission of any such names indicate disapproval. The Editor-in-Chief, the CPhA, and publisher do not accept any legal responsibility for any personal injury or other damage or loss arising from any use or misuse of the information and advice in this book.

Library and Archives Canada Cataloguing in Publication
    Canadian Pharmacists Association practical guide to drugs in Canada : understanding prescription and over-the-counter drug treatments for everyday ailments and diseases / Lalitha Raman-Wilms, editor-in-chief.

ISBN 978-1-55363-155-2

    1. Drugs – Popular works. I. Raman-Wilms, Lalitha II. Canadian Pharmacists Association III. Title: Practical guide to drugs in Canada.

RM301.15.P72 2011   615'.1   C2010-907388-6

Printed and bound in Singapore by Toppan Security Printing Pte. Ltd.
11 12 13 14   10 9 8 7 6 5 4 3 2 1

Discover more at
www.dk.com

TABLE OF CONTENTS

1 UNDERSTANDING AND USING DRUGS

2 COMMON AILMENTS, DISEASES, AND PREVENTIVE HEALTH ISSUES   23

3 PROFILES OF COMMON DRUGS AND SUPPLEMENTS

4 GLOSSARY AND INDEX

DRUG POISONING EMERGENCY GUIDE   197

INTRODUCTION

Every year, Canadians see their doctors for many different health concerns and are often prescribed drugs for their treatment. The tremendous pace of drug research often means multiple options for the treatment of various conditions. With more new drugs, and with many patients taking multiple medications, it is increasingly important to be vigilant to prevent potential adverse drug events. Patients and caregivers need to be more knowledgeable about the specifics of their medication therapies, including what has been prescribed, how the drugs work, expectations from the therapy, possible interactions and side effects, and how to monitor for long-term effectiveness and safety.

The Canadian Pharmacists Association *Practical Guide to Drugs in Canada* aims to provide information that can help in the understanding of common diseases and ailments, and the prescription and over-the-counter drugs used to treat them. The book addresses many common questions asked by patients, related to their conditions and drug therapy, by providing factual information in a clear and easy-to-read format

Part 1 explains what drugs are, how they work in the body, drug use in special risk groups such as children and pregnant women, and information on how best to manage your drug therapy. Part 2 provides an overview of some of the most common ailments, diseases, and preventive health issues for which Canadian doctors treat their patients. Each profile is dedicated to an ailment or disease, and describes what it is, what causes it, what can help the condition, and the types of drugs commonly used in managing the condition. In Part 3, detailed profiles of 100 common drugs are provided. Each drug profile includes information on doses, recommendations on how best to take the medication, available formulations, special precautions, and potential side effects. Also included in this section are profiles of common vitamins, minerals, and supplements. The glossary provides further explanations of terminology used in this book.

Our goal is that by providing you with a better understanding of common conditions and the drugs used to treat them, and alerting you to early signs of adverse drug effects, this guide will help you use your medications safely and effectively. This book is not intended to replace advice provided by your doctor or pharmacist but, rather, to help you to work in partnership with them. Your healthcare professionals can best explain the reasons why any drug has been prescribed for you and how it may affect you.

We hope that this book will enable you to improve your overall health through informed use of drug therapy.

Lalitha Raman-Wilms, PharmD, FCSHP
Editor-in-Chief

Jeff Poston, PhD, MRPharmS
Executive Director
Canadian Pharmacists Association

HOW TO USE THIS BOOK

The *Practical Guide to Drugs in Canada* has been planned and written to provide clear information and useful advice on medications, and the ailments that they treat, in a way that can be readily understood by a non-medical reader. It is intended to complement and reinforce the advice of your doctor and pharmacist.

The information you require, whether on the specific characteristics of an individual drug or on the description and treatment of a particular ailment, can be easily obtained without prior knowledge of the medical names of drugs or drug classification through the index.

How the book is structured
The book is divided into four parts. The first part, **Understanding and Using Drugs**, provides a general introduction to the effects of drugs and gives general advice on practical questions, such as the administration and storage of drugs. The second part, **Common ailments, diseases, and preventive health issues**, includes descriptions of the most common health concerns for which Canadian doctors treat their patients. Part 3, **Profiles of common drugs and supplements**, consists of 100 detailed profiles of commonly prescribed drugs, organized alphabetically by their generic names, along with profiles of common vitamins, minerals, and supplements. Part 4 contains a glossary of drug-related terms and a general index.

1 UNDERSTANDING AND USING DRUGS

The introductory part of the book, Understanding and Using Drugs, gives a grounding in the fundamental principles underlying the medical use of drugs. Covering such topics as classifications of drugs, how drugs work, and how to take them safely, it provides valuable background information that backs up the more detailed descriptions and advice given in Parts 2 and 3. You should read this section before seeking further specific information.

2 COMMON AILMENTS, DISEASES AND PREVENTIVE HEATH ISSUES

Grouped into ailments that affect each body system (for example, heart and circulation) or by major disease grouping (for example, common infections), this part of the book contains information on specific ailments, diseases, and other health issues. A brief explanation of each ailment or concern is given, along with information on what causes and what can help to treat the disease. Discussions on both lifestyle issues and drug treatments are given. Individual drugs used for treatment for each ailment are listed and cross-referenced to Part 3.

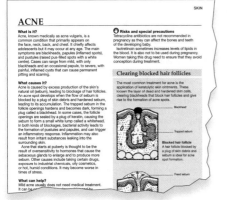

3 PROFILES OF COMMON DRUGS AND SUPPLEMENTS

This contains profiles of 100 drugs, written to a standard format to help you find specific information quickly and easily. Supplementary sections profile vitamins, minerals, and supplements.

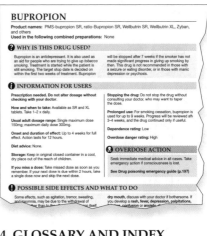

4 GLOSSARY AND INDEX

A glossary of terms explains technical words. The general index enables you to look up references throughout the book.

WHAT ARE DRUGS?

The health professions use the word "drugs" to refer to medicines – substances that can cure or arrest disease, relieve symptoms, ease pain, and provide other benefits. As of 2004, essential vitamins and minerals that may be given to correct deficiency diseases, and herbal products, are classified under Natural Health Products.

Powerful drugs often have marked side effects. Commonly used drugs with less potential to cause harm when used appropriately are sold over-the-counter (OTC) in pharmacies. Some OTC drugs can only be obtained with a pharmacist's consultation, and these are kept behind the pharmacy counter. Other drugs (those that cannot be used safely without medical supervision) require a doctor's prescription. Prescriptions for some drugs may be written by other health professionals as well.

A different use of the word "drugs" refers to those substances on which a person may become dependent. These range from mild stimulants such as caffeine (found in coffee) to powerful agents that alter mood and behaviour. Some addictive drugs have no medical use and cannot be obtained legally.

Where drugs come from
At one time, the only available drugs were substances extracted from plants, or, in some cases, animals. Herbalism, the study and medicinal use of plants, was practised by the Chinese more than 5,000 years ago and is becoming popular in many parts of the world today.

Virtually all the drugs in current use have been developed in the laboratory and are manufactured through various chemical processes. About a quarter of these are derived from plants or other organisms. Most drugs are synthetic chemical copies, but some are still extracted from natural sources. For example, the opioid drugs, including morphine, are made from a species of poppy. The main difference between drugs of plant origin and "herbal medicines" is that drugs have been thoroughly tested to prove that they work and are safe.

Some drugs can now be made through genetic engineering, in which the genes (which control a cell's function) of certain microorganisms are altered, changing the products of cell activity to the desired drug. For example, the hormone insulin can now be manufactured by genetically engineered bacteria. This could eliminate the need to extract insulin from animal pancreas glands, benefiting those people who experience adverse reactions to material derived from animal sources.

Purely synthetic drugs are either modifications of naturally occurring ones, with the aim of increasing effectiveness or safety, or drugs developed after scientific investigation of a disease process with the intention of changing it biochemically.

Developing and marketing new drugs
Pharmaceutical manufacturers find new products in a variety of ways. New drugs are usually developed for one purpose but quite commonly a variant will be found that will be useful for something entirely different.

All new drugs undergo a long, careful test period before they are approved for marketing by the Therapeutic Products Directorate (TPD) (see Testing and approving new drugs). Once approval has been given, the manufacturer can then market the drug under a brand or trade name. Technically, patent protection gives the manufacturer exclusive rights for 20 years, but this protection starts from when the drug is first identified. The time remaining after TPD approval can be much less than 20 years.

When patent protection ends, other manufacturers may produce the drug, although they must use a different brand name or the generic name (see How drugs are classified, facing page).

Testing and approving new drugs
Before a drug is cleared by the TPD, it undergoes a cautious, step-by-step period of testing, often lasting six to ten years. By law, a drug must be both safe and medically effective. Safety is established through various means, including tests on animals and human volunteers. Efficacy is proven through complex tests (including double-blind trials; see Placebo response, p.11) on groups of healthy and ill patients. The testing is done in various research institutions under government-approved procedures.

The approval process also involves weighing a new drug's risks against its benefits. A dangerous drug whose only potential might be the relief of an ordinary headache undoubtedly would not win approval. Yet an equally toxic drug, effective against cancer, might. Medical judgment is an important part of the approval process.

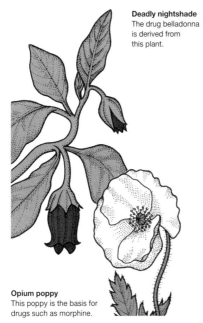

Deadly nightshade
The drug belladonna is derived from this plant.

Opium poppy
This poppy is the basis for drugs such as morphine.

HOW DRUGS ARE CLASSIFIED

The 5,000 or so substances loosely called drugs are described in many ways, depending on whether you are a pharmacologist, a doctor or pharmacist, a drug manufacturer or advertiser, or a federal or provincial regulator. For the purposes of this book, each drug is referred to by its generic or brand name, and is described according to its use, although a chemical description may be added to distinguish one group of drugs from others used to treat the same disorder (for example, benzodiazepine sleeping drugs).

Specific names

All drugs in general use rely on three terms: the generic, brand, and chemical names. The generic name, which is the official medical name for the basic active substance, is chosen by the USAN (US Adopted Name) Council, or is the British accepted name, or is one adopted in one of the world's major pharmacopoeias.

The brand name is chosen by the manufacturer, usually on the basis that it can be easily pronounced, recognized, or remembered. There may be several brands (each by a different manufacturer) containing the same generic substance. Differences between the brands may be slight but may relate to absorption rate, convenience, and digestibility. A drug may be available in generic form, as a brand-name product, or both. Some brand-name products contain several generic drugs. The chemical name is a technical description of the drug, and is not used in this book.

General terms

Drugs may be grouped according to chemical similarity, for example, the benzodiazepines. More often, though, drugs are classified according to use (antihypertensive) or biological effect (diuretic). Most drugs fit into one group, although many have multiple uses and are listed in several categories.

Legal classification

Besides specifying which drugs can be sold over-the-counter and which require a doctor's prescription, provincial and federal statutes and regulations govern the availability of many substances that have an abuse potential. The table below outlines the various categories of controlled drugs in Canada.

Categories of controlled drugs

Narcotic Drugs (Schedule N)	These drugs have a potential for abuse and can lead to serious physical and psychological dependence. They do, however, have accepted medical uses. In general, prescriptions for these agents cannot be renewed and a new prescription is required to be written by a doctor. Health care professionals refer to these agents as opioids. **Examples** Heroin (dispensed in hospitals only), methodone (authorized prescribers only), morphine, codeine, oxycodone, hydromorphone, and meperidine.
Schedule J	All the drugs in this group are restricted and illegal. All have a high potential for abuse and currently do not have an accepted medical use. They cannot be prescribed, except for marijuana; which is available legally for medical use only. **Examples** LSD, dimethyltryptamine (DMT), methylenedioxyamphetamine (MDA).
Controlled Drugs (Schedule G)	These drugs also possess a potential for abuse, and their use may lead to various forms of drug dependence. Records are kept of each doctor's prescribing. Prescriptions for Schedule G drugs can be refilled for a specified number of times. **Examples** Amphetamines, barbiturates, methylphenidate, diethylpropion.
Benzodiazepines and other Targeted Substances	These are drugs that have the potential for dependence and abuse, but are used quite commonly for many illnesses and conditions. A prescription can be issued in writing or can be transmitted by telephone to a pharmacist. Refills must be specified in the original prescription, indicating the specific date of refills and/or interval between refills. **Examples** Diazepam, alprazolam, lorazepam, bromazepam.
Prescription Drugs (Schedule 1 and F drugs)	These are drugs used to treat a wide variety of illnesses requiring a doctor's supervision. A prescription can be issued in writing or can be telephoned to a pharmacist. Repeat prescriptions are allowed. **Examples** Antibiotics, antihypertensive drugs, corticosteroids, antidepressants.
Non-prescription Drugs	These drugs are considered sufficiently safe to be sold over-the-counter in pharmacies and, for some products, in other retail stores. Most non-prescription drug products bear a Drug Identification Number (DIN). Some are available only through a pharmacist's consultation and are kept behind the counter. **Examples** Laxatives, antacids, mild analgesics (including those with a small amount of codeine combined with ASA or acetaminophen), iron tablets, dimenhydrinate, cough and cold preparations.

HOW DRUGS WORK

Thousands of effective drugs are available, and scientific knowledge regarding drugs and their actions has virtually exploded. Today's doctor and pharmacist understand the complexity of drug actions in the body, both beneficial and adverse. As a result of extensive research and clinical experience, the doctor and the pharmacist can now also recognize that some drugs interact harmfully with others, or with certain foods and alcohol.

DRUG ACTIONS

While the exact workings of some drugs are not fully understood, medical science provides clear knowledge as to what most of them do once they enter or are applied to the human body. Drugs serve different purposes: sometimes they cure a disease, sometimes they only alleviate symptoms. Their impact occurs in various parts of the anatomy. Although different drugs act in different ways, their actions generally fall into one of three categories.

Replacing chemicals that are deficient
To function normally, the body requires sufficient levels of certain chemical substances. These include vitamins and minerals, which the body obtains from food. A balanced diet usually supplies what is needed. But when deficiencies occur, various deficiency diseases result, such as scurvy (caused by a lack of vitamin C) and anemia (caused by iron, vitamin B_{12}, or folate deficiency).

Other deficiency diseases arise from a lack of various hormones which are the chemical substances produced by glands. Hormones act as internal "messengers." Diabetes mellitus, hypothyroidism, and Addison's disease all result from deficiencies of different hormones.

Deficiency diseases are treated with drugs that replace the substances that are missing or, in the case of some hormone deficiencies, with animal or synthetic replacements.

Interfering with cell function
Many drugs can change the way cells work by increasing or reducing the normal level of activity. Drugs that increase cell activity by mimicking the effect of the body's natural chemicals at receptor sites are called agonists, while drugs that reduce this activity by blocking receptor sites are called antagonists. Inflammation, for example, is due to the action of certain natural hormones and other chemicals on blood vessels and blood cells. Anti-inflammatory drugs block the action of the inflammatory components or slow their production.

Many such drugs do their work by altering the transmission system by which messages are sent from one part of the body to another. A message – such as to contract a muscle – originates in the brain and travels from nerve cell to nerve cell until it reaches the appropriate muscle. Many drugs can alter this process (see Receptor sites, below).

Acting against invading organisms or abnormal cells
Infectious diseases are caused by viruses, bacteria, protozoa, and fungi invading the body. We now have a wide choice of drugs that destroy these microorganisms, either by halting their multiplication or by killing them directly. Other drugs treat disease by killing abnormal cells produced by the human body – cancer cells, for example.

Receptor sites

Many drugs produce their effects through their action on special sites called receptors on the surface of body cells. Natural body chemicals such as neurotransmitters bind to these sites, initiating a response in the cell. A cell may have many types of receptors, each of which has an affinity for a different chemical in the body.

Drugs may also bind to receptors, either adding to the effect of the body's natural chemicals and enhancing cell response (agonists) or preventing such a chemical from binding to its receptor, and thereby blocking a particular cell response (antagonists).

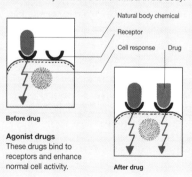

Agonist drugs
These drugs bind to receptors and enhance normal cell activity.

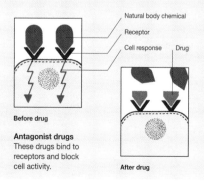

Antagonist drugs
These drugs bind to receptors and block cell activity.

THE EFFECTS OF DRUGS

Before a doctor selects a drug to be used in the treatment of a sick person, he or she carefully weighs the benefits (either a cure or relief of symptoms) and the risks (side effects or interactions).

Reaction time
Some drugs can produce rapid and spectacular relief from the symptoms of disease. Conversely, some drugs take much longer to produce a response. This can add to anxiety unless the individual is informed of the possibility of a delay in the onset of beneficial effects.

Side effects
The side effects of a drug (also referred to as adverse effects or adverse reactions) are its undesired effects. When drugs are taken, they are distributed throughout the body and their effects are unlikely to be restricted just to the organ or tissue we want them to affect. Other parts of the body contain receptor sites like those the drug is targeting. In addition, the drug molecule may fit other, different receptors well enough to activate or block them too.

Some side effects may gradually disappear as the body becomes used to the drug. If they persist, the dose may have to be reduced, or the time between doses may need to be increased. Reducing the dose will often reduce the severity of the side effect for those effects that are dose-related.

People are genetically different and, as a result, their response to drugs differs. For this reason, not everyone suffers the "common" side effects; but, occasionally, a new side effect, due to a rare and unsuspected genetic variation, will be discovered only after the drug has been taken by a large number of people. The phenomenon of these unusual side effects is called idiosyncrasy.

Other side effects that are not dose-related are allergic reactions. These reactions do not usually appear on the first exposure to the drug but on a subsequent occasion. The symptoms are similar to those caused by other allergens and, in extreme cases, may cause anaphylactic shock (see p.200).

Side effects of some drugs can be quite serious. Such drugs are given because they may be the only treatment for an otherwise serious illness or a fatal disease. But all drugs are chemicals, with a potential for producing serious, toxic reactions.

Beneficial vs. adverse effects
In evaluating the risk/benefit ratio of a prescribed drug, the doctor has to weigh the drug's therapeutic benefit against the possible side effects. For example, treating a life-threatening infection with an antibiotic that causes side effects of nausea, headache, and diarrhea would be acceptable, but the same side effects would be unacceptable in an over-the-counter drug for the relief of headaches.

Because some people are more at risk from adverse drug reactions than others (particularly those who have a history of drug allergy), the doctor normally checks whether there is any reason why a certain drug should not be prescribed (see Drug treatment in special risk groups, p.15). The pharmacist should also verify that the individual has no known contraindications to the drug.

Placebo response

The word placebo – Latin for "I will please" – is used to describe any chemically inert substance given as a substitute for a drug. Any benefit gained from taking a placebo occurs because the person taking it believes that it will produce good results.

New drugs are almost always tested against a placebo preparation in clinical trials as a way of assessing the efficacy of a drug before it is marketed. Volunteers are not told whether they have been given the active drug or the placebo. Sometimes the doctor is also unaware of which preparation an individual has been given. This is known as a double-blind trial. In this way, the purely placebo effect can be eliminated and the effectiveness of the drug determined more realistically.

Sometimes the mere taking of a medicine has a psychological effect that produces a beneficial physical response. It is most commonly seen with analgesics, antidepressants, and anti-anxiety drugs.

Dose and response

People respond in different ways to a drug, and often the dose has to be adjusted to account for a person's age, weight, or general health. Children and the elderly usually require different doses than adults.

The dose of any drug should be sufficient to produce a beneficial response but not so great that it will cause excessive adverse effects. The aim of drug treatment is to achieve a concentration of drug in the blood or tissue that lies between the lowest effective level and the maximum safe concentration. This is known as the therapeutic range. For certain drugs the therapeutic range is quite narrow, so the safety/effectiveness margin is small. Other drugs have a much wider therapeutic range.

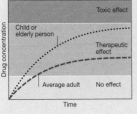

Dosage of drugs with a wide therapeutic range can vary considerably without altering the drug's effect. The effect of some drugs can be greater in children and the elderly.

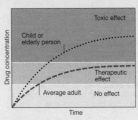

Dosage of drugs with a narrow therapeutic range must be carefully calculated to achieve the desired effect without toxicity. Children or the elderly require adjustment in doses.

DRUG INTERACTIONS

When different drugs are taken together, or when a drug is taken in combination with certain foods or with alcohol, effects different from those when the drug is taken alone may be produced. Sometimes this is beneficial, and doctors sometimes make use of interactions to increase the effectiveness of a treatment.

Other interactions, however, are unwanted and may be harmful. They may occur not only between prescription drugs, but also between prescription and over-the-counter drugs or herbal products. It is important to read warnings on drug labels and tell your doctor and pharmacist if you are taking any preparations – both prescription and over-the-counter, and even herbal or homeopathic remedies.

A drug may interact with another drug or with food or alcohol for a number of reasons (see below). For example, grapefruit juice can have an impact on the effect of some drugs.

Altered absorption

Alcohol and some drugs slow the digestive process that empties the stomach contents into the intestine. This may delay the absorption, and therefore the effect, of another drug. Other drugs may speed the rate at which the stomach empties and may, therefore, increase the rate at which another drug is absorbed and takes effect. Some drugs also combine with another drug or food in the intestine to form a compound that is not absorbed as readily.

Enzyme effects

Some drugs increase the production of enzymes in the liver that break down drugs, while others inhibit or reduce enzyme production. Thus, they affect the rate at which other drugs are activated or inactivated.

Excretion in the urine

A drug may reduce the kidneys' ability to excrete another drug, raising the drug level in the blood and increasing its effect.

Receptor effects

Drugs that act on the same receptor sites (see p.10) sometimes add to each other's effect on the body, or compete with each other in occupying certain receptor sites. For example, naloxone blocks receptors used by opioid drugs, thereby helping to reverse the effects of opioid overdose.

Similar or opposite effects

Drugs that produce similar effects (but act on different receptors) add to each others' actions. Often, lower doses are possible as a result, with fewer side effects. This is common practice in the treatment of high blood pressure and diabetes. Antibiotics are given together as the infecting organisms are less likely to develop resistance to the drugs. Drugs with antagonistic effects reduce the useful activity of one or both drugs. For example, some antidepressants oppose the effects of anticonvulsants.

Reduced protein binding

Some drugs circulate around the body in the bloodstream with a proportion of the drug attached to the proteins of the blood plasma. The amount of drug attached to the plasma proteins is inactive. If another drug is taken, some of the second drug may also bind to the plasma proteins and displace the first drug; more of the first drug is then active in the body.

Interaction between protein-bound drugs

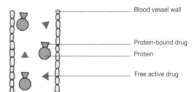

- Blood vessel wall
- Protein-bound drug
- Protein
- Free active drug

Protein-bound drugs taken alone
Drug molecules that are bound to proteins in the blood are unable to pass into body tissues. Only free drug molecules are active.

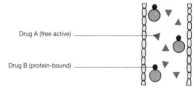

Drug A (free active)

Drug B (protein-bound)

Taken with another protein-bound drug
If a drug (B) with a greater ability to bind with proteins is also taken, drug (A) is displaced, increasing the amount of active drug.

Examples of important interactions

Adverse interactions between drugs may vary from a simple blocking of a drug's beneficial effect to a serious reaction between two drugs that may be life-threatening. Some of the more serious adverse interactions occur between the following:

Drugs that depress the central nervous system (opioids, sedating antihistamines, sleeping drugs, and alcohol). The effects of two or more of these drugs together may be additive, causing dangerous oversedation.

Drugs that lower blood sugar levels and such drugs as sulfonamides and alcohol. The drug interaction increases the effect of blood sugar-lowering drugs, thus further depressing blood sugar levels.

Oral anticoagulants and other drugs, particularly ASA and antibiotics. As these drugs may increase the tendency to bleed, it is essential to check the effects in every case.

Monoamine oxidase inhibitors (MAOIs). Many drugs and foods can produce a severe increase in blood pressure when taken with MAOIs. Such drugs include amphetamines and decongestants; foods include cheese, herring, chocolate, red wine, and beer. Some of the newer MAOIs, however, are much less likely to interact with food and drugs.

METHODS OF ADMINISTRATION

The majority of drugs must be absorbed into the bloodstream in order for them to reach the site where their effects are needed. The method of administering a drug determines the route it takes to get into the bloodstream and the speed at which it is absorbed into the blood.

When a drug is meant to enter the bloodstream it is usually administered in one of the following ways: through the mouth or rectum, by injection, or by inhalation. Drugs that are implanted under the skin or enclosed in a skin patch also enter the bloodstream.

When it is unnecessary or undesirable for a drug to enter the bloodstream in large amounts, it may be applied topically so that its effect is limited mainly to the site of the disorder, such as the surface of the skin or mucous membranes. Drugs are administered topically in a variety of preparations, including creams, sprays, drops, and suppositories. Most inhaled drugs also have a local effect on the respiratory tract.

Very often, a particular drug may be available in different forms. Many drugs are available both as tablets and injectable liquid. The choice between a tablet and an injection depends on a number of factors, including the severity of the illness, the urgency with which the drug effect is needed, the part of the body requiring treatment, and the patient's general state of health, in particular his or her ability to swallow.

ADMINISTRATION BY MOUTH

Giving drugs by mouth is the most common method of administration. Most of the drugs that are given by mouth are absorbed into the bloodstream through the walls of the intestine. The speed at which the drug is absorbed and the amount of active drug that is available for use depend on several factors, including the form in which the drug is given (for example, as a tablet or a liquid) and whether it is taken with food or on an empty stomach. If a drug is taken when the stomach is empty, it may act more quickly than a drug that is taken after a meal when the stomach is full.

Some drugs (like antacids, which neutralize stomach acidity) are taken by mouth to produce a direct effect in the stomach or digestive tract.

In-mouth administration
Products are available that are placed in the mouth but not swallowed. They are absorbed quickly into the bloodstream through the lining of the mouth, which has a rich supply of blood vessels. Sublingual tablets are placed under the tongue, wafers are placed on the tongue, and buccal tablets are placed in the pouch between the cheek and teeth.

How drugs pass through the body

Most drugs taken by mouth reach the bloodstream by absorption through the wall of the small intestine. Blood vessels supplying the intestine then carry the drug to the liver, where it may be broken down into a form that can be used by the body. The drug (or its breakdown product) then enters the general circulation, which carries it around the body. It may pass back into the intestine before being reabsorbed into the bloodstream. Some drugs are rapidly excreted via the kidneys; others may build up in fatty tissues in the body.

Certain insoluble drugs cannot be absorbed through the intestinal wall and pass through the digestive tract unchanged. These drugs are useful for treating bowel disorders, but if they are intended to have systemic effects elsewhere they must be given by intravenous injection.

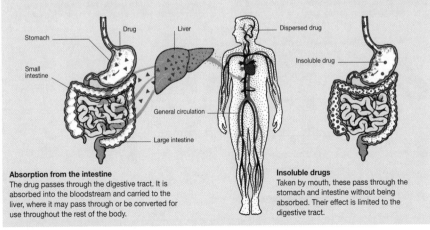

Absorption from the intestine
The drug passes through the digestive tract. It is absorbed into the bloodstream and carried to the liver, where it may pass through or be converted for use throughout the rest of the body.

Insoluble drugs
Taken by mouth, these pass through the stomach and intestine without being absorbed. Their effect is limited to the digestive tract.

RECTAL ADMINISTRATION

Drugs intended to have a systemic effect may be given in the form of suppositories inserted into the rectum, from where they are absorbed into the bloodstream. This method may be used to give drugs that might be destroyed by the stomach's digestive juices, or to administer drugs to people who cannot take medication by mouth, such as those who are suffering from nausea and vomiting.

Drugs may also be given rectally for local effect, either as suppositories (to relieve hemorrhoids) or as enemas (for ulcerative colitis).

INHALATION

Drugs may be inhaled to produce a systemic effect or a direct local effect on the respiratory tract.

Gases to produce general anesthesia are administered by inhalation and are absorbed into the bloodstream through the lungs, producing a general effect on the body, particularly the brain.

Bronchodilators, used to treat certain types of asthma, emphysema, and bronchitis, are a common example of drugs administered by inhalation for their direct effect on the respiratory tract, although some of the active drug also reaches the bloodstream.

ADMINISTRATION BY INJECTION

Drugs may be injected into the body to produce a systemic effect. One reason for injecting drugs is the rapid response that follows. Other circumstances that call for injection are when: a person is intolerant to the drug when taken by mouth; the drug would be destroyed by the stomach's digestive juices (insulin, for example); or the drug cannot pass through the intestinal walls into the bloodstream. Drug injections may also be given to produce a local effect, as is often done to relieve the pain of arthritis.

The three most common methods of injection are intramuscular (into a muscle), intravenous (into a vein), and subcutaneous (under the surface of the skin).

TOPICAL APPLICATION

In treating localized disorders such as skin infections and nasal congestion, it is often preferable to prescribe drugs in a form that has a topical, or localized, rather than a systemic effect. The reason is that it is much easier to control the effects of drugs administered locally and to ensure that they produce the maximum benefit with minimum side effects.

Topical preparations are available in a variety of forms, from skin creams, ointments, and lotions to nasal sprays, ear and eye drops, bladder irrigations, and vaginal suppositories. It is important when using topical preparations to follow instructions carefully, avoiding a higher dose than recommended or application for longer than necessary.

Slow-release and modified-release preparations

Some disorders can be treated with specially formulated preparations that can release the active drug slowly. Such preparations may be beneficial when it is inconvenient for a person to visit the doctor regularly, or when only small amounts of the drug need to be released into the body.

Slow release of drugs can be achieved by depot injections, transdermal patches, capsules and tablets, and implants. Modified-release tablets and capsules are a more advanced version in which release of the active ingredient is related to time.

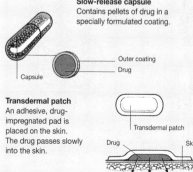

Slow-release capsule
Contains pellets of drug in a specially formulated coating.

Capsule
Outer coating
Drug

Transdermal patch
An adhesive, drug-impregnated pad is placed on the skin. The drug passes slowly into the skin.

Transdermal patch
Drug
Skin

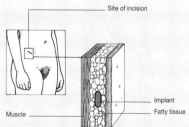

Site of incision

Muscle
Implant
Fatty tissue

Implants
A pellet containing the drug is implanted under the skin. By this rarely used method, a drug (usually a hormone) is slowly released into the bloodstream over a period of months.

DRUG TREATMENT IN SPECIAL RISK GROUPS

Different people tend to respond in different ways to drug treatment. Taking the same drug, one person may suffer adverse effects while another does not. However, doctors know that certain people are always more at risk from adverse effects when they take drugs; the reason is that in those people the body handles drugs differently, or the drug has an atypical effect. Those people at special risk include infants and children, women who are pregnant or breast-feeding, the elderly, and people with long-term medical conditions, especially those who have impaired liver or kidney function. Also at risk are those who are already taking regular medication and who may risk complications from a drug interaction when they take another drug (see p.12).

When doctors prescribe drugs for people at special risk, they take extra care to select appropriate medication, adjust dosages, and closely monitor the effects of treatment. If you think you may be at special risk, be sure to tell your doctor or pharmacist before taking any prescription or over-the-counter drugs.

INFANTS AND CHILDREN

Infants and children need a lower dosage of drugs than adults because of their relatively low body weight. However, children cannot simply be given a proportion of an adult dose as if they were small adults. Dosages need to be calculated in a more complex way, taking into account the child's age and weight, along with differences in body composition and the distribution and amount of body fat, and the state of development and function of organs such as the liver and kidneys at different ages. While newborn babies often have to be given very small doses of drugs, older children may need relatively large doses of some drugs compared to the adult dosage.

The liver
The liver's enzyme systems are not fully developed when a baby is born. This means that drugs are not broken down as rapidly, and may reach dangerously high concentrations in the baby's body. For this reason, many drugs are not prescribed for babies or are given in very reduced doses. In older children, because the liver is relatively large compared to the rest of the body, some drugs may need to be given in proportionately higher doses.

Liver ——

Kidneys ——

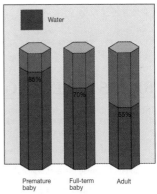

Water

85%

70%

55%

Premature baby   Full-term baby   Adult

The kidneys
During the first six months, a baby's kidneys are unable to excrete drugs as efficiently as an adult's kidneys. This may lead to a dangerously high concentration of a drug in the blood. The dose of certain drugs may therefore need to be reduced. Between one and two years of age, kidney function improves, and higher doses of some drugs may then be needed.

Body composition
The proportion of water in the body of a premature baby is about 85 percent of its body weight, that of a full-term baby is 70 percent, and that of an adult is only 55 percent. This means that drugs that stay in the body water will not be as concentrated in an infant's body as in an adult's, unless a higher dose relative to body weight is given.

PREGNANT WOMEN

Care is needed during pregnancy to protect the developing fetus. Drugs taken by the mother can cross the placenta and enter the baby's bloodstream. With certain drugs, and at certain stages of pregnancy, there is a risk of developmental abnormalities, retarded growth, or post-delivery problems affecting the newborn baby. In addition, some drugs may affect the health of the mother during pregnancy.

Many drugs are known to have adverse effects during pregnancy; others are known to be safe, but in a large number of cases there is no firm evidence to decide on risk or safety. If you are pregnant or trying to conceive, consult your doctor before taking any prescribed or over-the-counter medication. Your doctor will assess the potential benefits and risks to decide whether or not a drug should be taken. This is particularly important if you need to take medication regularly for a chronic condition such as epilepsy, high blood pressure, or diabetes.

Drugs such as marijuana, nicotine, and alcohol should be avoided during pregnancy. A high daily intake of caffeine should be reduced if possible.

Drugs and the stages of pregnancy
Pregnancy is divided into three three-month stages called trimesters. Depending on the trimester in which they are taken, drugs can have different effects on the mother, the fetus, or both. Some drugs may be considered safe during one trimester, but not during another. Doctors, therefore, often need to substitute one medication for another given during the course of pregnancy and/or labour.

The trimesters of pregnancy

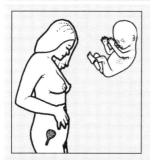

First trimester
During the first three months of pregnancy – the most critical period – drugs may affect the development of fetal organs, leading to congenital malformations. Very severe defects may result in miscarriage.

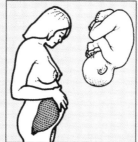

Second trimester
From the fourth to the sixth month some drugs may retard the growth of the fetus. This may also result in a low birth weight. Other drugs may affect the development of the nervous system.

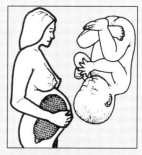

Third trimester
During the last three months of pregnancy, major risks include breathing difficulties in the newborn baby. Some drugs may also affect labour, causing it to be premature, delayed, or prolonged.

BREAST-FEEDING

The milk-producing glands in the breast are surrounded by a network of fine blood vessels. Small molecules of substances such as drugs can pass from the blood into the milk. This means that a breast-fed baby will receive small doses of whatever drugs the mother is taking. In many cases this is not a problem, because the amount of drug that passes into the milk is too small to have any significant effect on the baby. However, some drugs can produce unwanted effects on the baby. Antibiotics may sensitize the infant and consequently prevent their use later in life. Sedative drugs may make the baby drowsy and cause feeding problems. Moreover, some drugs may reduce the amount of milk produced by the mother.

Doctors usually advise breast-feeding women to take only essential drugs. When a mother needs to take regular medication while breast-feeding, her baby may also need to be closely monitored for possible adverse effects.

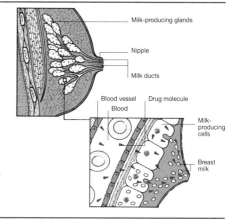

Milk-producing glands

Nipple

Milk ducts

Blood vessel   Drug molecule
Blood

Milk-producing cells

Breast milk

THE ELDERLY

Older people are particularly at risk when taking drugs. This is partly due to the physical changes associated with aging, and partly because many elderly people need to take several different drugs at the same time. They may also be at risk because they may be unable to manage their treatment properly, or they may lack the information to do so.

Physical changes

Elderly people have a greater risk of accumulating drugs in their body tissues because the liver is less efficient at breaking drugs down and the kidneys are less efficient at excreting them. Because of this, in some cases a smaller dose may be needed to produce a therapeutic effect without the side effects. (See also Liver and kidney disease, below.)

Older people usually have more chronic conditions and therefore take more drugs than younger people – many take three or more drugs at the same time. Apart from increasing the number of drugs in their systems, adverse drug interactions (see p.12) are more likely.

As people grow older, some parts of the body, such as the brain and nervous system, become more sensitive to drugs, thus increasing the likelihood of adverse reactions from drugs acting on those sites. A similar problem may occur due to changes in the body's ratio of body fat. Accordingly, doctors prescribe more carefully for older people, especially those with disorders that are likely to correct themselves in time.

Incorrect use of drugs

Elderly people often suffer harmful effects from their drug treatment when they may fail to take their medication regularly or correctly. This may happen because they have been misinformed about how to take it or received vague instructions. Problems arise sometimes because the elderly person cannot remember whether he or she has taken the drug and takes a double dose (see Exceeding the dose, p.22). Problems may also occur because the person is confused; this is not necessarily due to age or illness,

but can arise as a result of drug treatment, especially if an elderly person is taking a number of different drugs or a sedative.

Prescriptions for the elderly should be clearly and fully labelled, and/or information about the drug and its use should be provided either for the individual or for the person taking care of him or her. When appropriate, containers with memory aids should be used to dispense the medication in single doses.

Elderly people often find it difficult to swallow medicine in capsule or tablet form; they should always take capsules or tablets with a full glass or cup of liquid. A liquid medicine may be prescribed instead.

Effect of drugs that act on the brain

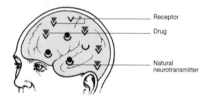

In young people
There are plenty of receptors to take up the drug as well as natural neurotransmitters.

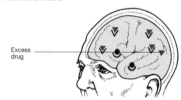

In older people
There are fewer receptors so that even a reduced drug dose may be excessive.

LIVER AND KIDNEY DISEASE

Long-term illness affects the way in which people respond to drugs. This is especially true of liver and kidney problems. The liver alters the chemical structure of many drugs that enter the body (see How drugs pass through the body, p.13) by breaking them down into simpler substances, while the kidneys excrete drugs in the urine. If the effectiveness of the liver or kidneys is reduced by illness, the action of drugs on the individual can be significantly altered. In most cases, people with liver or kidney disease will be prescribed a smaller number of drugs and lower doses. In addition, certain drugs may, in rare cases, damage the liver or kidneys. A doctor may be reluctant to prescribe such a drug to someone with already reduced liver or kidney function in order to avoid the risk of further damage.

Drugs and liver disease

Normally, drugs are processed by the liver before being excreted by the kidneys. Severe liver diseases, such as

cirrhosis and hepatitis, affect the way the body breaks down drugs, because the liver cannot process sufficient amounts of the drug. This can lead to a dangerous accumulation of certain drugs in the body. People suffering from these diseases should consult their doctor before taking any medication (including over-the-counter drugs) or alcohol. Some drugs must be avoided completely, since they could cause coma in someone with liver damage.

Drugs and kidney disease

People with poor kidney function are at risk from drug side effects. There are two reasons for this. First, drugs build up in the system because smaller amounts are excreted in urine. Second, kidney disease can cause protein loss through the urine, which lowers the level of protein in the blood. Some drugs bind to blood proteins, and if there are fewer protein molecules, a greater proportion of drug becomes free and active in the body.

MANAGING YOUR DRUG TREATMENT

A prescribed drug does not automatically produce a beneficial response. For a drug to have maximum benefit, it must be taken as directed by a doctor, pharmacist, or manufacturer. It is estimated that two out of every five people for whom a drug is prescribed do not take it properly, if at all. The reasons include failure to understand or remember instructions, fear of adverse reactions, and lack of motivation, often arising from the disappearance of symptoms.

It is your responsibility to take a prescribed drug at the correct time, and in the manner stipulated. To do this, you need to know where to obtain information about the drug (see Questioning your doctor, p.19) and to make certain that you fully understand the instructions.

The following pages describe the practical aspects of drug treatment, from obtaining a prescription and buying over-the-counter drugs to storing drugs and disposing of old medications safely. Problems caused by mismanaging drug treatment – overdosing, underdosing, or stopping the drug altogether – and long-term drug treatment are dealt with on pp.20–22. Information regarding specific drugs is given in Part 3.

OVER-THE-COUNTER DRUGS

Over-the-counter drugs, also called nonprescription, are those for which a prescription is not required. All are available from pharmacies (many only from pharmacies).

It is generally accepted that over-the-counter drugs are suitable for self-treatment and are unlikely to produce serious adverse reactions if taken as directed. But, as with all medicines, they can be harmful if they are misused. The same precautions should be taken when using any over-the-counter medicine as when using a drug prescribed by your doctor.

Using over-the-counter drugs
A number of minor ailments and problems, ranging from coughs and colds to minor cuts and bruises, can be adequately dealt with by taking or using over-the-counter medicines. However, when using these treatments, be sure to read the directions on the label and follow them carefully, particularly those advising on dosage and under what circumstances a doctor should be consulted. Most over-the-counter drugs are clearly labelled. They may warn of conditions under which the drug should not be taken, or advise you to consult a doctor if symptoms persist.

The pharmacist can usually recommend a suitable over-the-counter drug for your complaint, and can determine when an over-the-counter drug may not be effective or if self-treatment or prolonged treatment is not advisable. Always inform your pharmacist if you are taking any other drugs for another illness or condition.

It is important to speak to your doctor before buying over-the-counter drugs for children. Some symptoms, such as diarrhea in young children, should be treated only by a doctor since they may be caused by a serious condition.

PRESCRIPTION DRUGS

Drugs prescribed by a doctor are not necessarily "stronger" or more likely to have side effects than those you can buy without prescription. Indeed, doctors often prescribe drugs that are also available over-the-counter (OTC). Drugs that are available only on prescription are drugs whose safe use is difficult to ensure without medical supervision.

A prescribed drug treatment is usually started at the normal dosage for the disorder being treated. The dosage may later be adjusted (lowered or increased) if the drug is not producing the desired effect or if you experience adverse side effects. The doctor may also decide to switch to an alternative drug that may be more effective at treating the disorder.

Prescribing generic and brand-name drugs
When writing a prescription for a drug, the doctor often has a choice between a generic and a brand-name product. Although the active ingredient is the same, two versions of the same drug may look different and may act in slightly different ways due to different formulations. Generic drugs are often cheaper than brand-name products. For this reason, certain brand-name products are not available on certain drug plans. These are factors that a doctor must consider when writing a prescription.

Community pharmacists usually need to consider which drug is covered on your plan and may consult with you in substituting a generic name drug. Doctors may indicate "no substitution" on the prescription if they feel that the brand name product would be most suitable for treatment.

If you are prescribed a generic drug, the pharmacist can dispense whatever generic version of this drug is available. This means that your regular medication may vary in appearance each time you renew your prescription; always check with your pharmacist to reassure yourself that it is the correct drug.

Hospital pharmacies often dispense only generic versions of certain drugs. If your medication looks different, check with the pharmacist that you are receiving the correct drug.

Your prescription
Prescriptions usually have the same information. Your name and address will be listed, along with the name of the medication, the dose or strength, how much to take (the number of tablets or amount of liquid), and how frequently it should be taken. The prescription informs the pharmacist of the amount of the drug to be dispensed, and the information that should be put on the label.

In some cases, your doctor will indicate the number of refills of the medication that are allowed without having to obtain a repeat prescription. If treatment needs to be continued after the refills have been exhausted, usually you will have to see your doctor again, who will re-evaluate your situation.

Often, you will receive a Patient Information Leaflet, which gives details about the drug, its side effects, when not to use it, and so on. Compare this and the label on your medication with your doctor's instructions, and ask the pharmacist about any differences.

It is advisable for you to obtain all of your prescription drugs from the same pharmacy, so that your pharmacist can keep supplies of any unusual drugs you may be taking. If you need to take drugs that are prescribed by more than one doctor, or by your dentist, the pharmacist is able to call attention to possible harmful interactions. Doctors do ask if you are taking other medicines before prescribing, but your regular pharmacist provides valuable additional advice.

Questioning your doctor

Countless surveys unmistakably point to lack of information as the most common reason for failure of drug treatment. Be certain you understand the instructions for a drug before leaving your doctor's office, and don't leave with any questions unanswered.

Make a list of the questions you may want to ask before your visit, and make notes while you are there; it is easy to forget some of the instructions your doctor gives you during a consultation. You can check your instructions from the doctor with the pharmacist.

Your doctor should tell you the generic or brand name of the drug, exactly what condition or symptom it has been prescribed to treat, what dose you should take, how often to take it, and whether the prescription should be repeated. Be certain you

Prescription terms	
ac before meals	**qid** four times a day
ad lib freely	**s** without
AM morning	**sr** slow release
bid twice a day	**stat** at once
c with	**tab** tablet
cap capsule	**tid** three times a day
cc cubic centimetre	**top** apply topically
ext for external use	**ud** use as directed
gtt drops	**x** times
mg milligrams	
ml millilitres	
nocte at night	
pc after meals	
PM evening	
po by mouth	
prn as needed	

understand the instructions about how and when to take the drug (see also Taking your medication, below) and how long the treatment should last; some medications cause harmful effects if you stop taking them abruptly, or do not have beneficial effects unless the full course of drug treatment is completed.

Risks and special precautions

All drugs have side effects (see The effects of drugs, p.11). Ask your doctor what these are and what you should do if they occur. Also ask if there are any foods or other drugs you should avoid during treatment, whether the drug can cause drowsiness, and if you can drink alcohol while taking the drug.

TAKING YOUR MEDICATION

Among the most important aspects of managing your drug treatment is knowing how often the drug is to be taken. Should it be taken on an empty stomach? With food? Mixed with something? Specific instructions on such points are given in the individual drug profiles in Part 3.

When to take your drugs

Certain drugs, such as analgesics and drugs for migraine, are taken only as necessary, when warning symptoms occur. Others are meant to be taken regularly at specified intervals. The prescription or label instructions can be confusing, however. For instance, does four times a day mean once every six hours out of 24 – at 8 am, 2 pm, 8 pm, and 2 am? Or does it mean take at four equal intervals during waking hours – morning, lunchtime, late afternoon, and bedtime? Always ask your doctor or pharmacist for precise directions.

The actual time of day that you take a drug is generally flexible, so you can normally schedule your doses to fit your daily routine. This has the additional advantage of making it easier for you to remember to take your drugs. If the drug needs to be taken with

food, you would probably decide to take it with your breakfast, lunch, and dinner. Try to take your dose at the recommended intervals; if you take them too close together, the risk of side effects occurring is increased.

If you are taking several different drugs, ask your doctor or pharmacist if they can be taken together, or if they must be taken at different times in order to avoid any side effects or reduced effectiveness caused by an interaction between them.

How to take your drugs

If your prescription specifies taking your drug with food – or without food – it is very important to follow this instruction if you are to get the maximum benefit from your treatment.

Certain drugs should be taken on an empty stomach (usually one hour before or two hours after eating) so they will be absorbed more quickly into the bloodstream; others, such as ibuprofen, should be taken with food to avoid stomach irritation. Similarly, some foods need to be avoided. Milk and dairy products may inhibit the absorption of some drugs; fruit juices can break down certain antibacterial drugs in the stomach and thereby decrease their effectiveness;

TAKING YOUR MEDICATION continued

alcohol is best avoided with many drugs. (See also Drug interactions, p.12.) In some cases, you may be advised to eat foods rich in certain vitamins or minerals. But do not take supplements unless you are advised to do so by your doctor. If you use any of the salt substitutes (all of which contain potassium), remember to tell your doctor.

Tips on taking medicines
Whenever possible, take capsules and tablets with water while standing up or in an upright sitting position. This prevents them from becoming stuck in the esophagus, which can delay the action of the drug and may damage the esophagus.

When taking liquids, measure the dose carefully using a 5ml measuring spoon, dropper, children's medicine spoon, or oral syringe. Shake the bottle before measuring, or you may take improper dosages if the active substance has risen to the top or settled at the bottom of the bottle. A drink of cold water taken immediately before and after an unpleasantly flavoured medicine will often hide the taste.

Giving medicines to children

Some over-the-counter medicines are specifically prepared for children; others have labels that give both adult's and children's dosages. For the purposes of drug labelling, anyone 12 years of age or under is considered a child.

When giving over-the-counter medicines to children, always follow the instructions on the label exactly and never exceed the dosage recommended for a child. Never give a child even a small amount of a medicine intended for adult use without the advice of your doctor.

Do not deceive your child about the medicine, such as pretending that tablets are candies or that liquid medicines are soft drinks. Never leave a child's medicine within reach; he or she may be tempted to take an extra dose in order to hasten recovery.

MISSED DOSES

Missing a dose of your medication is usually not a cause for concern, but it can be a problem if you are taking the drug as part of a regular course of treatment. Ask your pharmacist how to deal with missed doses. For advice on individual drugs, consult the drug profile in Part 3.

When you miss a dose, the amount of drug in your body is lowered, and the effect of the drug may be diminished. You may therefore have to take other steps to avoid unwanted consequences. For example, if you forget to take an oral contraceptive pill, take the pill as soon as you remember, and for the next week use another form of contraception.

If you miss more than one dose of any drug you are taking regularly, you should tell your doctor. Missed doses are especially important with insulin and drugs for epilepsy.

Tell your doctor if you frequently forget to take your medication. He or she may be able to simplify your treatment schedule by prescribing a preparation

that contains several drugs, or a preparation that releases the drug slowly into the body over time, and only needs to be taken once or twice daily.

Remembering your medication

If you take several different drugs, it is useful to draw up a chart to remind yourself of when each drug should be taken. This will also help anyone who looks after you, or a doctor who is unfamiliar with your treatment.

Using a pill box is a handy way of making sure you take your tablets in the right order. There is a strip for each day of the week, and compartments for morning, afternoon, evening, and bedtime. Ask your pharmacist about this and other techniques to help you with organizing your medications.

ENDING DRUG TREATMENT

Ending drug treatment too soon can be a problem when you are taking a regular course of drugs. With medication that you take as required, you can stop treatment as soon as you feel better.

Advice on stopping individual drugs is given in the drug profiles in Part 3. Some general guidelines for ending drug treatment are given below.

Risks of stopping too soon
Suddenly stopping drug treatment before completing your course of medication may cause the original condition to recur or lead to other complications, including withdrawal symptoms. Even if you feel better, do not stop taking the drug unless your doctor advises you to do so.

Side effects
Do not stop taking a medication simply because it produces unpleasant side effects. Many adverse effects disappear or become bearable after a while. But if they do not, check with your doctor, who may want to reduce the dosage of the drug gradually or, alternatively, substitute another drug that does not produce the same side effects.

Gradual reduction
Some medications need to be reduced gradually to prevent a reaction when treatment ends. This is the case with long-term corticosteroid therapy as well as with dependence-inducing drugs.

STORING DRUGS

Once you have completed a medically directed course of treatment, you should not keep any unused drugs; take these to the pharmacist who will properly dispose of them for you. But most families will want to keep a supply of remedies for indigestion, headaches, or colds, for example. Such medicines should not be used if they show any signs of deterioration, or if their period of effectiveness has expired (see When to dispose of drugs, below).

How to store drugs
All drugs, including cough medicines, iron tablets, and oral contraceptives, should be kept out of the reach of children – a locked wall cabinet is ideal. The majority of drugs should be stored in a cool, dry place out of direct sunlight, even those in plastic containers or tinted glass. A few drugs should be stored in the refrigerator. Storage information for individual drugs is given in the drug profiles in Part 3.

Keep all drugs in the container in which you purchased them. If it is necessary to put them into other containers, such as special containers designed for the elderly, make sure you keep the original container with the label and any separate instructions for future reference.

Make certain that caps and lids are replaced and tightly closed after use; loose caps may leak and spill, or hasten deterioration of the drug.

When to dispose of drugs

Old drugs should be returned to the pharmacist for proper disposal. Always dispose of:

- Any drug that is past its expiry date.

- ASA and acetaminophen tablets that smell of vinegar.

- Tablets that are chipped, cracked, or discoloured, and capsules that have softened, cracked, or stuck together.

- Liquids that have thickened or discoloured, or that taste or smell different in any way from the original product.

- Tubes that are cracked, leaky, or hard.

- Ointments and creams that have changed odour, or changed appearance by discolouring, hardening, or separating.

- Any liquid needing refrigeration that has been kept for over two weeks.

LONG-TERM DRUG TREATMENT

People who suffer from chronic or recurrent disorders often need prolonged or lifelong treatment with drugs to control symptoms or prevent complications. Antihypertensive drugs for high blood pressure and insulin or oral antidiabetic drugs for diabetes mellitus are familiar examples. Long-term drug treatment may also be necessary to cure some diseases, such as tuberculosis, or to prevent a condition, such as malaria, from occurring and will have to be taken for as long as the individual is at risk.

Possible adverse effects
You may worry that taking a drug for a long period will reduce its effectiveness or that you will become dependent on it. However, most medicines continue to have the same effect indefinitely without necessitating an increase in dosage or change in drug. Similarly, for most drugs, taking a drug for more than a few weeks does not normally create dependence.

Changing drug treatment
There are a number of reasons for changing a drug. You may have had an adverse reaction, an improved preparation may have become available, or you may have new and different health concerns. If you wish to become pregnant, for example, you should ask your doctor right away if there is a need to switch to a different medication. If you contract a new illness, for which an additional drug is prescribed, your regular treatment may be altered.

Adjusting to long-term treatment
Establishing a daily routine for taking your medication will reduce the risk of a missed dose. Usually you should not stop taking your medication, even if there are side effects, without consulting your doctor. If you fear possible side effects from the drug, discuss this with your doctor.

Do not stop treatment because you feel well or your symptoms disappear. This can be dangerous; some diseases, like high blood pressure, have no noticeable symptoms, and others may recur or become worse. If you are uncertain about why you have to keep taking a drug, ask your doctor.

Only a few drugs require an alteration in habits, such as avoiding alcohol or certain foods. If you require a drug that makes you drowsy, do not drive a car or operate dangerous equipment.

If you are taking a drug that should not be stopped suddenly or that may interact with other drugs, carry a warning card or a bracelet such as MedicAlert® in case you need emergency medical treatment.

Monitoring treatment
Visit your doctor for periodic check-ups while on long-term treatment. He or she will check your underlying condition, monitor any adverse effects of treatment, and possibly measure levels of the drug in your blood. With insulin, you need to monitor blood levels each day.

If a drug is known to cause damage to an organ, tests may be done to check the function of the organ.

EXCEEDING THE DOSE

Most people associate drug overdoses with attempts at suicide or abuse of street drugs. However, drug overdoses can also occur among people who deliberately or inadvertently exceed the stated dose of a prescribed drug.

A single extra dose of most drugs is unlikely to be a cause for concern. Overdose of some drugs, however, is potentially dangerous even when the dose has been exceeded by only a small amount. Each of the drug profiles in Part 3 gives detailed information on the consequences of exceeding the dose, symptoms to look out for, and what to do. Each drug has an overdose danger rating of low, medium, or high to indicate the urgency with which medical help should be sought.

Taking an extra dose

People sometimes exceed the stated dose in the mistaken belief that by increasing dosage they will speed their cure, or by miscalculating the amount or forgetting that the dose has already been taken.

In some cases symptoms of poisoning may result, especially when liver or kidney function is impaired, causing the drug to build up in the blood. Symptoms of excessive intake may not be apparent for many days.

When and how to get help

If you honestly cannot remember whether or not you have taken your medicine, assume that you have missed the dose and follow the advice given in the individual drug profiles in Part 3 of this book. If you cannot find your drug listed, consult your doctor. Make a note to use some system in the future that will help you remember to take your medicine.

If you are looking after an elderly person on regular drug treatment who suddenly develops unusual symptoms such as confusion, drowsiness, or unsteadiness, consider the possibility of an inadvertent drug overdose and consult the doctor as soon as possible.

Deliberate overdose

Sometimes an excessive amount of a drug is taken with the intention of causing harm or even as a suicide attempt. Whether or not you think a dangerous amount of a drug has been taken, deliberate overdoses of this kind should always be brought to the attention of your doctor. Not only is it necessary to ensure that no physical harm has occurred as a result of the overdose, but the psychological condition of a person who takes such action should be assessed, especially when the person is elderly, has a physical illness, or is known to suffer from depression.

The effect of drug overdose on the body

The effect of drug overdose on the body depends on the type of drug involved. Some drugs produce an exaggeration of the desired effect, for instance overdose of tranquillizers leads to unconciousness.

With many drugs, the toxic overdose effects are unrelated to the action or side effects of the drug when it is taken in normal doses.

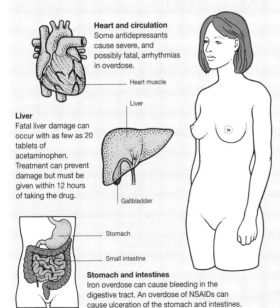

Heart and circulation
Some antidepressants cause severe, and possibly fatal, arrhythmias in overdose.

Heart muscle

Liver

Liver
Fatal liver damage can occur with as few as 20 tablets of acetaminophen. Treatment can prevent damage but must be given within 12 hours of taking the drug.

Gallbladder

Stomach

Small intestine

Stomach and intestines
Iron overdose can cause bleeding in the digestive tract. An overdose of NSAIDs can cause ulceration of the stomach and intestines.

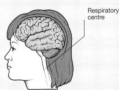

Respiratory centre

Brain
Depression of the respiratory centre in the brain is common with overdose of barbiturates and tranquillizers. ASA in overdose can result in convulsions.

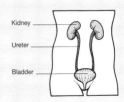

Kidney

Ureter

Bladder

Kidney
An overdose of NSAIDs, particularly in people who have impaired kidney function, can result in kidney failure.

COMMON AILMENTS, DISEASES, AND PREVENTIVE HEALTH ISSUES

The profiles in this section provide information on 37 of the most common issues that result in Canadians visiting their doctors every year. Some of these are ailments and diseases, for which treatment is sought to relieve symptoms or to provide a cure, and others are more preventive in nature, such as contraception or immunization against childhood diseases. They are generally grouped by the body system that they affect.

HOW TO UNDERSTAND THE PROFILES

For ease of reference, each profile is organized in a similar way, using mostly standard headings.

What is it?
Explains each disease, ailment, or issue, with a brief description of common symptoms.

What causes it?
Gives a brief summary of what causes the ailment or disease, how it is transmitted, and who is susceptible.

What can help?
Practical information on what you can do at home to relieve symptoms with natural remedies or over-the-counter drugs. Also explains which prescription drugs might be prescribed by your doctor.

Types of drugs
A list of the type of drugs that can help to relieve the ailment or condition, with brief explanations of their beneficial actions on the body.

RESPIRATORY SYSTEM

SINUSITIS

What is it?
The sinuses are the air filled cavities in the skull located behind the nose and eyes and in the cheeks and forehead. They are lined with a mucus-secreting membrane and connected to the nasal cavity by several narrow channels. Sinusitis occurs when the sinuses become blocked and inflamed. Symptoms can include headache, pain and tenderness in the face that tends to become worse when bending down, toothache, discoloured nasal discharge, and nasal congestion.

What causes it?
Sinusitis is usually caused by a viral infection, such as the common cold. If the channels connecting the nose to the sinuses become blocked due to the infection, mucus collects in the sinuses and can become infected with bacteria. Blockage of the channels is more likely in people with an abnormality in the nose, such as a deviated nasal septum or nasal polyps, or in people suffering from allergic rhinitis or cystic fibrosis.

What can help?
In many cases, sinusitis clears up without treatment. Symptoms of congestion can be relieved by a steam inhalation or a decongestant, and an over-the-counter analgesic may be taken for headaches. Your doctor may prescribe an antibiotic to clear up a secondary bacterial infection. Acute sinusitis usually clears up in a few weeks, but the symptoms of chronic sinusitis may last for a couple of months.

Types of drugs for sinusitis

- **Analgesics** are pain killers that can help to relieve headaches cause by blocked sinuses (see p.38).
- **Decongestants** are used to clear a stuffy nose and blocked sinuses. They work by reducing the swelling of the mucous membranes inside the nose and suppressing the production of mucus, which can block the channels connecting the nasal cavity to the sinuses (see p.28 for action of decongestants). Decongestants are used when home remedies are ineffective or when there is a particular risk from untreated congestion – for example, in people who suffer from recurrent middle-ear or sinus infections. Decongestants are available in the form of drops or sprays applied directly into the nose or they can be taken by mouth. Decongestants by mouth take a little longer to act, but their effect may also last longer.
- **Antibiotics** are prescribed to treat bacterial infections. Depending on the type of drug and the dosage, antibiotics are either bactericidal, killing organisms directly, or bacteriostatic, halting the multiplication of bacteria and enabling the body's natural defences to overcome the remaining infection. Antibiotics stop most common types of infection within days. It is important to complete the course of medication as it has been prescribed by your doctor, even if all your symptoms have disappeared. Failure to do this can lead to a resurgence of the infection in an antibiotic-resistant form.

⊙ **Risks and special precautions**
If used in excess, topical decongestants can cause rebound congestion; prevent this by using the minimum effective dose only when necessary. Decongestants taken by mouth may cause other side effects – consult with your pharmacist. These should be used cautiously in those with high blood pressure and other conditions.
The most common risk for antibiotics, especially with cephalosporins and penicillins, is a severe allergic reaction that can cause rashes and sometimes swelling of the face and throat. If this occurs, stop taking the drug and see your doctor. If you have had a previous allergic reaction to an antibiotic, inform your doctor and pharmacist – all other drugs in that class and related classes should be avoided.

Action of antibiotics

Penicillins and cephalosporins
Drugs from these groups are bactericidal – that is, they kill bacteria. They interfere with the chemicals needed by bacteria to form normal cell walls (below left). The cell's outer lining disintegrates and the bacterium dies (below right).

Bacterium

Drug | Cell wall | Disintegrating cell wall

Other drugs
These drugs alter chemical activity inside the bacteria, thereby preventing the production of proteins that the bacteria need to multiply and survive (below left). This may have a bactericidal effect in itself, or it may prevent reproduction (bacteriostatic action) (below right).

Drug

Protein | Unformed protein

✪ COMMON DRUGS

Analgesics	Topical decongestants
Acetaminophen ✳	Oxymetazoline
ASA ✳	Phenylephrine
Ibuprofen ✳	Xylometazoline
Antibiotics	**Oral decongestants**
Cefaclor	Phenylephrine
Cefixime	Pseudoephedrine ✳
Cephalexin ✳	
Ciprofloxacin ✳	
Clindamycin	
Erythromycin	✳ See Part 3

29

Risks and special precautions
If needed, a brief explanation of any special cautions regarding this condition and certain drug groups used to treat it.

Action of drugs
An illustrated explanation of how the drug achieves its beneficial effects.

Common drugs
A list of some of the most common drugs used to treat the condition. An asterisk indicates a profile in Part 3.

GLAUCOMA

What is it?
Glaucoma is the name given to a group of conditions in which the pressure in the eye builds up to an abnormally high level. This compresses the blood vessels that supply the nerve connecting the eye to the brain (optic nerve) and may result in irreversible nerve damage and permanent loss of vision. The most common type is **chronic glaucoma.** It often has no symptoms until late in the disease, when it is probable that your vision has been permanently affected. Late stage symptoms include loss of the outer edges of vision (peripheral vision) and eventual blurring of objects that are straight ahead. **Acute glaucoma** can occur suddenly; symptoms include sudden blurring of vision, a red and painful eye, seeing haloes around lights, headaches, nausea, and vomiting.

What causes it?
Fluid is continually secreted into the front of the eye to maintain the tissue and the shape of the eye. This fluid normally drains away through the trabecular meshwork, a structure found in the passage between the iris and the edge of the cornea that forms the drainage angle. In chronic (or open-angle) glaucoma, the trabecular meshwork gradually becomes blocked, preventing the drainage of the fluid and causing pressure inside the eye to build up slowly. The reasons for this blockage are not fully understood, but genetic factors may be involved.

In acute (or closed-angle) glaucoma, the iris bulges forward and blocks the drainage angle suddenly, causing fluid pressure to build in the eye. It is more common in farsighted people, the elderly, and sometimes runs in families. The drainage angle may also narrow suddenly following injury or after taking certain drugs, for example, anticholinergic drugs.

What can help?
Seek medical treatment immediately for any symptoms of acute glaucoma to prevent total loss of vision. If it is detected, immediate drug treatment will be given to bring down the pressure in the eye. Laser treatment or surgery is then carried out to prevent a recurrence of the problem so that long-term drug treatment is seldom required. Symptoms usually disappear after surgery, but some loss of peripheral vision may remain.

Chronic glaucoma is treated with drugs to reduce the pressure in the eye. These drugs will prevent further deterioration of vision but cannot restore damage that has already been sustained, and therefore these drugs may be required lifelong. If drugs are ineffective, surgery may be required.

Types of drugs for glaucoma

- **Beta blockers** in the form of eyedrops are used to reduce the production of fluid inside the eye.

- **Prostaglandin analogues** increase the outflow of fluid from inside the eye.

- **Miotic or cholinergic agonist eyedrops** constrict the pupil, which pulls the iris away from the cornea, opening the drainage angle to improve fluid drainage.

- **Adrenergic agonists** and **carbonic anhydrase inhibitors** reduce fluid production in the eye.

🞶 COMMON DRUGS

Miotic or Cholinergic agonist
Pilocarpine
Carbonic anhydrase inhibitors
Brinzolamide
Dorzolamide
Methazolamide

| ✱ See Part 3 |

Prostaglandin analogues
Bimatoprost
Latanoprost ✱
Tavoprost
Beta blockers
Betaxolol
Timolol
Adrenergic agonists
Apraclonidine
Epinephrine

Action of drugs for glaucoma

Miotics
These act on the circular muscle in the iris to reduce the size of the pupil. This relieves any obstruction to the flow of fluid by pulling the iris away from the cornea.

Beta blockers
The fluid-producing cells are stimulated by signals passed through beta receptors. Beta blocking drugs prevent the transmission of signals through these receptors, thereby reducing the stimulus to produce fluid.

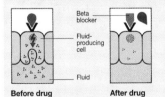

Before drug   After drug

Carbonic anhydrase inhibitors
These block carbonic anhydrase, an enzyme involved in the production of fluid in the eye.

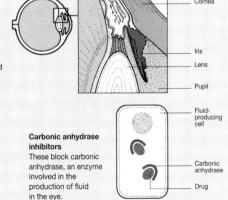

ACNE

What is it?
Acne, known medically as acne vulgaris, is a common condition that primarily appears on the face, neck, back, and chest. It chiefly affects adolescents but it may occur at any age. The main symptoms are blackheads, papules (inflamed spots), and pustules (raised pus-filled spots with a white centre). Cases can range from mild, with only blackheads and an occasional papule, to severe, with painful, inflamed cysts that can cause permanent pitting and scarring.

What causes it?
Acne is caused by excess production of the skin's natural oil (sebum), leading to blockage of hair follicles. An acne spot develops when the flow of sebum is blocked by a plug of skin debris and hardened sebum, leading to its accumulation. The trapped sebum in the follicle openings hardens and becomes dark, forming a plug called a blackhead. In some cases, the follicle openings are sealed by a plug of keratin, causing the sebum to form a small white lump called a whitehead. In both kinds of blockages, bacterial activity leads to the formation of pustules and papules, and can trigger an inflammatory response. Inflammation may also result from irritant substances leaking into the surrounding skin.

Acne that starts at puberty is thought to be the result of oversensitivity to hormones that cause the sebaceous glands to enlarge and to produce more sebum. Other causes include taking certain drugs, exposure to industrial chemicals, oily cosmetics, or hot, humid conditions. It may become worse in times of stress.

What can help?
Mild acne usually does not need medical treatment. It can be controlled by regular washing and by moderate exposure to sunlight or ultraviolet light (discuss with your doctor). Over-the-counter antibacterial soaps and lotions are limited in use and may cause irritation. Acne can also be treated with a topical preparation that has a keratolytic or antibacterial effect. A course of antibiotics by mouth may be prescribed if the topical preparations are ineffective. Estrogen drugs, such as an estrogen-containing oral contraceptive, may also have a beneficial effect on acne.

Risks and special precautions
Tetracycline antibiotics are not recommended in pregnancy as they can affect the bones and teeth of the developing baby.

Isotretinoin sometimes increases levels of lipids in the blood. It is also not to be used during pregnancy. Women taking this drug need to ensure that they avoid conception during treatment.

Clearing blocked hair follicles

The most common treatment for acne is the application of keratolytic skin ointments. These loosen the layer of dead and hardened skin cells, clearing blackheads that block hair follicles and give rise to the formation of acne spots.

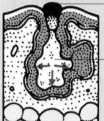

Blackhead

Trapped sebum

Blocked hair follicle
A hair follicle blocked by a plug of skin debris and sebum is ideal for acne spot formation.

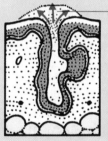

Freed sebum

Cleared hair follicle
Once the follicle is unblocked, sebum can escape and air can enter, thereby limiting bacterial activity.

Types of drugs for acne

- **Topical keratolytic preparations** loosen the dead cells on the skin surface and unblock hair follicles. These include **benzoyl peroxide** and **salicylic acid**.

- **Topical antibacterial preparations** counter bacterial activity in the skin, helping to reduce redness and inflammation. Benzoyl peroxide also has an antibacterial effect.

- **Antibiotics** can be used in topical preparations or taken orally. They work by reducing bacteria and inflammation on the skin.

- Other drugs, such as **isotretinoin**, reduce sebum production.

COMMON DRUGS

Topical treatments
Adapalene
Benzoyl peroxide
Isotretinoin
Salicylic acid
Tazarotene
Tretinoin
Triclosan
Oral and/or topical antibiotics
Clindamycin
Doxycycline
Erythromycin

Minocycline
Tetracycline
Other oral drugs
Cyproterone/ethinyl estradiol (women)
Isotretinoin
Levonorgestrel/ethinyl estradiol (women)

DERMATITIS

What is it?
Dermatitis, commonly called **eczema**, is a skin condition causing a dry, itchy rash that may be red, inflamed, blistered, and crusty. The most common type, **atopic dermatitis**, may appear in infancy, but many children grow out of it. However, flare-ups can occur throughout adolescence and into adulthood. Atopic dermatitis commonly appears in patches, typically on the hands or feet, and in skin creases. The skin in these areas can become thickened as a result of continuous scratching. Contact dermatitis is an inflammatory reaction to irritants.

What causes it?
The cause of atopic dermatitis is not known, but it can run in families and is often associated with a family history of asthma or allergic rhinitis. Flare-ups are sometimes linked to stress, temperature change, or an allergic reaction to certain foods. Exposure to skin irritants, such as detergents, and to excess moisture, can also contribute to flare-ups – this is why dermatitis is common on the hands and feet. In some individuals, certain drugs either taken orally or applied topically can cause an eczema-type of reaction.

What can help?
Protecting your skin from known irritants and from getting excessively dry can help to avoid flare-ups. Avoid immersing your hands in water for long periods, and protect your hands with PVC gloves or emollient cream before cleaning, gardening, or other activities that can irritate your skin. Cotton clothing should be worn next to the skin. Cosmetic moisturizers should be avoided because they usually contain perfumes and other sensitizers. Use emollient creams frequently during the day to soften and moisten the skin.

Topical corticosteroids may be prescribed to help control a flare up. Oral antihistamines (p.33) may be used to treat a particularly itchy rash (topical antihistamines make the skin more sensitive and are not usually recommended). Coal tar may help to relieve symptoms.

🅗 COMMON DRUGS

Emollient and cooling preparations
Aqueous creams and lotions
Calamine lotion
Emulsifying ointment
Hydrating creams and lotions

Antihistamines (see also p.33)
Chlorpheniramine
Diphenhydramine ✳
Hydroxyzine
Corticosteroids
Clobetasone
Hydrocortisone
Other drugs
Coal tar

✳ See Part 3

Types of drugs for eczema

- **Topical corticosteroids** are absorbed into the tissues to relieve itching and inflammation. The least potent one that is effective is given. Hydrocortisone 1% is often used in 12-week courses.

- **Antihistamines** block the action of histamine, a chemical present in all cells that dilates the blood vessels in the skin, causing redness and swelling of the surrounding tissue. Antihistamines also prevent histamine from irritating the nerve fibres, which causes itching.

- **Oral or topical antibiotics** destroy the bacteria sometimes present in broken, oozing, or blistered skin.

Action of corticosteroids on the skin

Skin inflammation
Irritation of the skin, caused by allergens or irritant factors, provokes white blood cells to release substances that dilate the blood vessels. This makes the skin hot, red, and inflamed.

Drug action
Applied to the skin surfaces, corticosteroids are absorbed into the underlying tissue. There they inhibit the action of the substances that cause inflammation, allowing the blood vessels to return to normal and reducing the swelling.

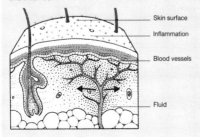

Skin surface
Inflammation
Blood vessels
Fluid

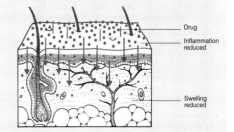

Drug
Inflammation reduced
Swelling reduced

COMMON COLD

What is it?
The common cold is a viral infection, usually of the upper airways, which includes the nose and throat. Symptoms may include congested and runny nose, mild headache, sore throat, sneezing, and a cough.

What causes it?
Colds are caused by more than 200 highly contagious viruses. These viruses are easily transmitted in minute airborne droplets from the coughs or sneezes of infected people, or by hand-to-hand contact with objects that have been contaminated by the virus, such as a cup, towel, or door knob. Colds can occur at any time of the year, but infections are more frequent in the fall and winter. Children are more susceptible to colds because they have an underdeveloped immune system and because viruses spread very quickly in communities such as daycares or schools.

What can help?
The common cold usually resolves within two weeks, although a cough may last longer. There is no cure, but some simple non-drug strategies can help minimize the symptoms. Get enough rest and drink plenty of liquids. A cold humidifier, especially at night, may be helpful to clear nasal congestion. Some people find that taking large quantities of vitamin C can prevent or treat a cold infection, but there is no clinical evidence to support this. Certain over-the-counter drugs can help to relieve cold symptoms.

⏱ Risks and special precautions
For children under 6 years of age, consult a doctor or pharmacist before using a cough or cold product. If used in excess, topical decongestants can cause rebound congestion; prevent this by using the minimum effective dose only when necessary for no longer than 2 or 3 days. Decongestants taken by mouth may cause other side effects – consult with your pharmacist.

Action of cough remedies

Cough remedies are divided into two main groups: those that alter the consistency or production of phlegm (expectorants), and those that suppress the coughing reflex (opioid and non-opioid cough suppressants). Both are taken by mouth. Expectorants are supposed to help bring up phlegm. Cough suppressants act on the coughing centre in the brain.

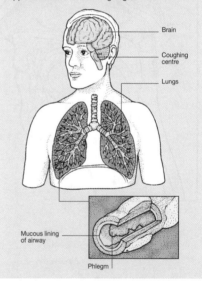

Brain

Coughing centre

Lungs

Mucous lining of airway

Phlegm

☣ COMMON DRUGS

Analgesics
Acetaminophen ✳
ASA ✳
Ibuprofen ✳
Oral decongestants
Phenylephrine
Pseudoephedrine ✳
Topical decongestants
Oxymetazoline
Phenylephrine
Xylometazoline

Expectorants
Guaifenesin
Opioid cough suppressants
Codeine ✳
Hydrocodone
Non-opioid cough suppressant
Dextromethorphan ✳

✳ See Part 3

Types of drugs for the common cold

- **Analgesics** are pain killers that can help to relieve mild headaches (see p.38).

- **Decongestants** are used to clear a stuffy nose and blocked sinuses. They work by reducing the swelling of the mucous membranes inside the nasal passages and suppressing the production of mucus. Decongestants are used when non-drug strategies are ineffective or when there is a particular risk from untreated congestion – for example, in people who suffer from recurrent middle-ear or sinus infections. Decongestants are available in the form of drops or sprays applied directly into the nasal passages or they can be taken by mouth. Decongestants by mouth take a little longer to act, but their effect may last longer; they also result in more side effects.

- **Cough remedies** may help to relieve some symptoms, but overall there is little evidence that these drugs are effective. Remedies are available to either help you cough up phlegm (expectorants), or to relieve a dry, irritating cough (suppressants). Cough suppressants are usually not recommended for a productive cough, as this may prevent you from getting rid of excess infected phlegm and may delay your recovery. All cough suppressants may have a generally sedating effect and commonly cause drowsiness and other side effects. Speak to your doctor or pharmacist for advice.

COMMON COLD continued

Action of decongestants

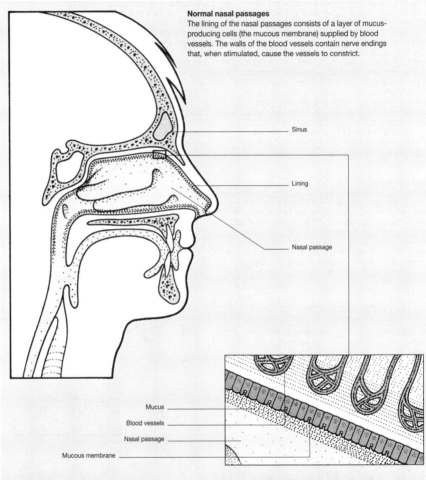

Normal nasal passages
The lining of the nasal passages consists of a layer of mucus-producing cells (the mucous membrane) supplied by blood vessels. The walls of the blood vessels contain nerve endings that, when stimulated, cause the vessels to constrict.

Sinus

Lining

Nasal passage

Mucus

Blood vessels

Nasal passage

Mucous membrane

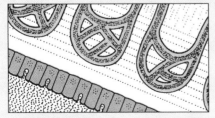

Congested nasal lining
When the blood vessels enlarge in response to infection or irritation, increased amounts of fluid pass into the mucous membrane, which swells and produces more mucus.

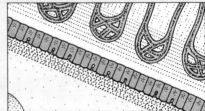

Effect of decongestants
Decongestants enhance the action of chemicals that stimulate constriction of the blood vessels. Narrowing of the blood vessels reduces swelling and mucus production.

SINUSITIS

What is it?
The sinuses are the air filled cavities in the skull located behind the nose and eyes and in the cheeks and forehead. They are lined with a mucus-secreting membrane and connected to the nasal cavity by several narrow channels. Sinusitis occurs when the sinuses become blocked and inflamed. Symptoms can include headache, pain and tenderness in the face that tends to become worse when bending down, toothache, discoloured nasal discharge, and nasal congestion.

What causes it?
Sinusitis is usually caused by a viral infection, such as the common cold. If the channels connecting the nose to the sinuses become blocked due to the infection, mucus collects in the sinuses and can become infected with bacteria. Blockage of the channels is more likely in people with an abnormality in the nose, such as a deviated nasal septum or nasal polyps, or in people suffering from allergic rhinitis or cystic fibrosis.

What can help?
In many cases, sinusitis clears up without treatment. Symptoms of congestion can be relieved by a steam inhalation or a decongestant, and an over-the-counter analgesic may be taken for headaches. Your doctor may prescribe an antibiotic to clear up a secondary bacterial infection. Acute sinusitis usually clears up in a few weeks, but the symptoms of chronic sinusitis may last for a couple of months.

Types of drugs for sinusitis

- **Analgesics** are pain killers that can help to relieve headaches cause by blocked sinuses (see p.38).

- **Decongestants** are used to clear a stuffy nose and blocked sinuses. They work by reducing the swelling of the mucous membranes inside the nose and suppressing the production of mucus, which can block the channels connecting the nasal cavity to the sinuses (see p.28 for action of decongestants). Decongestants are used when home remedies are ineffective or when there is a particular risk from untreated congestion – for example, in people who suffer from recurrent middle-ear or sinus infections. Decongestants are available in the form of drops or sprays applied directly into the nose or they can be taken by mouth. Decongestants by mouth take a little longer to act, but their effect may also last longer.

- **Antibiotics** are prescribed to treat bacterial infections. Depending on the type of drug and the dosage, antibiotics are either bactericidal, killing organisms directly, or bacteriostatic, halting the multiplication of bacteria and enabling the body's natural defences to overcome the remaining infection. Antibiotics stop most common types of infection within days. It is important to complete the course of medication as it has been prescribed by your doctor, even if all your symptoms have disappeared. Failure to do this can lead to a resurgence of the infection in an antibiotic-resistant form.

Risks and special precautions
If used in excess, topical decongestants can cause rebound congestion; prevent this by using the minimum effective dose only when necessary. Decongestants taken by mouth may cause other side effects – consult with your pharmacist. These should be used cautiously in those with high blood pressure and other conditions.

The most common risk for antibiotics, especially with cephalosporins and penicillins, is a severe allergic reaction that can cause rashes and sometimes swelling of the face and throat. If this occurs, stop taking the drug and see your doctor. If you have had a previous allergic reaction to an antibiotic, inform your doctor and pharmacist – all other drugs in that class and related classes should be avoided.

Action of antibiotics

Penicillins and cephalosporins
Drugs from these groups are bactericidal – that is, they kill bacteria. They interfere with the chemicals needed by bacteria to form normal cell walls (below left). The cell's outer lining disintegrates and the bacterium dies (below right).

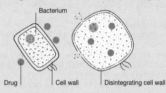

Bacterium

Drug | Cell wall | Disintegrating cell wall

Other antibiotics
These drugs alter chemical activity inside the bacteria, thereby preventing the production of proteins that the bacteria need to multiply and survive (below left). This may have a bactericidal effect in itself, or it may prevent reproduction (bacteriostatic action) (below right).

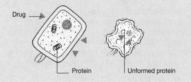

Drug

Protein | Unformed protein

COMMON DRUGS

Analgesics	Topical decongestants
Acetaminophen *	Oxymetazoline
ASA *	Phenylephrine
Ibuprofen *	Xylometazoline
Antibiotics	**Oral decongestants**
Cefaclor	Phenylephrine
Cefixime	Pseudoephedrine *
Cephalexin *	
Ciprofloxacin *	
Clindamycin	
Erythromycin	

* See Part 3

ASTHMA

What is it?

Asthma is a chronic lung disease characterized by episodes in which the bronchioles (airways) constrict due to over-sensitivity. The attacks are usually, but not always, reversible; asthma is also known as reversible airways obstruction. Breathlessness is the main symptom. Wheezing, coughing, and chest tightness are common. Asthma sufferers can have attacks during the night and may wake up with breathing difficulty. The illness varies in severity, and it can range from very mild to life-threatening attacks.

What causes it?

Asthma is caused by inflammation and constriction of the bronchioles in the lungs. Sometimes the inflammation causing the constriction is due to an identifiable allergen in the atmosphere, such as house dust mites, but often there is no obvious trigger. Asthma triggered by an allergic reaction tends to occur in childhood, and it may develop in association with eczema or hay fever. Rarely, certain foods, such as milk, eggs, nuts, and wheat, can provoke an allergic asthmatic reaction. Some people who have asthma are sensitive to aspirin and NSAIDs; taking them may trigger an attack. Other factors that may cause an attack include cold air, exercise, smoke, and emotional stress.

What can help?

Some people with asthma do not need treatment if they manage to avoid the factors that trigger their symptoms. However, there are often so many triggers that it can be difficult to avoid them all, and for this reason drug treatment is often necessary. Drugs called "relievers" can be used to control an occasional attack, while "preventers/controllers" are used as continuous, preventative treatment. Sometimes these drugs are combined. Inhaling a drug directly into the lungs is the best way of getting benefit without excessive side effects.

Types of drugs for asthma

- **Bronchodilators** act by relaxing the muscles surrounding the bronchioles, which eases the passage of air into the lungs. A sympathomimetic bronchodilator can be used in inhaler form to relieve an attack. Anticholinergic bronchodilators are slower acting, and are used as preventative treatment.

- **Corticosteroids** reduce inflammation inside of the bronchioles, and also reduce the amount of mucus produced, which helps to clear the airways. An inhaled corticosteroid may be used to prevent attacks. Corticosteroids usually start to improve exercise capacity of the asthma sufferer within a few days.

- **Leukotriene antagonists** work by stopping leukotrienes, which occur naturally in the body, and thus decreasing inflammation in the bronchioles. Leukotriene antagonists may be prescribed when inhaled corticosteroids cannot be used in an individual; they are less effective in severe cases when patients are taking high doses of other drugs.

- **Omalizumab**, a monoclonal antibody, may be prescribed in those with moderate to severe persistent asthma to improve asthma control.

Risks and special precautions

Dry powder inhalations can cause a reflex bronchospasm as the powder hits the lining of the airways; this can be avoided by using a short-acting sympathomimetic first. Inhaled corticosteroids may encourage fungal growth in the mouth and throat (thrush); minimize this risk by using a spacer and/or by rinsing the mouth with water after each use. High doses of inhaled steroids may, over time, suppress adrenal gland function, reduce bone density, and increase the risk of glaucoma. Sympathomimetics and theophylline taken by mouth may affect heart rate, and should be prescribed with caution to people with heart problems, high blood pressure, or an overactive thyroid gland.

Different types of inhaler

A wide range of different types of inhaler is available and the most commonly prescribed ones are shown here. Although every inhaler works on the same broad principle to deliver the drug directly to the bronchioles through a mouthpiece, there are individual differences in the actions required. Therefore, it is important to read the instructions carefully and practise using the inhaler before you need it in an emergency. Some inhalers are activated by taking in a breath, and these may be easier for some people to use. If you have trouble operating an inhaler, you can ask your doctor for a spacer device; this requires less coordination between releasing the drug and breathing in, and is particularly suitable for children and the elderly. Always check how to use your particular device with the pharmacist.

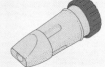

⊗ COMMON DRUGS

Sympathomimetics	**Xanthines**
Formoterol ✳	Oxtriphylline
Salbutamol ✳	Theophylline
Salmeterol ✳	**Corticosteroids**
Terbutaline	Beclomethasone
Anticholinergics	Budesonide
Ipratropium	Ciclesonide
Tiotropium ✳	Fluticasone ✳
Leukotriene	Prednisone ✳
antagonists	**IgE neutralizing**
Montelukast	**antibody**
Zafirlukast	Omalizumab
	Other drugs
	Ketotifen
	Sodium cromoglycate

✳ See Part 3

Action of bronchodilators

When the bronchioles are narrowed following contraction of the muscle layer and swelling of the mucous lining, the passage of air is impeded. Bronchodilators act on the nerve signals that govern muscle activity. Sympathomimetics (or Beta$_2$-agonists) and xanthines encourage the muscle layer of the bronchioles to relax. Anticholinergics stop muscle contractions and reduce production of mucus.

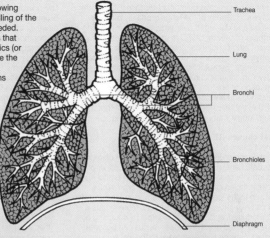

Trachea

Lung

Bronchi

Bronchioles

Diaphragm

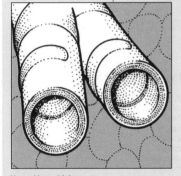

Normal bronchioles
The muscle surrounding the bronchioles is relaxed, thus leaving the airway open.

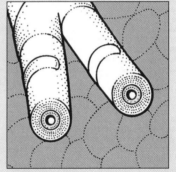

Asthma attack
The bronchiole muscle contracts and the lining swells, narrowing the airway.

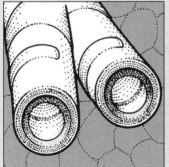

After drug treatment
The muscles relax, thereby opening the airway, but the lining remains swollen.

CHRONIC OBSTRUCTIVE PULMONARY DISEASE

What is it?
In chronic obstructive pulmonary disease (COPD), the airways and tissues of the lungs gradually become inflamed and damaged over time, causing increasing shortness of breath. COPD is usually made up of two different lung conditions, chronic **bronchitis** and **emphysema**, and either one of these conditions can be dominant. Symptoms, which may take several years to develop, include chronic coughing, increasing production of sputum, frequent chest infections, wheezing, and shortness of breath. Some people with COPD eventually become so short of breath that they can no longer carry out simple daily activities.

What causes it?
In most cases of COPD, the cause is smoking. Atmospheric pollution also contributes to the disorder. Occupational exposure to dust, noxious gases, or other lung irritants can worsen existing COPD. In bronchitis, smoke irritation causes the lining of the bronchioles (airways) in the lungs to thicken, narrowing the passages that carry air into and out of the lungs. More mucus is also produced, and is difficult to expel by coughing due to the narrowed airways. Excess mucus can become infected, causing further damage to the lungs. In emphysema, smoke and other airborne pollutants damage the tissues of the alveoli (air sacs), causing them to lose their elasticity and become enlarged. These damaged air sacs can no longer efficiently transfer oxygen from the lungs into the bloodstream. Rarely, emphysema can also be caused by an inherited condition called alpha$_1$-antitrypsin deficiency.

What can help?
See your doctor right away if you suspect that you have COPD. Damage to the lungs from bronchitis and emphysema is usually irreversible. If you smoke, give up smoking (see p.45) permanently to delay the progress of COPD. Keep your environment as free as possible from smoke, pollution, dust, dampness, and cold. If possible, take part in a rehabilitation program that includes exercise, relaxation breathing, and energy conservation techniques. Your doctor will probably prescribe certain drugs to ease shortness of breath and other symptoms. Learn the signs of a chest infection and see your doctor right away for treatment if one develops. It is advisable to get vaccinated against influenza each winter. Your doctor may also recommend pneumococcal vaccine; in some individuals who are more at risk, this may be repeated in 5 to 10 years.

✋ Risks and special precautions
Dry powder inhalations can cause a reflex bronchospasm as the powder hits the lining of the airways; this can be avoided by using a short-acting sympathomimetic first. Inhaled corticosteroids may encourage fungal growth in the mouth and throat (thrush); minimize this risk by using a spacer and/or by rinsing the mouth with water after each use. High doses of inhaled steroids may, over time, suppress adrenal gland function, reduce bone density, and increase the risk of glaucoma. Sympathomimetics and theophylline taken by mouth may affect heart rate, and should be prescribed with caution to people with heart problems, high blood pressure, or an overactive thyroid gland.

Using an inhaler

Inhalers are used to deliver drugs to relieve or prevent the symptoms of COPD. Many people are prescribed a reliever and a preventer drug and these may come in different types of inhaler, depending on the drugs that are given. Although every inhaler works on the same broad principle to deliver the drug directly to the bronchioles through a mouthpiece, there are individual differences in the actions required. See page 30 for the mostly commonly prescribed types of inhaler.

❸ COMMON DRUGS

Sympathomimetics	Corticosteroids
Fenoterol	Beclomethasone
Formoterol ✻	Budesonide
Salbutamol ✻	Fluticasone ✻
Salmeterol ✻	Prednisone ✻
Terbutaline	**Antibiotics**
Anticholinergics	Amoxicillin ✻
Ipratropium	Azithromycin ✻
Tiotropium ✻	Clarithromycin ✻
Xanthines	Sulfamethoxazole-
Oxtriphylline	trimethoprim ✻
Theophylline	

✻ See Part 3

Types of drugs for COPD

- **Bronchodilators** are prescribed in inhaled form to widen the bronchioles and improve breathing. Bronchodilators can either be taken when they are needed in order to relieve an attack of breathlessness that is in progress, or on a regular basis to prevent such attacks from occurring. There are three main groups of bronchodilators: sympathomimetics (or Beta$_2$-agonists), anticholinergics, and xanthine drugs. Sympathomimetic drugs are mainly used for rapid relief of breathlessness; anticholinergic and xanthine drugs are used long term. See p.30-1 for action of bronchodilators and types of inhalers.

- **Corticosteroids**, usually as an inhaler, may also be prescribed for patients with advanced COPD who have frequent exacerbations. The drug reduces inflammation and mucus production in the bronchioles.

- **Antibiotics** may be prescribed during acute exacerbations to treat respiratory infections.

ALLERGIES

What is it?
An allergy is an extreme reaction of the body's immune system to a normally harmless substance, called an allergen. After exposure to the allergen, the immune system develops a hypersensitivity to the substance, and during subsequent exposures, an allergic reaction occurs. Common types of allergic conditions include **allergic rhinitis** (hay fever, p.30), **eczema** (p.26), and **hives**. Symptoms may include an itchy sensation in the nose and throat, sneezing, blocked and runny nose, itchy and watery eyes, hives, skin rash, and swelling of the lips, tongue, or throat. **Anaphylaxis** is a serious systemic allergic reaction that occurs when an allergen reaches the bloodstream, causing a sudden drop in blood pressure and narrowing of the airways.

What causes it?
When the body encounters an allergen, the immune system releases a chemical known as histamine. Histamine can produce a rash, swelling, narrowing of the airways, and a drop in blood pressure. Hay fever is caused by allergic reaction to allergens such as inhaled grass pollen, house-dust mites, animal fur, and feathers. Asthma may result from the action of leukotrienes rather than histamine. Anaphylaxis can be triggered by insect stings, or certain types of drugs or food.

What can help?
Most environmental allergies are mild and can be treated with self-help remedies or drugs. If you suffer from hay fever, maintain an allergen-free environment as much as possible by avoiding furry pets, replacing feather pillows and quilts with those containing synthetic stuffing, removing dust collecting items from your house, and keeping windows and doors closed during pollen season. Foods and drugs that cause allergic reactions should be avoided.

Drugs can be used to inhibit the immune response to allergens and to relieve symptoms of allergies. If you suffer from anaphylaxis, carry an emergency injection of epinephrine with you at all times; the condition can be fatal if not treated immediately. You may also wish to wear a medical bracelet documenting such a serious allergy.

Sites of action

Antihistamines act on a variety of sites and systems throughout the body. Their main action is on the muscles surrounding the small blood vessels that supply the skin and mucous membranes.

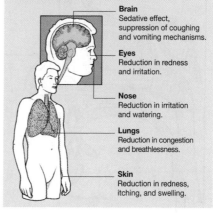

Brain
Sedative effect, suppression of coughing and vomiting mechanisms.

Eyes
Reduction in redness and irritation.

Nose
Reduction in irritation and watering.

Lungs
Reduction in congestion and breathlessness.

Skin
Reduction in redness, itching, and swelling.

COMMON DRUGS

Antihistamines
Generally non-sedating
Cetirizine ✳
Desloratadine
Fexofenadine
Loratadine
Sedating
Brompheniramine
Chlorpheniramine
Cyproheptadine
Diphenhydramine ✳
Hydroxyzine
Promethazine
Anti-allergic eye preparations
Emedastine

Ketotifen
Levocabastine
Lodoxamide
Nedocromil
Olopatadine
Sodium cromoglycate
Drug used for serious allergic reaction
Epinephrine (EpiPen®, EpiPen® Jr, Twinject®)
Decongestants
(see p.27)
Corticosteroids
Fluticasone ✳
Mometasone

Types of drugs for allergies

- **Antihistamines** block the action of histamine. This helps prevent the dilation of the blood vessels in the skin, nose and eyes, thus reducing the redness, watering, and swelling. The anticholinergic action of these drugs also reduces the secretions from tear glands and nasal passages. Some antihistamines cause drowsiness – avoid driving or operating machinery.

- **Decongestants** (see p.28) work by clearing the nose in allergic rhinitis.

- **Leukotriene antagonists** block the action of leukotrienes, which are substances that occur

naturally in the body and seem to play an important part in asthma (p.30).

- **Bronchodilators** (see p.31) act to widen the airways of those with asthma.

- **Corticosteroids** are given by inhaler to treat allergic rhinitis and asthma. They are also applied as a lotion to skin affected by eczema (p.26).

- **Epinephrine** is given as an emergency injection to stop an anaphylactic reaction.

ALLERGIES continued

Action of antihistamines

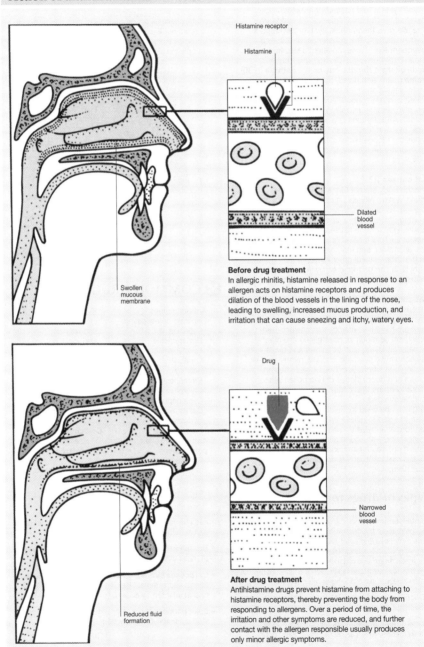

Histamine receptor

Histamine

Dilated blood vessel

Swollen mucous membrane

Before drug treatment
In allergic rhinitis, histamine released in response to an allergen acts on histamine receptors and produces dilation of the blood vessels in the lining of the nose, leading to swelling, increased mucus production, and irritation that can cause sneezing and itchy, watery eyes.

Drug

Narrowed blood vessel

Reduced fluid formation

After drug treatment
Antihistamine drugs prevent histamine from attaching to histamine receptors, thereby preventing the body from responding to allergens. Over a period of time, the irritation and other symptoms are reduced, and further contact with the allergen responsible usually produces only minor allergic symptoms.

ANEMIA

What is it?

Anemia is a deficiency or an abnormality of hemoglobin or in the number of red blood cells. Hemoglobin is the component of red blood cells that binds with oxygen from the lungs and carries it through the circulatory system to the body tissues. The oxygen-carrying capacity of the blood is thus reduced, and the tissues of the body may not receive enough oxygen. Mild anemia may cause no symptoms. As anemia progresses, the individual may feel easily fatigued, experience shortness of breath during mild exertion, and have a rapid heart rate. The person may appear pale. Severe anemia can increase the risk of chronic heart failure as the heart has to work harder to supply blood to the rest of the body. Symptoms depend on the age of the individual, how quickly anemia develops, and any other medical conditions the individual may have.

What causes it?

There are many types of anemia. The most common form is iron-deficiency anemia, which results from low levels of iron in the body. Iron is needed in the formation of healthy red blood cells, and is also involved in the uptake of oxygen by the cells and the conversion of blood sugar to energy. Iron levels may be low due to persistent bleeding; causes may include heavy menses, bleeding from the stomach lining due to ulcers, or cancer of the bowel. Insufficient iron in the diet can also cause iron-deficiency anemia; vegans are particularly at risk. The condition is more likely to develop if an individual needs higher levels of iron than normal – for example, pregnant women or children during a growth spurt. Some disorders, such as celiac disease, prevent the absorption of iron from the diet and can lead to iron deficiency. Some drugs can also cause anemia, either due to an immune reaction, effect on blood-forming cells, or by causing peptic ulcers.

What can help?

A blood test is required to make a diagnosis of anemia and to determine the underlying cause. Your doctor will treat any underlying disorder that is causing the iron-deficiency anemia, such as a stomach ulcer (p.71) or celiac disease. With insufficient dietary iron intake, changing the diet to include iron-rich foods, such as liver, chicken, eggs, and fish, can help. Iron is better absorbed from animal sources, but leafy green vegetables, dried fruit, wholegrain bread and pasta, nuts, and dried legumes are also good sources. Foods containing vitamin C can enhance iron absorption. An iron supplement may be prescribed if dietary measures are unsuccessful or for those who have a disorder that prevents absorption of iron from the diet.

The role of iron in transporting oxygen

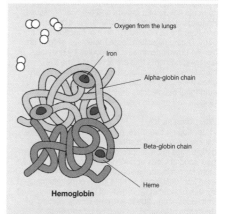

Hemoglobin

Red blood cells

Each red blood cell contains millions of molecules of hemoglobin, each made up of four protein chains (two alpha- and two beta-globin) and four heme, an iron-bearing red pigment.

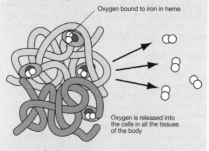

Oxyhemoglobin

How hemoglobin carries oxygen

The oxygen from the lungs enters the red blood cells in the blood stream. The oxygen then combines with the heme within the hemoglobin, which is carried around the body. In areas that need oxygen, the oxyhemoglobin releases its oxygen and reverts to hemoglobin.

Types of drugs for iron-deficiency anemia

- **Iron supplements** provide extra iron that can be absorbed by the digestive tract (see p.36 for how nutrients are absorbed). There are many different types of iron salts that can be used such as ferrous sulfate or ferrous gluconate (see p.182).

✚ COMMON DRUGS

Iron supplements (see p.182)
  Ferrous fumarate
  Ferrous gluconate

Ferrous sulfate
Iron dextran
Iron sucrose

NUTRITIONAL DEFICIENCIES

What is it?
Nutritional deficiencies occur when the body lacks essential elements that are obtained by food. Food provides energy (as calories) and materials called nutrients needed for growth and renewal of tissues. Protein, carbohydrate, fat, vitamins and minerals, and fibre are all needed for normal function of the body. During digestion, large molecules of food are broken down into smaller molecules by enzymes, releasing nutrients that are absorbed into the bloodstream. Particular vitamins and minerals are often necessary for this process. Symptoms of nutritional deficiencies may include weight loss, fatigue, and muscle weakness.

What causes it?
In developing countries, nutritional deficiencies are usually the result of a shortage of food. Nutritional deficiencies in developed countries often result from poor food choices or dietary restrictions and usually stem from a lack of a specific vitamin or mineral, such as in iron-deficiency anemia (p.35) or rickets (caused by lack of vitamin D). A general deficiency may result from poor eating due to extreme illness, dieting, or deliberate starvation, as caused by some eating disorders. Deficiencies may occur when nutritional needs increase, such as in growth spurts in childhood or during pregnancy.

Some nutritional deficiencies may be caused by a disorder, such as Crohn's or celiac disease, that inhibits the body's ability to absorb nutrients from food (malabsorption) or to utilize them once they have been absorbed. Malabsorption may be caused by lack of an enzyme or an abnormality of the digestive tract.

What can help?
If poor eating is the cause of nutritional deficiency, a change to a well-balanced diet may resolve the problem. Psychological problems that result in poor eating, such as anorexia nervosa or depression, will need treatment. Specific vitamin and mineral deficiencies are usually treated with appropriate supplements. Malabsorption disorders may require changes in diet or long-term use of supplements. Supplements should never be used as a substitute for a balanced diet.

🖐 Risks and special precautions
Supplements can be taken without risk by most people. Do not exceed the recommended dosage for supplements. Overdosage has at best no therapeutic value and at worst it may incur the risk of serious harmful effects. Overdoses of single vitamin or mineral supplements can be harmful because an excess of one vitamin or mineral may increase the requirements for others; hence, they should be used only on medical advice.

Types of supplements

- **Vitamins** are complex chemicals that are essential for a variety of body functions. With the exception of vitamin D, which is produced in the body when the skin is exposed to sunlight, the body cannot manufacture these substances itself, and therefore we need to include them in our diet. Most vitamins are required in very small amounts and each vitamin is present in one or more foods (see the table on page 37).

- **Minerals** are elements – the simplest form of substances – many of which are essential in trace amounts for normal metabolic processes. A balanced diet usually contains all of the minerals that the body requires; mineral deficiency diseases, except iron-deficiency anemia, are uncommon.

🔀 COMMON SUPPLEMENTS

Vitamins	Minerals
Cobalamin (B12) ✳	Calcium ✳
Folic acid ✳	Iron ✳
Niacin (B3) ✳	Magnesium
Pyridoxine (B6)	Potassium
Riboflavin (B2)	Selenium
Thiamine (B1)	Zinc
Vitamin A ✳	
Vitamin C ✳	✳ See Part 3
Vitamin D ✳	

Absorption of nutrients

Food passes through the mouth, esophagus, and stomach to the small intestine. The lining of the small intestine secretes many enzymes and is covered by tiny projections (villi) that enable nutrients to pass into the blood.

Malabsorption
Enzyme action breaks food down into molecules that can be absorbed. Lack of certain enzymes may cause malabsorption of nutrients. Other causes include flattened villi and scars on the intestine.

Inside the intestine
Nutrients pass through the intestinal lining into the blood.

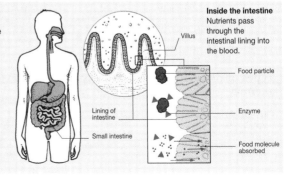

Villus

Food particle

Enzyme

Food molecule absorbed

Lining of intestine

Small intestine

Main food sources of vitamins and minerals

The table below indicates which foods are especially good sources of particular vitamins and minerals. Selecting foods from a variety of categories helps to maintain adequate intake for most people, without a need for supplements. Remember that processed and overcooked foods are likely to contain fewer vitamins than fresh, raw, or lightly cooked foods.

Vitamins

	Red meat	Poultry	Liver	Milk	Cheese	Butter/margarine	Eggs	Fish	Cereals and bread	Green vegetables	Root vegetables	Legumes	Nuts	Fruit	Other	
Biotin			●				●					●	●			Especially peanuts. Cauliflower and mushrooms are good sources.
Folic acid			●				●			●					●	Wheat germ and mushrooms are rich sources.
Niacin as nicotinic acid	●	●	●				●	●				●	●			Protein-rich foods such as milk and eggs contain tryptophan, which can be converted to niacin in the body.
Pantothenic acid			●				●	●								Each food group contributes some pantothenic acid.
Pyridoxine	●	●	●				●	●	●							Especially white meat (poultry), fish, and wholegrain cereals.
Riboflavin		●	●	●			●		●			●	●	●		Found in most foods.
Thiamine	●		●					●				●	●			Brewers yeast, wheat germ, and bran are also good sources.
Vitamin A		●	●	●	●	●	●			●	●				●	Especially fish liver oil, dark green leafy vegetables such as spinach, and orange or yellow-orange vegetables and fruits such as carrots, apricots, and peaches.
Vitamin B12	●		●	●	●		●	●								Obtained only from animal products, especially liver and red meat.
Vitamin C										●	●				●	Especially citrus fruits, tomatoes, potatoes, broccoli, strawberries, and melon.
Vitamin D				●		●	●	●								Fish liver oils, margarine, and milk are the best sources, but the vitamin is also produced when the skin is exposed to sunlight.
Vitamin E						●	●		●	●			●	●		Vegetable oils, wholegrain cereals, and wheat germ are the best sources.
Vitamin K										●	●					Found in small amounts in fruits, seeds, root vegetables, dairy and meat products.

Minerals

	Red meat	Poultry	Liver	Milk	Cheese	Butter/margarine	Eggs	Fish	Cereals and bread	Green vegetables	Root vegetables	Legumes	Nuts	Fruit	Other	
Calcium				●	●					●		●	●			Dark green leafy vegetables, soy bean products, and nuts are good non-dairy alternatives. Also present in hard, or alkaline, water supplies.
Chromium	●			●								●	●			Especially unrefined wholegrain cereals.
Copper	●	●	●				●	●	●			●	●			Especially shellfish, wholegrain cereals, and mushrooms.
Fluoride								●								Primarily obtained from fluoridated water supplies. Also in seafood and tea.
Iodine				●	●			●	●							Provided by iodized table salt, but adequate amounts can be obtained without using table salt from dairy products, saltwater fish, and bread.
Iron	●	●	●				●	●	●	●						Especially liver, red meat, and enriched or whole grains.
Magnesium			●					●	●	●		●	●			Dark green leafy vegetables such as spinach are rich sources. Also present in alkaline water supplies.
Phosphorus	●	●	●	●	●		●	●	●	●	●	●	●	●	●	Common food additive. Large amounts found in some carbonated beverages.
Potassium								●	●		●				●	Best sources are fruits and vegetables, especially oranges, bananas, and potatoes.
Selenium	●		●	●			●	●								Seafood is the richest source. Amounts in most foods are variable, depending on soil where plants were grown and animals grazed.
Sodium	●	●	●	●	●	●	●	●	●	●	●	●	●	●	●	Present in all foods, especially table salt, processed foods, potato chips, crackers, and pickled, cured, or smoked meats, seafood, and vegetables. Also present in softened water.
Zinc	●				●		●	●				●				Highest amounts in wholegrain breads and cereals.

PAIN

What is it?

Pain is an unpleasant sensation that hurts, and can cause feelings of discomfort, distress, or agony, depending on its severity. It can either be **acute** (intense and short-lived) or **chronic** (lasting much longer and recurring). Pain is a very individual experience and is your body's way of telling you something is wrong.

What causes it?

Damage to body tissues as a result of disease or injury is detected by nerve endings that transmit signals to the brain, causing the sensation of pain. Most acute pain goes away once the painful stimulus is removed, or the injury has healed. The severity of pain can be affected by the psychological state of the individual, so that pain is worsened by anxiety and fear, for example. Often a reassuring explanation of the cause of discomfort makes pain easier to bear.

What can help?

Pain is not a disease but a symptom, and long-term relief depends on treatment of the underlying cause. For example, toothache can be relieved by drugs but can be cured only by appropriate dental treatment. If the underlying disorder is irreversible, such as some rheumatic conditions, long-term pain treatment may be necessary.

Analgesics are drugs that relieve pain. Anti-anxiety drugs (see p.43) are helpful when pain is accompanied by anxiety, and some of these drugs are also used to reduce painful muscle spasms. Antidepressant drugs (see p.41) act to block the transmission of impulses signalling pain and are particularly useful for nerve pains (neuralgia), which do not always respond to analgesics. Other medications used to treat nerve pains include anticonvulsant drugs like valproic acid, gabapentin, or pregabalin.

Risks and special precautions

When treating pain with an over-the-counter preparation, seek medical advice if pain persists for longer than 48 hours, recurs, or worsens significantly. Opioid analgesics produce feelings of euphoria, which can lead to abuse and addiction, especially when used inappropriately, and are dangerous when taken in overdose. They may prevent clear thought, and may cause nausea, vomiting, constipation, drowsiness, and depressed breathing.

Types of Analgesics

- **Non-opiod analgesics** are usually the first pain relievers recommended by doctors, the most common being acetaminophen or ASA. These drugs block production of prostaglandins, a chemical produced when there is damage to tissue that sends a signal via the nerve endings to the brain. These drugs can be used for everyday aches and pains, such as headaches, joint pains and fever. This type of analgesics also includes **non-steroidal anti-inflammatory drugs (NSAIDs)**, which are useful for reducing pain and fever as well as inflammation.

- **Opioid analgesics** are related to opium, and act directly on the brain to stop the transmission of pain signals between brain cells. They are the strongest analgesics and are used to treat pain arising from surgery, serious injury, and cancer. These drugs can relieve severe pain during terminal illnesses, in part due to their ability to produce a state of relaxation and euphoria. Morphine is the best known of the opioid analgesics. In addition to the powerful opioids, there are some less powerful analgesics in this group that are used to relieve mild to moderate pain, including hydrocodone and codeine.

- **Combined analgesics** are made up of mild opioids, such as codeine, and non-opioids, such as acetaminophen or NSAIDs. These mixtures may add the advantages of analgesics that act on the brain to the benefits of those acting at the site of pain. Another advantage of combining analgesics is that the reductions in dose of the components may reduce the side effects of the preparation. Combinations can be helpful in reducing the number of tablets taken during long-term treatment.

Sites of action

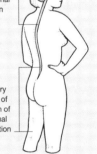

Acetaminophen and the opioid drugs act on the brain and spinal cord to reduce pain perception

Non-steroidal anti-inflammatory drugs (NSAIDs) act at the site of pain to prevent the stimulation of nerve endings and on the spinal cord to decrease pain perception

COMMON DRUGS FOR PAIN

Cannabinoids
Cannabis Sativa Extract
(Cannabidiol, Delta-9-
tetrahydro-cannabinol)
Opioids
Codeine *
Fentanyl *
Hydromorphone
Methadone
Morphine *
Oxycodone *
Cox-2 Selective Inhibitor
Celecoxib *

NSAIDs
ASA *
Diclofenac *
Ibuprofen *
Ketoprofen
Meloxicam
Naproxen *
Piroxicam
Other non-opioids
Acetaminophen *

| * See Part 3 |

Action of analgesics

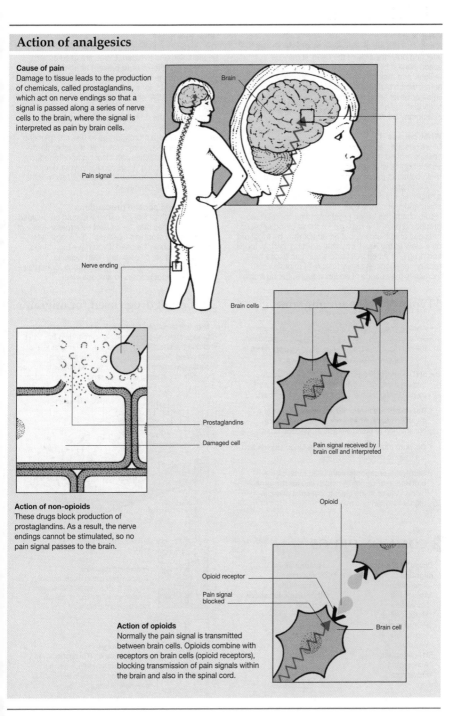

Cause of pain
Damage to tissue leads to the production of chemicals, called prostaglandins, which act on nerve endings so that a signal is passed along a series of nerve cells to the brain, where the signal is interpreted as pain by brain cells.

Brain

Pain signal

Nerve ending

Brain cells

Prostaglandins

Damaged cell

Pain signal received by brain cell and interpreted

Action of non-opioids
These drugs block production of prostaglandins. As a result, the nerve endings cannot be stimulated, so no pain signal passes to the brain.

Opioid

Opioid receptor

Pain signal blocked

Brain cell

Action of opioids
Normally the pain signal is transmitted between brain cells. Opioids combine with receptors on brain cells (opioid receptors), blocking transmission of pain signals within the brain and also in the spinal cord.

MIGRAINE

What is it?
A migraine is a recurrent severe headache sometimes affecting only one side of the head. It may be accompanied by nausea, vomiting, and a sensitivity to light, and may be preceded by warning signs, called auras, which can include visual signs such as flashing lights or other sensory signs such as numbness and tingling in the arms. Speech may be impaired, or the attack may be disabling.

What causes it?
Migraines are caused by changes in the blood vessels around the brain and scalp. A migraine attack begins when blood vessels surrounding the brain constrict (become narrower), producing the typical migraine warning signs. The next stage of a migraine attack occurs when blood vessels in the scalp and around the eyes dilate (widen). As a result, chemicals called prostaglandins are released, producing pain. The reasons for these blood vessel changes are unknown, but an attack may be triggered by a blow to the head, physical exertion, certain foods and drugs, or emotional factors such as excitement, tension, or shock. A family history of migraine also increases the chance of an individual suffering from it.

What can help?
The factors that trigger a migraine attack should be identified and avoided. Drugs are used either to relieve symptoms or to prevent attacks. In most people, migraine headaches can be relieved by a mild analgesic, for example, acetaminophen, ibuprofen, or ASA, or a stronger one like naproxen, ergotamine, or a triptan. An anti-emetic (p.73) may be taken with the drug if nausea and vomiting accompany the migraine. If the attacks occur more often than once a month, drugs to prevent migraine may be taken every day. However, a susceptibility to migraine headaches can clear up spontaneously, and if you are taking drugs regularly, your doctor may recommend that you stop them after a few months to see if this has happened.

🤚 Risks and special precautions
Preparations that contain caffeine should be avoided since headaches may be caused by excessive use of caffeine or on stopping treatment. 5HT₁ agonists should not usually be used if you have high blood pressure, angina, or coronary heart disease. You should not take more of the medications for migraine than your doctor advises in any one week.

Types of drugs for migraine

- **Analgesics** (see p.39) are used to relieve migraine symptoms. They work by blocking prostaglandins, the chemical released as the blood vessels dilate in the scalp and around the eyes.

- **5HT₁ agonist drugs** are used to relieve acute attacks if analgesics are not effective. They work by narrowing dilated blood vessels in the scalp.

- **Beta blockers** (see p.52) are used to prevent a migraine attack. They work by preventing the constriction of blood vessels around the brain.

- **Calcium channel blockers** dilate blood vessels and are used to prevent migraines.

- **Serotonin antagonists** are used to block the production of serotonin, which causes the large blood vessels in the brain to constrict and can trigger the start of a migraine.

🔘 COMMON DRUGS

Drugs to prevent migraine	Other drugs
Amitriptyline	Rizatriptan
Atenolol ✱	Sumatriptan
Flunarizine	Zolmitriptan
Metoprolol ✱	**Other drugs to relieve migraine**
Propranolol ✱	Acetaminophen ✱
Topiramate ✱	ASA ✱
Verapamil ✱	Ergotamine
5HT₁ agonists	Ibuprofen ✱
Almotriptan	Naproxen ✱
Frovatriptan	

✱ See Part 3

Action of drugs used for migraine

Migraine is caused by the action of chemicals in the bloodstream on blood vessels surrounding the brain and in the scalp. In the first stage of a migraine attack, the blood vessels surrounding the brain constrict, causing warning signs. In the second stage, the blood vessels in the scalp dilate, causing a severe headache.

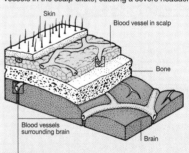

Skin
Blood vessel in scalp
Bone
Blood vessels surrounding brain
Brain

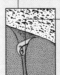

Constricted blood vessel

Preventing migraine
Migraine-preventing drugs block the action of chemicals that cause constriction of the blood vessels surrounding the brain.

Dilated blood vessel

Relieving migraine
Ergotamine and 5HT₁ agonists taken during a migraine attack return the dilated blood vessels in the scalp to their normal size.

DEPRESSION

What is it?
Most individuals may experience occasional episodes of sadness or feeling down. However, those who experience extreme sadness or a feeling of despair over several weeks may be suffering from depression, and medical attention is needed. Additional symptoms may include difficulty sleeping (sleeping too much or insomnia), significant lack of energy and desire to carry out their usual routine, and changes in appetite leading to weight gain or loss.

What causes it?
Depression is thought to be caused by an imbalance in the level of certain chemicals in the brain called neurotransmitters, which affect mood by stimulating brain cells. Some people, including those with a personal or a family history of depression, are at risk of developing depression. Significant life stressors, such as death of someone close or a serious illness, can trigger an episode, but sometimes an episode of depression can occur for no apparent cause. Some women may be susceptible to this condition shortly after giving birth; this is called post-partum depression.

What can help?
Minor depression does not usually require drug treatment. Cognitive behavioural therapy, psychological counselling, and support in coming to terms with the cause of the depression may be all that is needed. Moderate or severe depression, in addition to counselling, usually requires drug treatment, which is effective in most cases. Antidepressant drugs work by increasing the level of certain neurotransmitters in the brain. With proper treatment, a first depressive episode may resolve over several months. However, future episodes may require longer treatment. Treatment should not be stopped without consultation with your doctor as, if stopped too soon, symptoms may reappear.

Risks and special precautions
Ongoing monitoring of individuals with depression, by their doctor and other care providers, with regards to feelings of self-harm is important. Overdose of TCAs and MAOIs can be dangerous, and both are prescribed with caution for people with heart problems or epilepsy. People taking MAOIs are given a list of prohibited foods and drugs (for example, cheese, meat, yeast extracts, and red wine).

Bipolar disorder

Changes in mood are normal. However, bipolar disorder can result in a person's mood swings becoming grossly exaggerated, with peaks of elation, mania, or hypomania, alternating with clinical depression. Manic episodes are treated with drugs such as lithium, divalproex or newer antipsychotics. Lithium or lamotrigine can be helpful with depression associated with bipolar disorder, as it lifts the depression and lessens the frequency of mood swings.

Types of antidepressants

- **Tricyclics** (TCAs) and **venlafaxine** block the reabsorption of the neurotransmitters serotonin and norepinephrine (noradrenaline), increasing the levels of these neurotransmitters in the brain. TCAs cause some drowsiness, which is useful for sleep problems in depression.

- **Selective serotonin re-uptake inhibitors** (SSRIs) act by blocking the reabsorption of serotonin. The SSRIs generally have fewer side effects and are better tolerated than the TCAs. SSRIs are especially effective in people who are anxious as well as depressed, or who suffer from certain phobias or obsessive-compulsive disorder. Some SSRIs may cause drowsiness and should be taken at bedtime.

- **Mirtazapine** is an antidepressant used in the treatment of mild to moderate depression and is as effective as other antidepressants. It can cause drowsiness and weight gain.

- **Monoamine oxidase inhibitors** (MAOIs) act by blocking the breakdown of neurotransmitters, mainly serotonin and norepinephrine (noradrenaline). Older MAOIs are used much less frequently today as these often require certain food restrictions.

- **Bupropion** is an antidepressant that is also used as an aid in smoking cessation (see p.45).

COMMON DRUGS

Tricyclics	MAOIs
Amitriptyline	Moclobemide
Clomipramine	Phenelzine
Desipramine	Tranylcypromine
Imipramine	**Other drugs**
Nortriptyline	Bupropion ✳
SSRIs	Desvenlafaxine
Citalopram	Duloxetine
Escitalopram	Mirtazapine ✳
Fluoxetine ✳	Trazodone
Fluvoxamine ✳	Venlafaxine ✳
Paroxetine ✳	
Sertraline	

✳ See Part 3

41

DEPRESSION continued

Action of antidepressants

Normally, the brain cells release sufficient quantities of excitatory chemicals (known as neurotransmitters) to stimulate neighbouring cells. The neurotransmitters are constantly reabsorbed into the brain cells where they are broken down by an enzyme called monoamine oxidase. In depression, fewer neurotransmitters are released. The levels of neurotransmitters in the brain are raised by antidepressant drugs.

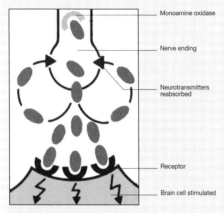

Monoamine oxidase

Nerve ending

Neurotransmitters reabsorbed

Receptor

Brain cell stimulated

Normal brain activity
In a normal brain neurotransmitters are constantly being released, reabsorbed, and broken down.

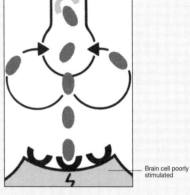

Brain cell poorly stimulated

Brain activity in depression
The brain cells release fewer neurotransmitters than normal, leading to reduced stimulation.

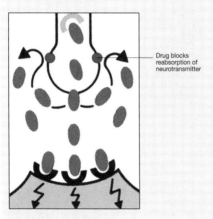

Drug blocks reabsorption of neurotransmitter

Action of TCAs and SSRIs
TCA and SSRI drugs increase the levels of neurotransmitters by blocking their reabsorption.

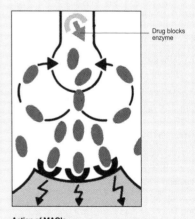

Drug blocks enzyme

Action of MAOIs
MAOIs increase the neurotransmitter levels by blocking the action of the enzyme (monoamine oxidase) that breaks them down.

ANXIETY

What is it?
Anxiety is an unpleasant feeling that is typically characterized by nervousness, apprehension, and fear. It is often not caused by any real danger, and can be accompanied by physical symptoms such as shaking, palpitations, and headaches. It is a normal reaction to stress, but in excessive amounts it can be debilitating.

What causes it?
Anxiety is generally a reaction to too much stress. Clinically, anxiety arises when the balance of certain chemicals in the brain is disturbed. The fearful feelings increase brain activity, stimulating the sympathetic nervous system and often triggering any physical symptoms.

What can help?
Tackling the underlying problem through counselling and perhaps psychotherapy offers the best hope of a long-term solution. Anti-anxiety drugs (also called anxiolytics) are prescribed for short-term relief of severe anxiety and nervousness caused by psychological problems, but these drugs cannot resolve the causes. The drugs can also be used to relax people before uncomfortable medical procedures. Antidepressants, such as selective serotonin reuptake inhibitors (SSRIs), are effective for generalized anxiety disorder. These drugs take a few weeks to be effective and are usually prescribed for longer-term therapy. Benzodiazepines may be used for more immediate relief of anxiety.

✋ Risks and special precautions
Do not combine benzodiazepines with alcohol and other substances. There is a risk of psychological and physical dependence, especially when used regularly in higher doses. This risk, however, is minimal when used appropriately for short periods under medical supervision. If used for a period of longer than two weeks, the drugs should be withdrawn gradually under medical supervision to avoid withdrawal symptoms such as excessive anxiety, nightmares, and restlessness.

Types of anti-anxiety drugs

- **Benzodiazepines and related drugs** depress activity in the part of the brain that controls emotion by blocking transmission of electrical impulses and thus reducing communication between brain cells. This prevents the excessive brain activity that causes anxiety. The drugs' sedative effects also help relieve insomnia, which often accompanies anxiety.

- **Buspirone** also prevents excessive brain activity, but does not cause drowsiness. Its effect is not felt for at least two weeks after starting treatment.

- **Selective serotonin re-uptake inhibitors** (SSRIs) act by blocking the reabsorption of serotonin (see p.42). The SSRIs generally have fewer side effects.

- **Beta blockers** are used intermittently for specific task-related anxiety. They block the stimulation of the heart, digestive system, and other organs by the sympathetic nervous system (see p.52).

Action of benzodiazepines and related drugs

The reticular activating system (RAS) in the brain stem controls the level of mental activity by stimulating higher centres of the brain controlling consciousness. Benzodiazepines and related drugs depress the RAS, relieving anxiety. In larger doses they depress the RAS sufficiently to cause drowsiness and sleep.

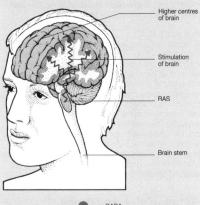

Higher centres of brain

Stimulation of brain

RAS

Brain stem

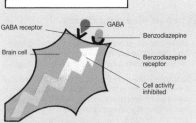

GABA receptor

GABA

Benzodiazepine

Brain cell

Benzodiazepine receptor

Cell activity inhibited

Action of brain cells in the RAS
Brain cell activity is normally inhibited by GABA, a chemical that binds to specialized cell receptors. Brain cells also have receptors for benzodiazepines. The drug binds to its receptor and promotes the inhibitory effect of GABA, which depresses brain cell activity in the RAS.

💊 COMMON DRUGS

Benzodiazepines	Beta blockers
Alprazolam ✳	Atenolol ✳
Clonazepam	Metoprolol ✳
Diazepam	Propranolol ✳
Lorazepam ✳	**Antidepressants**
Oxazepam	Citalopram
Other	Clomipramine
Buspirone	Desipramine
	Paroxetine ✳
	Sertraline
	Venlafaxine ✳

✳ See Part 3

INSOMNIA

What is it?
Difficulty in getting to sleep or staying asleep for a normal period over many days is called insomnia. Most people suffer from sleepless nights from time to time, but persistent sleeplessness can be problematic, resulting in excessive fatigue and a general inability to cope.

What causes it?
Occasional sleepless nights are usually as a result of a temporary worry or discomfort from a minor illness. Ongoing sleeplessness can be caused by psychological problems including anxiety or depression, or by pain arising from a physical disorder.

What can help?
For occasional sleeplessness, simple remedies to promote relaxation – for example, taking a warm bath or a hot milk drink before bedtime – are usually the best form of treatment. Sleeping drugs (also known as hypnotics) are normally prescribed only when these self-help remedies have failed, and when lack of sleep is beginning to affect general health. These drugs are used to reestablish the habit of sleeping. They should be used in the smallest dose and for the shortest possible time (usually not for more than three weeks). Long-term treatment of sleeplessness depends on resolving the underlying cause of the problem. Alcohol is not recommended to get to sleep as it can cause disturbed sleep and can affect the normal sleep cycle.

Risks and special precautions
Do not to use sleeping drugs every night – they become less effective over time and can produce physical dependence when taken regularly for more than a few weeks or in large doses. Rarely, psychological dependence can also develop. Some benzodiazepines may produce minor side effects, such as daytime drowsiness, which can impair the ability to drive or operate machinery. Some people may experience a variety of hangover effects the following day. Elderly people are likely to become confused, and selection of an appropriate drug is important. Sleeping drugs should be stopped gradually under your doctor's supervision.

COMMON DRUGS

Benzodiazepines
Flurazepam
Lorazepam ✳
Nitrazepam
Oxazepam
Temazepam
Triazolam

Other non-benzodiazepine sleeping drugs
Zopiclone

✳ See Part 3

Types of sleeping drugs

Most sleeping drugs promote sleep by reducing brain activity, allowing one to fall asleep more easily. However, the nature of the sleep can be affected by the drug.

- **Benzodiazepines** are the most commonly used class of sleeping drugs as they have comparatively few side effects and are relatively safe in overdose. They are also used to treat anxiety (see p.43).

- Other **non-benzodiazepine sleeping drugs**, such as zopiclone, work in a similar way to benzodiazepines. It is not intended for long-term use.

- Widely used to treat allergic symptoms (see p.33), **antihistamines** such as diphenhydramine also cause drowsiness. They are sometimes used to promote sleep but can cause adverse effects and are not recommended in some individuals, especially in older people.

- **Antidepressant drugs** may be used to promote sleep in those who are depressed (see p.41), as they can also effectively treat the underlying depressive illness.

The effects of drugs on sleep patterns

Normal sleep can be divided into three types: light sleep, deep sleep, and dream sleep. The proportion of time spent in each type of sleep changes with age and is altered by sleeping drugs. Dramatic changes in sleep patterns also occur in the first few days following abrupt withdrawal of sleeping drugs after regular, prolonged use.

Normal sleep
Young adults spend most sleep time in light sleep with roughly equal proportions of dream and deep sleep.

Drug-induced sleep has less dream sleep and less deep sleep with relatively more light sleep.

Sleep following drug withdrawal
There is a marked increase in dream sleep following withdrawal of drugs used regularly for a long time.

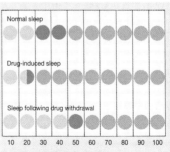

Normal sleep

Drug-induced sleep

Sleep following drug withdrawal

10 20 30 40 50 60 70 80 90 100
Percentage of total sleep time

● Dream sleep   ● Deep sleep   ● Light sleep

TOBACCO ADDICTION

What are the issues?
Tobacco is most commonly smoked in cigarettes but can be smoked in cigars and pipes, inhaled as snuff, or chewed. However it is used, tobacco is addictive and harmful to health. Nicotine addiction is the number one cause of preventable death in Canada.

Health risk from smoking is related to nicotine, as well as the many cancer-causing chemicals in tobacco smoke (see p.46 for effects of tobacco use). Nicotine in tobacco is largely responsible for tobacco addiction in over one-third of the population who are cigarette smokers. In regular tobacco users, nicotine temporarily increases alertness, concentration, relieves tension and fatigue, and counters boredom. Most people who start go on to smoke regularly, and most become physically dependent on nicotine, and psychologically dependent on the process of smoking. Stopping can produce temporary withdrawal symptoms that include nausea, headache, diarrhea, increased appetite, drowsiness, fatigue, irritability, restlessness, depressed mood, an inability to concentrate, and craving for cigarettes.

What can help?
Disease and damage can be prevented by not smoking, or quitting smoking before you begin to develop a heart or lung condition. If a disease has already been diagnosed, quitting smoking immediately can prevent further damage to health. You are never too old to benefit from giving up smoking.

How to quit
If you need help to quit smoking, consult with your doctor and pharmacist. Aids such as nicotine gum, lozenges, patches, or inhalers, or prescription medications such as bupropion or varenicline can help with withdrawal symptoms.

If you plan on quitting on your own, plan in advance how you will stop – you may decide to quit completely all at once or taper off slowly. Make a list of your reasons for quitting, and a list of the most common reasons why you smoke. You may smoke as a habit in certain situations or at certain times of the day, so an alteration in these rituals may help. There are many smokers' cessation programs and resources available to help you with this; your pharmacist can assist in obtaining this information. Also, plan ways to cope with temptation and withdrawal symptoms and tell your family and friends so that they can offer support. Dispose of all cigarettes, lighters, and ashtrays, and distract yourself with other enjoyable activities.

Help with quitting

Visit the following websites for further helpful information on quitting:

- Canadian Lung Association: http://www.lung.ca/ protect-protegez/tobacco-tabagisme/quitting-cesser/how-comment_e.php

- Public Health Agency of Canada: http://www.phac-aspc.gc.ca/chn-rcs/tobacco-tabagisme-eng.php?rd=tobacco_tabac_eng

✋ Risks and special precautions
Nicotine replacement therapy should not be used with other nicotine-containing products, including cigarettes. Nicotine in any form should not be used during pregnancy or while breast-feeding. Discuss with your doctor if you have long-term liver or kidney problems, diabetes mellitus, thyroid disease, circulation or heart problems, a peptic ulcer, pheochromocytoma, or any skin disorders. Quitting smoking may increase the blood levels of some drugs, such as warfarin and theophylline. Discuss with your doctor or pharmacist.

Types of nicotine replacement therapies

Addiction to nicotine is the main reason that people fail in their goal to quit smoking. Nicotine replacement therapies provide a method for people to get nicotine without smoking, thus reducing withdrawal symptoms.

- **Nicotine patches** are applied directly to the skin. The strength of the patch is gradually reduced until complete abstinence is achieved, usually after about 3 months.

- **Nicotine chewing gum or lozenges** can be used whenever the urge to smoke occurs.

- **Nicotine inhalers** come equipped with cartridges that regulate each dosage.

- **Bupropion**, which is also used as an antidepressant, is effective in helping with smoking cessation. This drug is not recommended in those with a history of seizures , anorexia or bulimia. **Varenicline**, a non-nicotine medication, can also be helpful. This drug is not to be used with nicotine products and during pregnancy. For effective cessation of smoking, these drugs should be used along with behavioural programs.

💊 COMMON DRUGS

Bupropion ✳
Nicotine ✳
Varenicline ✳

| ✳ See Part 3 |

TOBACCO ADDICTION continued

Effects of tobacco use

Tobacco smoke contains several substances that are toxic or irritating to the body – most notably nicotine, tar, carbon monoxide, and carcinogenic (cancer-causing) substances. Nicotine narrows the blood vessels and increases the heart rate and blood pressure. Tar in tobacco smoke irritates and inflames lung tissues.

- **Damage to the respiratory system** is caused by substances in tobacco smoke that irritate the mucous membranes that line the air passages to the lungs, causing them to produce more mucus and leading to the characteristic "smoker's cough." This may lead to chronic obstructive pulmonary disease (see p.32), or increase the risk for cancer of the lungs, nasopharynx, or larynx.

- **Damage to the vascular system** is caused by nicotine and carbon monoxide, which can lead to atherosclerosis (p.47), high blood pressure (p.48), stroke (p.55), and coronary artery disease. In women over 35, smoking combined with oral contraceptive use can increase the risk of heart attack (p.51) and stroke.

- **Damage to other systems** is also common with tobacco use. Smokers are at an increased risk of developing cancer of the mouth and esophagus. Tobacco smoke can aggravate peptic ulcers (p.72), reduce fertility in men and women, and cause accelerated skin changes, such as wrinkling, or earlier menopause in women (p.70). Pregnant women who smoke are likely to have a low birthweight baby, and the baby is at greater risk of illness or death just after birth.

- **Second-hand smoking** is the term given to inhaling the smoke from other people's cigarettes. Secondhand smoke is a mixture of smoke from burning cigarettes and that exhaled by smokers. It irritates the eyes, nose, and throat, and may cause headaches and nausea. People who are regularly exposed to secondhand smoke are at a greater risk of developing lung cancer and cardiovascular diseases, asthma (p.30), allergies (p.33), and infections such as sinusitis (p.29) and acute bronchitis (p.32). Children of smokers are particularly at risk.

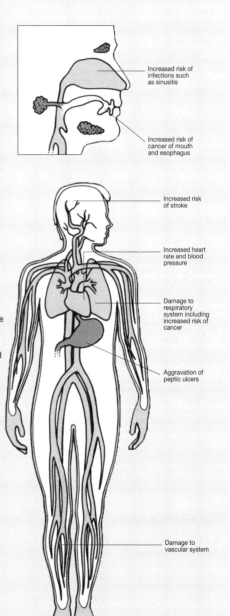

Increased risk of infections such as sinusitis

Increased risk of cancer of mouth and esophagus

Increased risk of stroke

Increased heart rate and blood pressure

Damage to respiratory system including increased risk of cancer

Aggravation of peptic ulcers

Damage to vascular system

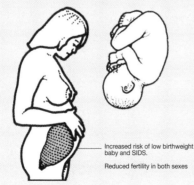

Increased risk of low birthweight baby and SIDS.

Reduced fertility in both sexes

HIGH CHOLESTEROL

What is it?
The blood contains several types of fats, or lipids, which are necessary for normal body function. However, certain types of fats can be damaging if present in excess, in particular certain types of cholesterol. Low-density lipoprotein (LDL) is considered a "bad" cholesterol; if present in large amounts, it can increase the risk of developing **atherosclerosis**, in which fatty deposits called atheroma build up in the arteries, restricting and disrupting the flow of blood. This can lead to cardiovascular disease and an increased likelihood of the formation of abnormal blood clots, causing potentially fatal disorders such as stroke and heart attack. In contrast, high-density lipoprotein (HDL) is a "good" cholesterol that can protect against cardiovascular disease. An individual suffering from high cholesterol may have high levels of LDL and possibly other damaging fats, including triglycerides. Some may also have low levels of the protective HDL.

What causes it?
Atherosclerosis is most common in Western countries where people tend to eat a diet high in fat and calories. Other lifestyle issues are linked to high cholesterol levels, including lack of exercise, smoking, and obesity. Some disorders, such as diabetes mellitus, are associated with high lipids such as triglycerides, regardless of diet or lifestyle. Certain inherited disorders also result in high levels of fat in the bloodstream.

What can help?
For most people, adopting a low-fat diet is sufficient to reduce the amount of "bad" LDL cholesterol and the risk of developing atherosclerosis. Quitting smoking, exercising regularly, and maintaining your recommended weight can also help. Lipid-lowering drugs are generally prescribed only when dietary measures have failed, and should be combined with a healthy lifestyle and a low-fat diet for maximum benefit. The drugs may be given at an earlier stage to individuals at increased risk of atherosclerosis, such as those with diabetes and people already suffering from circulatory disorders. Drugs, such as statins, can decrease LDL, which helps prevent accumulation of fatty deposits in the arteries. Lipid-lowering drugs do not correct the underlying cause of raised levels of fat in the blood, so it is usually necessary to continue with dietary measures and drug treatment indefinitely. Stopping treatment can lead to a return of high blood lipid levels. Your total cholesterol, LDL, and HDL are usually monitored.

🎯 COMMON DRUGS

Fibrates	**Nicotinic acid**
Fenofibrate	Niacin ✳
Gemfibrozil ✳	**Drugs that bind to bile**
Statins	**salts**
Atorvastatin ✳	Cholestyramine
Fluvastatin	Colestipol
Lovastatin ✳	**Other drugs acting on**
Pravastatin ✳	**the liver**
Rosuvastatin ✳	Omega-3 acid ethyl
Simvastatin ✳	esters ✳
Cholesterol absorption	Omega-3 oils
inhibitor	
Ezetimibe ✳	

Types of lipid-lowering drugs

- **Drugs that act on the liver** alter the way in which the liver converts fatty acids in the blood into different types of lipids, including cholesterol and triglycerides. These drugs include **fibrates, niacin, statins, and fish oil preparations.**

- **Drugs that bind to bile salts** produced by the liver prevent the absorption of cholesterol from the bowel.

✳ See Part 3

Action of lipid-lowering drugs

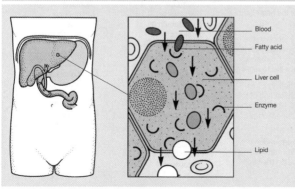

Blood
Fatty acid
Liver cell
Enzyme
Lipid

Drugs that act on the liver
Fatty acids in the blood are normally converted into lipids by enzyme activity in the liver (left). Several drugs alter the way fatty acids are taken into the liver cells and others alter the enzyme activity in the liver to prevent the manufacture of lipids.

HIGH BLOOD PRESSURE

What is it?

Blood pressure is the force exerted by the blood against the walls of the arteries. It varies naturally with activity, rising during exercise or stress and falling during rest. It also varies among individuals and normally increases with age. Two measurements of blood pressure are usually taken: one indicates the force when the ventricles are contracting (this is the larger number) and the second is when the ventricles are relaxed (smaller number of the two). An ideal blood pressure is stated as a pressure of 120mm/80mm. If an individual has higher than normal blood pressure on at least three separate occasions, he or she may have a condition called **hypertension**. This condition puts strain on the heart and arteries, and can result in damage to the delicate tissues. Hypertension does not usually cause any symptoms, but severely raised blood pressure may produce headaches and palpitations. It is important to reduce high blood pressure because it can have serious consequences, including stroke, heart attack, heart failure, and kidney damage.

What causes it?

Often there is no obvious cause of hypertension. Lifestyle and genetic factors may contribute to this condition. It is more common in middle aged and elderly people, due to arteries that have become more rigid with age. People who are overweight, smoke, or drink large amounts of alcohol are more likely to develop hypertension, and a stressful lifestyle may aggravate the condition.

Also at risk are those with diabetes, people with pre-existing heart damage, and those whose blood contains a high level of fat (cholesterol). Some conditions, such as kidney disease, certain hormonal disorders, and pregnancy, can lead to high blood pressure. High blood pressure is more common among those of African-American background than among Caucasians, and in countries where the diet is high in salt.

Types of antihypertensive drugs

- **Diuretic drugs** help to turn excess body water into urine. This reduces the amount of water in the bloodstream, and in turn reduces the total volume of blood and the pressure in the blood vessels.

- **Beta blockers** stop the stimulating action of norepinephrine, the main "fight or flight" hormone. This reduces the speed and force of the heart beat. See p.52 for action of beta blockers.

- **Calcium channel blockers** work by blocking the passage of calcium through muscle cells, which is needed to cause muscles to contract. This causes the muscle layer in the blood vessel walls to relax.

- **ACE inhibitors** act by blocking the activity of an enzyme in the blood that causes constriction of the blood vessels. These drugs are useful in those who also suffer from diabetes. See p.52 for action of ACE inhibitors.

- **Vasodilators**, including alpha blockers, widen the blood vessels by relaxing the muscles surrounding them, thereby reducing the workload on the heart. See p.53 for action of vasodilators.

What can help?

Mild hypertension can be controlled by reducing alcohol and salt consumption, losing weight, exercising regularly, and quitting smoking. In addition to these lifestyle changes, one or more antihypertensive drugs may be prescribed. These drugs usually work by either dilating the blood vessels or by reducing blood volume, and it may take some time to find the right combination and dosage. The drugs are not a cure and may need to be taken indefinitely.

Action of antihypertensive drugs

Each type of antihypertensive drug acts on a different part of the body to lower blood pressure.

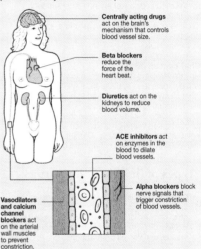

Centrally acting drugs act on the brain's mechanism that controls blood vessel size.

Beta blockers reduce the force of the heart beat.

Diuretics act on the kidneys to reduce blood volume.

ACE inhibitors act on enzymes in the blood to dilate blood vessels.

Alpha blockers block nerve signals that trigger constriction of blood vessels.

Vasodilators and calcium channel blockers act on the arterial wall muscles to prevent constriction.

⊗ COMMON DRUGS

ACE inhibitors
  Enalapril ✳
  Lisinopril
  Ramipril ✳
Angiotensin II blockers
  Candesartan ✳
  Losartan ✳
  Valsartan ✳
Beta blockers
  Atenolol ✳
  Metoprolol ✳
  Propranolol ✳
Calcium channel blockers
  Amlodipine ✳
  Diltiazem ✳
  Nifedipine
  Verapamil ✳

Centrally acting antihypertensives
  Clonidine
  Methyldopa
Diuretics
  Chlorthalidone
  Furosemide ✳
  Hydrochlorothiazide ✳
  Triamterene
Alpha blockers
  Doxazosin
  Prazosin
  Terazosin ✳
Vasodilators
  Hydralazine

✳ See Part 3

ARRHYTHMIA

What is it?

The heart contains two upper and two lower chambers, which are known as the atria and ventricles. The pumping actions of these two sets of chambers are normally coordinated by electrical impulses that ensure that the heart beats with a regular rhythm. If this coordination breaks down, the heart will beat abnormally, either irregularly, or faster or slower than usual. The general term for abnormal heart rhythm is arrhythmia. Two types of arrhythmias are **tachycardias**, in which the heart rate is too high, and **bradycardias**, in which the rate is too low. A common type of tachycardia that affects the atria is call atrial fibrillation (AF). Some individuals may not feel any symptoms with AF while others may experience palpitations, light-headedness and shortness of breath. Arrhythmia affecting the ventricles can sometimes be life-threatening. An ECG will usually help confirm the type of arrhythmia.

What causes it?

Arrhythmias may occur as a result of a birth defect, coronary heart disease, or other less common heart disorders. A variety of more general conditions, including overactivity of the thyroid gland, can disturb heart rhythm, as can certain drugs such as caffeine, some drugs with an anticholinergic effect, and drugs used in other heart conditions. AF can sometimes occur without a clearly identifiable cause in adults.

What can help?

Minor disturbances of heart rhythm are common and do not usually require drug treatment. However, if the pumping action of the heart is seriously affected, the circulation of blood throughout the body may become inefficient, and drug treatment may be necessary. Drugs may be taken to treat individual attacks of tachycardia, or they may be taken on a regular basis to prevent or control abnormal heart rhythms. A pacemaker may be inserted if needed to restore a normal heart beat in the case of bradycardia. Those with chronic AF are usually prescribed drugs to slow the heart rate. In addition, as they are at a higher risk for stroke, an anticoagulant is usually prescribed.

Types of anti-arrhythmic drugs

- **Beta blockers** help to prevent attacks of tachycardia, including AF, by slowing the force and speed of the heart beat. See p.52 for action of beta blockers.

- **Digitalis** works by slowing yet increasing the force of the heart's muscle contractions, which improves the efficiency of each heart beat.

- **Calcium channel blockers** act to slow the heart's contractions and to regulate the heart beat.

- **Amiodarone** is an anti-arrhythmic drug that is used for both atrial and ventricular arrhythmias and is usually also used when other drugs are not effective. There are several other anti-arrhythmic agents such as quinidine, lidocaine, disopyramide and procainamide, but these are not commonly used.

Risks and special precautions

Anti-arrhythmic drugs may further disrupt heart rhythm under certain circumstances and are used only when the benefit outweighs the risks.

Amiodarone may accumulate in the tissues over time, and may lead to light-sensitive rashes, changes in thyroid function, and lung problems. Those taking amiodarone should be followed closely by their cardiologist.

Sites of drug action

Anti-arrhythmic drugs either slow the flow of electrical impulses to the heart muscle, or inhibit the muscle's ability to contract. Beta blockers reduce the ability of the pacemaker to pass electrical signals to the rest of the heart. Digoxin reduces the passage of signals from the atrioventricular node. Calcium channel blockers interfere with the ability of the heart muscle to contract by impeding the flow of calcium into muscle cells. Other drugs, such as quinidine and disopyramide, reduce the sensitivity of muscle cells to electrical impulses.

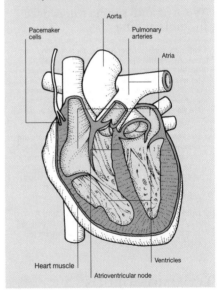

COMMON DRUGS

Beta blockers	**Digitalis**
Metoprolol ✳	Digoxin
Propranolol ✳	**Other drugs**
Sotalol	Amiodarone
Calcium channel	Disopyramide
blockers	Lidocaine
Diltiazem ✳	Procainamide
Verapamil ✳	Quinidine
	Warfarin ✳
✳ See Part 3	

ANGINA

What is it?

Angina is chest pain, or chest discomfort, produced when the heart muscle receives insufficient oxygen. The most common type of angina is called **stable angina**, which is usually brought on by exertion or emotional stress and is relieved by rest. Symptoms include a dull, heavy, constricting sensation in the centre of the chest, and a discomfort that spreads into the throat and down one or both arms. Angina affects both sexes, but is less common in women before menopause. If you experience angina, see your doctor immediately – the condition can lead to an increased risk of heart attack if left untreated. If you experience a sudden worsening of angina, or angina at rest, or persistent discomfort not relieved by nitroglycerin, seek immediate medical help.

What causes it?

Angina is usually caused by coronary artery disease, the narrowing of the blood vessels (coronary arteries) that transport blood and oxygen to the heart muscle. The blood flow through the arteries may be sufficient for the heart while it is at rest, but becomes inadequate during exertion. As a result, the heart muscle is starved of oxygen and toxic substances build up in the heart, causing a constrictive, cramp-like pain. In the most common type of angina (stable angina), narrowing of the coronary arteries results from deposits of fat – called atheroma – on the walls of the arteries, causing the condition called athersclorosis (see p.47). The deposits build up more rapidly in the arteries of people with high cholesterol and high blood pressure, smokers, people who eat a high-fat diet, and people suffering from diabetes mellitus.

What can help?

Eating a low fat diet, quitting smoking, and losing weight can all help to improve the symptoms of angina. Drug treatment is also often necessary, both to treat the pain and to reduce the number and severity of attacks. Drugs can often control angina for many years, but they cannot cure the disorder. When severe angina cannot be controlled by drugs, a procedure to open up the arteries or bypass surgery to increase the blood flow to the heart, may be recommended.

Types of anti-angina drugs used in stable angina

- **Nitrates**, such as nitroglycerin, are fast acting and are prescribed for people who suffer from only occasional episodes of stable angina. The drug is taken at the first signs of an attack, or before an activity that is known to bring on an attack. This is available as a sublingual tablet or a spray. Nitrates are also available as a topical ointment and as a longer-acting oral tablets.

- **Beta blockers, long-acting nitrates,** and **calcium channel blockers** are used as regular medication to prevent attacks for people who suffer more frequent or severe attacks of stable angina. The introduction of adhesive patches to administer nitrates through the patient's skin has extended the duration of the action of nitroglycerin, making treatment easier.

- **Lipid-lowering drugs, ACE-inhibitors,** and **ASA** may be recommended in those with stable angina to improve long-term prognosis. Lipid-lowering drugs called statins are usually used.

Action of anti-angina drugs

Nitrates and calcium channel blockers work by dilating blood vessels. Blood is more easily pumped through the dilated vessels, reducing the strain on the heart.

Beta blockers and some calcium channel blockers reduce heart muscle stimulation during exercise or stress by interrupting signal transmission in the heart. Decreased heart muscle stimulation means less oxygen is required, reducing the risk of angina attacks.

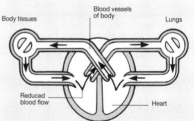

Before drug

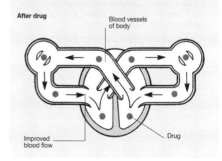

After drug

🅧 COMMON DRUGS

Beta blockers	Nitrates
Atenolol ✳	Isosorbide dinitrate/
Metoprolol ✳	mononitrate
Propranolol ✳	Nitroglycerin ✳
Calcium channel	**Other drugs**
blockers	ASA ✳
Amlodipine ✳	Atorvastatin ✳
Diltiazem ✳	Enalapril ✳
Felodipine	Pravastatin ✳
Nifedipine	Ramipril ✳
Verapamil ✳	Simvastatin ✳

✳ See Part 3

HEART ATTACK

What is it?
A heart attack, or a myocardial infarction, happens when there is a loss of blood supply to part of the heart muscle, due to a blockage in a coronary artery. Symptoms include severe, crushing pain in the centre of the chest that may spread up the neck and down the left arm, pallor and sweating, shortness of breath, and nausea. Some patients may not have these symptoms and may instead feel an extreme heaviness in the chest. Heart attacks can be fatal, so call for medical attention immediately if these symptoms develop.

What causes it?
Heart attacks are usually a result of coronary artery disease, which causes the narrowing of the coronary arteries that supply the heart muscle with fresh oxygenated blood. The narrowing is often caused by atherosclerosis (see p.47), in which fatty deposits build up in the arteries, restricting and disrupting the flow of blood and leading to the formation of plaque. The plaque may rupture and the resulting thrombus may partially or completely block blood flow through the artery, leading to a heart attack. People at risk include those who smoke, have a high-fat diet and high blood cholesterol levels, get little exercise, and are overweight. Those with a family history (parents, siblings) of heart disease are also at risk.

What can help?
The immediate goal of treatment is to relieve pain and restore the blood supply to the heart muscle in order to minimize damage to the heart. Call for medical assistance immediately; they may instruct you to chew on an ASA tablet if possible, which will thin the blood to prevent further clotting. After admission to the critical care unit, a powerful analgesic such as morphine may be given to alleviate the pain and nitroglycerin to help open the blood vessels, along with a thrombolytic drug to dissolve the thrombus with a complete blockage. An ACE inhibitor may be given to improve prognosis. Surgery may be needed to remove a blockage. Other drugs that may be used include a beta blocker, an antiplatelet agent, and an anticoagulant.

Long-term care to reduce the risk of another heart attack will involve lifestyle changes, such as maintaining a low-fat diet, quitting smoking, reducing weight, and starting an exercise program. Prior to discharge, a beta blocker, an ACE inhibitor, an antiplatelet agent, and a statin will likely be prescribed. Discuss follow-up visits with your doctor.

🖑 Risks and special precautions
Beta blockers are prescribed with caution for people who have asthma, bronchitis, or other forms of respiratory disease, and those who are subject to heart failure. They are not commonly prescribed for people who have poor circulation in the limbs. Diabetics who need to take beta blockers should be aware that they may notice a change in the warning signs of low blood sugar; in particular, they may find that symptoms such as palpitations and tremor are suppressed. Beta blockers should not be stopped suddenly after prolonged use; this may provoke a sudden heart attack or a marked rise in blood pressure. Treatment should be withdrawn gradually under medical supervision. See p.54 for risks and special precautions for anticoagulant drugs.

Types of drugs for heart attack

- **Thrombolytic drugs** are used to dissolve clots that have already formed. They are usually given in hospital intravenously to clear a blocked blood vessel. The sooner they are given after the start of symptoms, the more likely they are to reduce the size and severity of a heart attack. See pp.54–5 for action of thrombolytic drugs and risks and special precautions.

- **Antiplatelet drugs** are taken regularly by people with a tendency to form clots in the arteries. They reduce the tendency of platelets to stick together when blood flow is disrupted. The most commonly used antiplatelet drug is ASA, which can be taken immediately when the symptoms of a heart attack present, or as a regular drug treatment after a heart attack to prevent further clots. See p.55 for action of antiplatelet drugs.

- **Beta blockers** are given after a heart attack to reduce the likelihood of abnormal heart rhythms or further damage to the heart muscle. They reduce the force and speed of the heart beat.

- **ACE inhibitors** are given after a heart attack to minimize further damage to the heart muscle. Both beta blockers and ACE inhibitors can also help decrease blood pressure.

🟢 COMMON DRUGS

Antiplatelet drugs	Injected anticoagulants
Abciximab	Dalteparin (see Heparin)
ASA ✳	Enoxaparin (see Heparin)
Clopidogrel ✳	Heparin ✳
Eptifibatide	**Oral anticoagulant**
Beta blockers	Warfarin ✳
Atenolol ✳	**Thrombolytic drugs**
Metoprolol ✳	Alteplase
Timolol	Reteplase
	Tenecteplase

✳ See Part 3

HEART ATTACK continued

Action of beta blockers

Beta blockers are drugs that interrupt the transmission of stimuli through the beta receptors of the body. By occupying the beta receptors, beta blockers nullify the stimulating action of norepinephrine (noradrenaline), the main fight or flight hormone. As a result, they reduce the force and speed of the heart beat and prevent the dilation of the blood vessels surrounding the brain and leading to the extremities.

Types of beta receptor
There are two types of beta receptors: beta 1 and beta 2. Beta 1 receptors are located mainly in the heart muscle; beta 2 receptors are found both in the airways and blood vessels. Cardioselective drugs act mainly on beta 1 receptors; non-cardioselective drugs act on both types of receptor.

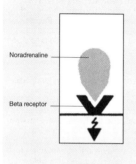

Noradrenaline

Beta receptor

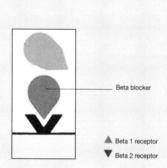

Beta blocker

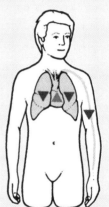

▲ Beta 1 receptor

▼ Beta 2 receptor

ACE Inhibitors

The ACE (angiotensin-converting enzyme) inhibitors are powerful vasodilators. They act by blocking the action of an enzyme in the bloodstream that is responsible for converting a chemical called angiotensin I into angiotensin II. Angiotensin II encourages constriction of the blood vessels, and its absence permits them to dilate (see below).

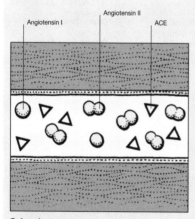

Angiotensin I

Angiotensin II

ACE

Before drug
Angiotensin I is converted by the enzyme into angiotensin II. The blood vessel constricts.

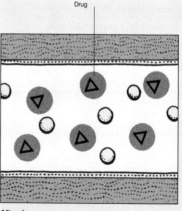

Drug

After drug
ACE inhibitors block enzyme activity, thereby preventing the formation of angiotensin II. The blood vessel dilates.

HEART FAILURE

What is it?
Heart failure is the term given when the heart's ability to pump efficiently is reduced. It can either be sudden (acute heart failure) or a long-standing inefficiency (chronic heart failure). Information on chronic heart failure is included here. The symptoms of **chronic heart failure** are often vague and develop gradually, and can include fatigue, shortness of breath aggravated by exertion or lying flat, loss of appetite, nausea, swelling of the hands and feet, and confusion.

What causes it?
In chronic heart failure, the heart is unable to pump blood around the body effectively, leading to a buildup of fluid in the lungs and body tissues (edema). Chronic heart failure can be caused by any condition that damages the heart, such as coronary artery disease or persistent high blood pressure (p.48). Other conditions that can lead to chronic heart failure include chronic obstructive pulmonary disease (p.32), heart valve disorders, or obesity. People with diabetes mellitus (p.76) may be at risk of developing chronic heart failure.

What can help?
Chronic heart failure can be treated with diuretics, vasodilators, ACE inhibitors, digoxin, and aldosterone antagonists, and in certain cases, beta blockers. Treatment will also be given for any underlying cause

of the heart failure. Lifestyle changes, including maintaining a healthy diet and weight, avoiding strenuous exercise, quitting smoking, and reducing salt intake, can also help.

🔩 COMMON DRUGS

Loop diuretics	**Nitrates**
Furosemide *	Isosorbide dinitrate/
Potassium-sparing	mononitrate
diuretics	Nitroglycerin *
Amiloride	**Calcium channel**
Spironolactone	**blockers**
Triamterene	Amlodipine *
Thiazides	**Angiotensin II blockers**
Chlorthalidone	Candesartan *
Hydrochlorothiazide *	Irbesartan
ACE inhibitors	Losartan *
Captopril	Valsartan *
Enalapril *	**Other drugs**
Fosinopril	Digoxin
Lisinopril	Hydralazine
Perindopril	
Ramipril *	
Alpha blockers	
Prazosin	
Terazosin *	⬚ * See Part 3

Types of drugs for heart failure

- **Diuretic drugs** help to turn excess body water into urine. As the urine is expelled, body tissues become less water-swollen, and heart action improves because it has a smaller volume of blood to pump.

- **Vasodilators** widen the blood vessels by relaxing the muscles surrounding them, thereby reducing the workload on the heart.

- **ACE inhibitors** act by blocking the activity of an enzyme in the blood that causes constriction of the blood vessels. See p.52 for action of ACE inhibitors.

- **Beta blockers** are prescribed to some individuals with heart failure, once their condition is stable. They reduce strain on the heart and can improve long term survival. See p.52 for action of beta blockers.

- **Digoxin** strengthens the heart's pumping action by increasing the force of each muscle contraction, relieving many of the symptoms that result from poor heart function.

Action of vasodilators

The diameter of blood vessels is governed by the contraction of the surrounding muscle. The muscle contracts in response to signals from the sympathetic nervous system. Vasodilators encourage the muscles to relax, thus increasing the size of blood vessels. Each type of vasodilator acts on a different part of the mechanism controlling blood vessel size in order to prevent contraction of the surrounding layer of muscles.

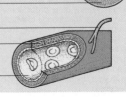

Constricted blood vessel

Dilated blood vessel

Muscle band

Alpha blockers interfere with
nerve signals to the muscles

Calcium channel blockers
act directly on the **muscle**
to inhibit contraction

ACE inhibitors block enzyme
activity in the **blood**

STROKE

What is it?

A stroke damages a part of the brain due to an interruption in its blood supply. Symptoms include weakness or numbness on one side of the body, loss of control of fine movements, dizziness, blurry vision, slurred speech, and difficulty in finding words. There is usually little or no warning before a stroke. Immediate admission to the hospital is essential to prevent permanent brain damage or death. If the symptoms disappear within 24 hours, the condition is known as a transient ischemic attack, which is a warning sign of a possible future stroke – although it has no after effects, it should not be ignored.

What causes it?

Strokes are generally caused by blood clots that block an artery supplying blood to the brain. When a blood clot forms in an artery in the brain, it is called cerebral thrombosis. Cerebral embolism occurs when a fragment of a blood clot that has formed elsewhere in the body travels in the blood and lodges in an artery supplying the brain. These clots can form as a result of injury or surgery. Cerebral hemorrhage occurs when an artery supplying the brain ruptures and blood seeps out into the surrounding tissue. Cerebral thrombosis or blood clots are more likely to form in those with atherosclerosis (p.47), heart rhythm (p.49) or heart valve disorders, recent myocardial infarction (p.51), high blood pressure (p.48), sickle cell anemia, and diabetes mellitus (p.76). Lifestyle issues that increase risk of stroke include a high-fat diet and smoking.

What can help?

If you suspect that a person has had a stroke, he or she should be taken to the hospital immediately to find the cause and start treatment. Once emergency procedures have been performed and the cause of the stroke determined, a drug treatment plan to dissolve or prevent blood clots will be devised by a doctor. Other treatment for stroke can include physiotherapy, speech therapy, and occupational therapy. Management of conditions that increase the risk of a stroke, such as high cholesterol and high blood pressure, can reduce the risk of another stroke. Lifestyle changes, such as starting a low-fat diet and quitting smoking, can also help.

Types of drug for stroke

- **Thrombolytic drugs,** also known as fibrinolytics, are used to dissolve clots that have already formed. They are usually given in hospital intravenously to clear a blocked artery. The sooner they are given after the start of symptoms, the more likely they are to reduce the size and severity of a cerebral thrombosis or embolism.

- **Anticoagulants** are used in preventing a stroke caused from heart rhythm problems. An oral anticoagulant such as warfarin is usually used and takes effect after a few days. Oral anticoagulants may also be given after injury or surgery (in particular, heart valve replacement) when there is a high risk of embolism.

- **Antiplatelet drugs** are taken regularly by people with a tendency to form clots in the fast-flowing blood of the heart and arteries. The most widely used antiplatelet drug is ASA, which is also an analgesic.

🛈 Risks and special precautions

The most common problems with the use of thrombolytics are increased susceptibility to bleeding and bruising. Allergic reactions may occur and can include rashes, breathing difficulty, or general discomfort.

A common problem experienced with oral anticoagulants is that overdosage may lead to bleeding from the nose or gums, or in the urinary tract. For this reason, the dosage needs to be carefully calculated; regular blood tests are performed to ensure that the clotting mechanism is correctly adjusted. The action of oral anticoagulant drugs may be affected by many other drugs. It may therefore be necessary to alter the dosage of anticoagulant when other drugs also need to be given. People who have been prescribed oral anticoagulants should carry a warning list of drugs that they should not be given. In particular, none of the anticoagulants should be taken with ASA except on the direction of a doctor. Always check with your doctor or pharmacist before taking any other drug.

💊 COMMON DRUGS

Antiplatelet drugs	Thrombolytic drugs
ASA ✳	Alteplase
Clopidogrel ✳	Reteplase
Dipyridamole	Tenecteplase
Ticlopidine	**Oral anticoagulant**
	Warfarin ✳

✳ See Part 3

Action of thrombolytic drugs

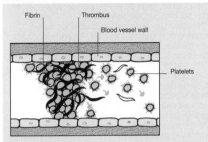

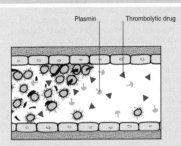

Before drug
When platelets accumulate in a blood vessel and bind together with strands of fibrin, the resultant blood clot, which is known as a thrombus, cannot be dissolved either by antiplatelet drugs or anticoagulant drugs.

After drug
Thrombolytic drugs boost the action of plasmin, an enzyme that breaks up the strands of fibrin, allowing the accumulated platelets to disperse and restoring normal blood flow.

Action of anticoagulant drugs

Anticoagulant drugs block the action of certain blood clotting factors that convert fibrinogen into fibrin, the protein that binds platelets into blood clots.

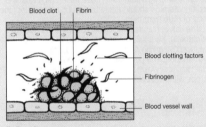

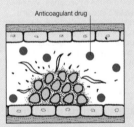

Before drug

After drug

Action of antiplatelet drugs

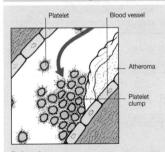

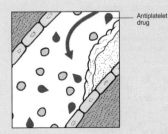

Before drug
Where the blood flow is disrupted by an atheroma in the blood vessels, platelets tend to clump together.

After drug
Antiplatelet drugs reduce the ability of platelets to stick together and so prevent clot formation.

INFECTIOUS DISEASES

What are they?

Infectious diseases are illnesses that are transmitted from an infected person to another who has no immunity against the specific illness. Once exposed to the germ, the immune system fights off these diseases by creating specific antibodies that attack the infecting organisms. Many infectious diseases, including most of the common viral infections, occur only once during a person's lifetime. The reason is that the antibodies produced in response to the disease remain afterwards, prepared to repel any future invasion as soon as the first infectious germs appear. The duration of such immunity varies, but it can last a lifetime. Examples of infectious diseases include influenza (p.59), measles, chicken pox, tetanus, meningitis, hepatitis B, and HIV/AIDS.

What causes them?

Infectious diseases result from microbial agents, such as viruses, bacteria, fungi, protozoa, and parasites. These infectious organisms enter the body by direct contact with another person's skin, saliva, or blood, or through sexual contact. They may also spread from person to person in food, water, or air. Many infectious diseases have been eliminated in developed countries through the use of vaccines, but they are much more common in developing countries.

What can help?

Protection against many infectious diseases can now be provided artificially by the use of vaccines. Vaccines provoke the immune system into creating antibodies that help the body to resist specific infectious diseases. Many vaccines (known as live vaccines) are made from artificially weakened forms of the disease-causing germ. But even these weakened germs are effective in stimulating sufficient growth of antibodies. Other vaccines rely either on inactive (or killed) disease-causing germs, or inactive derivatives of these germs,

but their effect on the immune system remains the same. Another type of immunization, called passive immunization, relies on giving appropriate antibodies after the infection has occurred.

Newborn babies receive antibodies for many diseases from their mothers, but this protection lasts only for about three months. Most children from 2 months to 15 years are vaccinated against common childhood infectious diseases. In addition, travellers to many countries, especially in the tropics, are advised to be vaccinated against the diseases common in those regions. Rabies, yellow fever, and hepatitis B vaccines may be required for remote areas. Effective lifelong immunization can sometimes be achieved by a single dose of the vaccine. However, in many cases reinforcing doses, commonly called booster shots, are needed later in order to maintain reliable immunity.

Risks and special precautions

Serious reactions to vaccines are rare and, for most children, the benefits from the protection far outweigh the risks. Children who have had seizures may be advised against vaccinations for pertussis (whooping cough) or measles. Children who have any infection more severe than a common cold will not be given any routine vaccination until they have recovered.

Live vaccines should not be given during pregnancy because they can affect the developing baby, nor to those whose immune systems are weakened by disease or drug treatment. Those taking high doses of corticosteroids should delay their vaccinations until the end of drug treatment.

The risk of high fever following the DPT (combined diphtheria, pertussis, and tetanus) vaccine can be reduced by giving acetaminophen at the time of vaccination. The pertussis vaccine may rarely cause a mild seizure, which is brief, usually associated with fever, stops without treatment, and causes no lasting effects.

Active and passive immunization

Active immunization

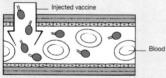

Injected vaccine

Blood

Before infection
A vaccine containing altered forms of the infection is injected.

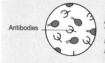

Antibodies

Antibody formation
The vaccine causes antibodies to form against the infection.

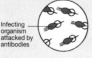

Infecting organism attacked by antibodies

Immunity
Invasion of the body by a similar organism causes antibodies to form as a result of the vaccine and eliminate the infection.

Passive immunization

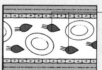

Infecting organisms

After infection
Passive immunization is needed when the infection has entered the blood.

Injected antibodies

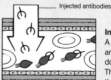

Immune globulin injection
A serum containing antibodies extracted from donated blood is injected. This helps the body to fight the infection.

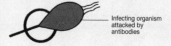

Infecting organism attacked by antibodies

COMMON VACCINATIONS

Disease	Age at which vaccination is given	How given	General information
Diphtheria	2 months, 4 months, 6 months, 18 months, 4–6 years.	Injection	Infants: given with tetanus, pertussis, and polio vaccines (DTaP-IPV). In later life immunity may diminish. Adults: booster every 10 years.
Tetanus	2 months, 4 months, 6 months, 18 months, 4–6 years.	Injection	Infants: given with diphtheria, pertussis, and polio (DTaP-IPV). Protection lasts 5–10 years. Booster shots given for injuries likely to result in tetanus infection. Adults: booster every 10 years.
Acellular pertussis	2 months, 4 months, 6 months, 18 months, 4–6 years.	Injection	Preferable to use products in which diptheria toxin is combined with acellular pertussis. Preschool booster. Adults: give one dose as Tdap if not previously received.
Polio	2 months, 4 months, 6 months, 18 months, 4–6 years.	Injection	Many doctors may recommend a booster every 10 years, especially if primary series during childhood is not complete, and especially for people who are travelling to countries where polio is still prevalent. Single booster dose recommended for those at high risk of exposure.
Haemophilus influenzae type b (Hib)	2 months, 4 months, 6 months, 18 months.	Injection	Routinely given in infancy to prevent serious disease up to the age of 4 years.
Rubella (German measles)	12 months and at 18 months or 4–6 years.	Injection	Given in infancy with measles and mumps vaccines (MMR). Rubella is important because it can damage the fetus if it affects a woman in early pregnancy.
Measles	12 months and at 18 months or 4–6 years.	Injection	Given with mumps and rubella vaccines (MMR) in infancy.
Mumps	12 months and at 18 months or 4–6 years.	Injection	Given with measles and rubella vaccines (MMR) in infancy.
Influenza	Recommended for all children 6–23 months. Also children and adults of any age who are at risk of serious illness or death if they develop influenza and their household carers, health care workers, as well as those wishing to be protected against influenza, and all adults 65 years of age and over.	Injection	Long-term immunity against all forms of influenza is impossible. Annual vaccinations are needed to protect against the latest strains. Also given to individuals capable of transmitting influenza to those at high risk (e.g. health care workers). Safe in pregnant and breast-feeding women.
Hepatitis A	Single dose for people any age who are at risk. Booster 6–12 months after initial shot.	Injection	Given to people travelling to areas of poor hygiene or where hepatitis infection is likely and to those exposed at school or work.
Hepatitis B	3 inoculations any age, with the second and third shots 1 and 6 months after the first.	Injection	Efficacy is checked by a blood test. Recommended for at risk groups, such as health-care providers, intravenous drug users, and long-stay travellers. Adolescents (11–15 years) may be given a 2-dose regimen of adult formulation.
Pneumococcal pneumonia	2 months, 4 months, 6 months, and at 12–15 months of age (pneumococcal conjugate vaccine). Single dose for people any age who are at risk and adults 65 years of age and over (pneumococcal polysaccharide).	Injection	Given to persons at risk of contracting pneumococcal pneumonia. This includes people who have had their spleen removed, immunodeficient persons, or those with chronic liver or lung disease or diabetes mellitus. Single booster dose after 5 years recommended in those at high risk.
Meningococcal meningitis A/C/Y/W-135	Recommended for all children in early adolescence. Single dose for people any age who are at risk. Schedule depends on age of individual.	Injection	Given to persons at risk of contracting meningitis; for example to travellers to the "Meningitis belt" of tropical and subtropical countries where there is a high risk of meningitis infection, also contacts of cases in Canada.
Meningococcal meningitis C	Schedule depends on age of individual.	Injection	Given in infancy to protect against one of the most common types of childhood meningitis.
Typhoid	Single dose for people any age who are at risk.	Injection	Travellers to areas with poor sanitation.

URINARY TRACT INFECTION

What is it?

In a urinary tract infection (UTI), the lining of the bladder becomes inflamed due to a bacterial infection. Symptoms include a continual urge to urinate, although often nothing is passed, pain or burning on urinating, and lower abdominal pain.

What causes it?

The condition is most often caused by *Escherichia coli*, a bacterium that normally lives in the intestines. Infection normally occurs when bacteria enter the bladder through the urethra (the tube from the bladder to the outside of the body), often during sex or when the anus is wiped after a bowel movement. Women have a shorter urethra, and are therefore more at risk of developing an infection. Incomplete emptying of the bladder can also increase the risk of developing a UTI because the retained urine can harbor bacteria.

What can help?

Urinary tract infections are treated with antibiotics and antibacterials. Once appropriate antibiotic treatment is started, symptoms are commonly relieved within a few hours. For maximum effect, all drug treatments prescribed for urinary tract infections need to be completed as prescribed and accompanied by increased fluid intake. An analgesic may be taken to relieve pain until the treatment starts to take effect.

People who are prone to UTIs can help prevent further attacks by drinking plenty of water throughout the day, emptying the bladder frequently, especially after sexual intercourse, and wiping from front to back after a bowel movement. Some people find that increasing the acidity of the urine, thereby making it hostile to bacteria, can also help – ascorbic acid (vitamin C) and acidic fruit juices such as cranberry juice have this effect.

🖐 Risks and special precautions

Inform your doctor or pharmacist if you have suffered an adverse reaction to an antibiotic or antibacterial; some (especially cephalosporins and penicillins) can cause a severe allergic reaction.

Prolonged treatment with antibiotics can lead to overgrowth of Candida (thrush) in the mouth, vagina, or bowel, or a rare but serious disorder known as pseudomembranous colitis (most commonly linked to the lincosamides class of antibiotics), which causes violent, bloody diarrhea.

Types of drugs for UTIs

* **Antibiotics** work by either destroying bacteria directly, or by halting the multiplication of bacteria and enabling the body's natural defences to overcome the remaining infection. There are several classes – penicillins (such as amoxicillin), sulfamethoxazole-trimethoprim, and quinolones (such as norfloxacin) are particularly effective for UTIs. See p.29 for action of antibiotics.

* **Antibacterials** are similar to antibiotics, and function by preventing growth and multiplication of bacteria. Sulfonamindes are especially useful for treating UTIs because high concentrations of the drug reach the urine. The drugs usually take several days to eliminate bacteria – your doctor may recommend additional medication to alleviate any discomfort.

🔴 COMMON DRUGS

Antibiotics	Antibacterials
Amoxicillin ✳	Ciprofloxacin ✳
Cephalexin ✳	Levofloxacin ✳
Gentamicin	Norfloxacin ✳
Tetracycline	Sulfamethoxazole-
Tobramycin	trimethoprim ✳
	Trimethorpin

✳ See Part 3

Action of sulfonamides

Before drug treatment
Folic acid, a chemical that is necessary for the growth of bacteria, is produced within bacterial cells by an enzyme that acts on a chemical called para-aminobenzoic acid.

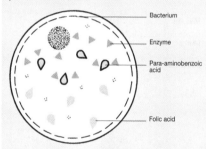

After drug treatment
Sulfonamides interfere with the function of the enzyme. This prevents folic acid from being formed. The bacterium is therefore unable to function properly and dies.

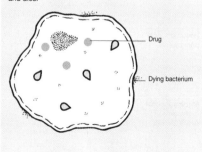

INFLUENZA

What is it?
Influenza, also known as the flu, is a highly contagious viral infection that mainly affects the upper respiratory tract. Symptoms usually develop in about 2 days after infection, and include high fever, sweating, shivering, aching muscles, exhaustion, sneezing, stuffy or runny nose, sore throat, and cough.

What causes it?
Influenza is caused by two main types of influenza viruses: A and B. The type A virus, in particular, frequently mutates and produces new strains to which few people have immunity. It tends to occur in epidemics in the winter, and is easily transmitted by airborne droplets from coughs and sneezes of infected people, or through touching of objects contaminated with respiratory secretions which can then be transmitted to mucous membranes. The type B virus can be associated with sporadic outbreaks, such as in nursing homes.

What can help?
The natural defences of the body are usually strong enough to overcome an influenza infection. Rest in bed, drink plenty of fluids, and relieve a fever with a cool sponge bath. Over-the-counter drugs can be taken to ease pain and lower fever. Antiviral drugs can sometimes be taken to prevent infection, or to treat it once it has occurred. These are most effective if they are given within 48 hours or sooner of the onset of symptoms. Babies, young children, the elderly, or those with chronic heart or lung conditions or reduced immunity are at increased risk of serious complications from influenza. A doctor should be seen immediately if flu symptoms appear in any of these groups. Being immunized yearly against influenza is recommended (see pp.56-7).

⚠ Risks and special precautions
Some of the antivirals may affect the kidneys adversely and doses may need to be adjusted based on kidney function. Some antiviral drugs can adversely affect the activity of normal body cells, particularly those in the bone marrow. Speak to your doctor or pharmacist about the drug you are taking.

✪ COMMON DRUGS

Amantadine	**Analgesics (p.38)**
Oseltamivir ✱	**Decongestants (p.27)**
Zanamivir	**Cough remedies (p.27)**

✱ See Part 3

Action of antivirals

This simplified illustration shows the way influenza viruses spread by infecting host cells.

Influenza virus   Host cell

 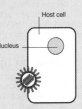
Nucleus

Genes (RNA)

Influenza virus invades host cell.

Virus breaks apart, releasing its genes, which then enter the host cell's nucleus.

Once inside the nucleus, the virus's genes replicate themselves by the thousands.

The genes leave the host cell's nucleus and reform into new influenza viruses.

The viruses leave the host cell, and move on to infect new cells.

Antivirals work by preventing the influenza virus from breaking apart inside the host cell and releasing its genes, or by slowing or stopping the reformed viruses from leaving the host cell.

Types of drugs for influenza

- **Antivirals** stop the spread of viruses by altering the cell's genetic material (DNA) so that the virus cannot use it to multiply. Other drugs stop multiplication of viruses by blocking enzyme activity within the host cell, or by preventing the virus from entering the host cell in the first place.

- **Analgesics** can be taken to relieve aching muscles and lower fever (see p.38).

- **Decongestants** may be used to relieve a blocked or runny nose (see p.27). Talk to your doctor or pharmacist before taking any.

- **Cough remedies** can be taken to relieve bothersome dry cough. However, productive cough should usually not be suppressed; discuss with your doctor and pharmacist (see p.27).

OTHER COMMON INFECTIONS

What are they?
The human body provides a suitable environment for the growth of many types of microorganisms, including bacteria, viruses, fungi, yeasts, and protozoa. Microorganisms can be transmitted from person to person in many ways: direct contact, inhalation of infected air, and consumption of contaminated food or water. Not all microorganisms cause disease; and those that do are normally eliminated by the body's immune system before they can multiply in sufficient numbers to cause serious disease. But if the body has little or no natural immunity to the invading organism, or the number of invading microbes is too great for the body's immune system to overcome, an infection can occur. An immune system weakened or destroyed by a disease, such as AIDS, can result in severe infections.

Some common infections

- **Pneumonia** is an infection that causes the alveoli (air sacs) of the lungs to become inflamed and filled with fluid. As a result, it is harder for oxygen to pass across the walls of the alveoli into the bloodstream. The infection can result from bacterium, viruses, fungi, or protozoa. Most adult cases of pneumonia are caused by the bacterium *Streptococcus pneumoniae*, and can develop as a complication of a viral infection of the upper respiratory tract, such as a common cold (see p.27). Other pneumonia-causing bacterium, such as *Staphylococcus aureus*, can infect people who are already in the hospital with another illness. The elderly and young children are particularly at risk. Symptoms include a cough that may produce bloody sputum, chest pain that worsens on inhaling, shortness of breath at rest, high fever, delirium, or confusion. Severe pneumonia can be life-threatening.

  Treatment: Mild pneumonia in otherwise healthy people can be treated at home with analgesics to reduce fever and chest pain, and antibiotics or antifungals to treat the infection. Severe cases will be treated in the hospital.

- **Eye infections** are the most common disorders to affect the eye. **Conjunctivitis** is a common infection in which the conjunctiva, the membrane covering the white of the eye and the inside of the eyelid, becomes inflamed and irritated. It is usually caused by bacterium or by a virus, including those responsible for the common cold or cold sores. It is easily spread by hand-to-eye contact. Symptoms include redness of the eye, gritty sensation in the eye, swollen eyelids, and discharge from the eye that is either thick and yellowish or clear and watery.

  Treatment: Symptoms of conjunctivitis can be relieved by bathing the eye with artificial tears. Wash hands well after touching the eye to avoid spreading the infection, and do not share towels or facecloths. Antibiotic eyedrops may be prescribed.

  Stye is another common infection that causes a painful, pus-filled swelling at the root of an eyelash. Most styes are caused by *Staphylococcus aureus*, a bacterium found on the skin of many healthy people. Adults are less likely than children to develop styes, but wearing makeup or contact lenses can increase the risk.

  Treatment: Styes usually rupture, drain, and heal without treatment within a few days. To avoid spreading the infection, wash hands well after touching the eye, and do not share towels or facecloths. A topical or oral antibiotic may be prescribed if the stye does not clear up on its own.

- **Ear infections** most often affect the middle and outer ear rather than the inner ear. **Otitis externa**, commonly known as swimmer's ear, is an inflammation of the ear canal, caused by a bacterial, viral, or fungal infection. It often develops after swimming because of persistent moisture in the ear canal which increases the risk of infection, and can also occur in people who work in a hot, humid environment, or who wear hearing aids. Symptoms include itching and pain within the ear canal, and discharge of pus from the ear.

  Treatment: Depending on the cause, antibiotic or antifungal eardrops may be prescribed. If the infection is severe, oral antibiotics may be given. Analgesics can be taken for the pain.

  Otitis media is an inflammation of the middle ear, usually as a result of a bacterial or viral infection. The condition can occur when a viral infection, such as a common cold (see. p.27) or influenza (see p.59) spreads from the throat to the middle ear. It is more common in children, and can cause the eardrum to rupture. Symptoms include pain in the ear, partial hearing loss, fever, and bloodstained discharge from the ear if the eardrum ruptures.

  Treatment: Oral antibiotics may be prescribed and analgesics given to relieve the pain.

- **Skin infections** can occur when infectious organisms enter the skin, either through a natural opening such as a hair follicle, or through skin damaged by a cut, burn, insect bite, or a condition such as eczema (see p.26)

  Athlete's foot is a fungal infection of the foot, producing cracked, sore, itchy, and peeling skin between the toes. It is caused by several types of fungi that thrive in warm, humid conditions and can be picked up by walking barefoot in communal areas, such as locker rooms and poolsides.

  Treatment: An over-the-counter antifungal preparation can be used on the affected area. Wash the feet at least once a day and dry them thoroughly between the toes to prevent the infection from recurring.

  Warts, also called verrucae, are small growths of thickened and sometimes darkened skin, caused by human papillomaviruses. They usually occur on the hands and feet and are generally harmless. Warts on the soles of the feet are called plantar warts. Warts are transferred by direct contact with an infected person or from virus particles on recently shed flakes of skin.

Treatment: Most warts disappear without treatment, but this can take months or even years. There are many over-the-counter preparations that will remove warts. If the wart persists, see your doctor, who may remove the wart by freezing, scraping, or burning it off.

Cold sores are painful clusters of blisters usually caused by herpes simplex virus type 1. Most people have been infected with this virus by the time they reach adulthood; the virus remains dormant and may be reactivated to produce cold sores, usually near the lips. An outbreak can be triggered by wind, sunburn, fatigue, stress, the common cold, and fever.

Treatment: Antiviral creams can help prevent an outbreak if applied at the first sign of a flare-up. Oral antiviral drugs may be prescribed in some cases. People with recurrent cold sores should protect themselves from trigger factors such as sunburn.

Types of infecting organisms

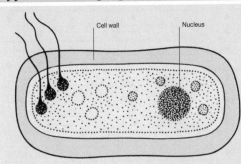

Cell wall   Nucleus

Bacteria
A typical bacterium (left) consists of a single cell that has a protective wall. Some bacteria are aerobic – that is, they require oxygen – and therefore are more likely to infect surface areas such as the skin or respiratory tract. Others are anaerobic and multiply in oxygen-free surroundings such as the bowel or deep puncture wounds.

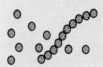

Cocci (spherical)
Streptococcus (above) can cause sore throats and pneumonia.

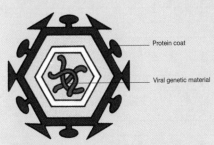

Bacilli (rod-shaped)
Mycobacterium tubercolosis (above) causes tubercolosis.

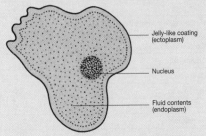

Spirochaete (spiral-shaped)
This group includes bacteria that cause syphilis and gum infections.

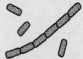

Protein coat

Viral genetic material

Jelly-like coating (ectoplasm)

Nucleus

Fluid contents (endoplasm)

Viruses
These infectious agents are smaller than bacteria and consist simply of a core of genetic material surrounded by a protein coat. A virus can multiply only in a living cell by using the host tissue's replicating material.

Protozoa
These single-celled parasites are slightly bigger than bacteria. Many protozoa live in the human intestine and are harmless. However, some types cause malaria, sleeping sickness, and dysentery.

OTHER COMMON INFECTIONS continued

Uses of antibiotics

The table below is not intended to be comprehensive, but shows which common drugs in each class of antibiotic are used for the treatment of infections in different parts of the body. For the purposes of comparison, this table also includes (in the Other drugs category) some antibacterial drugs. This table is not intended to be a guide to prescribing but indicates the possible applications of each drug. Some drugs have a wide range of possible uses; this table concentrates on the most common ones.

Antibiotic	Ear, nose, throat, and mouth	Respiratory tract	Skin and soft tissue	Gastrointestinal tract	Eye	Kidney and urinary tract	Brain and nervous system	Heart and blood	Bones and joints	Genital tract
Penicillins										
Amoxicillin *	•	•	•			•		•	•	•
Amoxicillin/clavulanic acid	•	•	•			•		•		
Cloxacillin	•		•					•	•	
Penicillin G	•	•	•		•			•	•	•
Penicillin V	•	•	•							
Cephalosporins										
Cefaclor	•	•				•				
Cefazolin		•	•			•			•	
Cefprozil	•	•	•							
Cefuroxime	•	•	•							•
Cephalexin *		•	•			•				
Macrolides										
Azithromycin *	•	•	•							•
Clarithromycin *	•	•	•	•						
Erythromycin	•	•	•	•	•			•		•
Tetracyclines										
Doxycycline	•	•				•				•
Minocycline	•	•	•			•				•
Aminoglycosides										
Gentamicin		•	•	•	•	•		•	•	
Tobramycin		•	•		•	•			•	
Sulfonamide combination										
Sulfamethoxazole-trimethoprim (Co-trimoxazole) *		•				•				
Other drugs										
Clindamycin		•	•	•					•	
Fusidic acid			•					•	•	
Metronidazole	•		•	•			•	•	•	•
Quinolones										
Ciprofloxacin *		•		•		•				•
Levofloxacin *		•								
Norfloxacin *						•				

* See Part 3

ARTHRITIS

What is it?
The term arthritis covers a group of inflammatory and degenerative conditions that cause stiffness, swelling, and pain in the joints. **Osteoarthritis**, the most common form, is the gradual degeneration of the cartilage, which acts as a cushion, covering the bone ends within joints. It most often involves the knees, hips, and hands. The joint pain often worsens with exercise and improves with rest. Inflammation may sometimes be associated with osteoarthritis.

Rheumatoid arthritis is a systemic autoimmune condition which commonly affects joints, but can also affect other body systems. It causes the affected joints to become stiff, swollen, and eventually deformed. This disorder usually appears in the small joints of the hands and feet but may develop in any joint.

What causes it?
There is often no obvious cause for osteoarthritis, but there are factors that may increase the likelihood of developing the disorder. Wear of the cartilage occurs most often in joints that have been damaged repeatedly by strenuous activity or by multiple minor injuries. It is common in former athletes. Being overweight can also increase the risk of developing the condition due to the stress that this puts on the joints, especially the knee joint.

Rheumatoid arthritis is an autoimmune disorder in which the body produces antibodies that attack the synovial membrane covering the joints, and in some cases, other body tissues such as the eyes, lungs, heart, and blood vessels.

What can help?
If you have chronic arthritis, you may be able to manage your symptoms to maintain an active lifestyle. Gentle, regular exercise or physiotherapy can help to relieve stiffness, improve mobility, reduce weight, and strengthen muscles that support the joints. In osteoarthritis of the knee, corrective shoe inserts (orthotics) after a professional assessment can help relieve knee pain in some cases. Joint pain can be relieved by applying heat or cold to the affected area. An analgesic or a non-steroidal anti-inflammatory drug (NSAID) may be prescribed to relieve pain and swelling. A corticosteroid may also be injected directly into the affected joint for the same result. For rheumatoid arthritis, antirheumatic drugs may slow the disease process and limit permanent joint damage. There is no cure for either of these forms of arthritis.

Risks and special precautions
The main risk from NSAIDs is that, occasionally, they can cause ulcers and bleeding in the stomach or duodenum. They should therefore be avoided by people who have had peptic ulcers. Most NSAIDs are not recommended for those who are pregnant or breast-feeding, those with kidney or liver abnormalities, a hypersensitivity to other drugs, or a bleeding disorder. DMARDs can have potentially severe side effects. There are important health cautions in using BRMs, which need to be discussed with your doctor.

Types of drugs for arthritis

- **Acetaminophen** is the initial drug of choice for pain associated with osteoarthritis and in those with ongoing pain. It may need to be taken regularly (see also pp.38-9).

- **Non-steroidal anti-inflammatory drugs** (NSAIDs) relieve the pain, stiffness, and inflammation of painful conditions affecting the muscles, bones, and joints (see also pp.38-9).

- **Disease-modifying antirheumatic drugs** (DMARDs) are used in rheumatoid arthritis to decrease disease progression, and include immunosuppressants, gold-based drugs, and others. It is thought that they reduce the body's immune response and therefore prevent any further joint damage and disability.

- **Biological Response Modifiers** (BRM) may be considered for those with aggressive, debilitating rheumatoid arthritis. BRMs are administered by injection and may need to be given daily, weekly, or every 2 weeks, depending on the agent.

- **Corticosteroids** are sometimes used in the treatment of osteoarthritis (locally in the joint) and rheumatoid arthritis (locally or by mouth), but only for limited periods as they can have significant side effects when taken over prolonged periods.

COMMON DRUGS

NSAIDs
ASA *
Celecoxib *
Diclofenac *
Ibuprofen *
Ketoprofen
Naproxen *
Piroxicam
ANTIRHEUMATIC DRUGS
Immunosuppressants
Azathioprine
Cyclosporine
Cyclophosphamide
Leflunomide
Methotrexate *
Gold-based drugs
Auranofin
Sodium aurothiomalate (Myochrysine)

Biological Response Modifiers
Abatacept
Adalimumab
Anakinra
Etanercept
Infliximab
Rituximab
Other drugs
Acetaminophen *
Hydroxychloroquine
Penicillamine
Prednisone *

* See Part 3

ARTHRITIS continued

Action of antirheumatic drugs

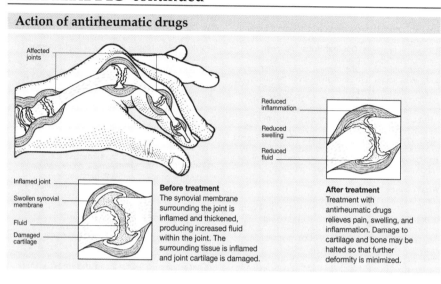

Before treatment
The synovial membrane surrounding the joint is inflamed and thickened, producing increased fluid within the joint. The surrounding tissue is inflamed and joint cartilage is damaged.

After treatment
Treatment with antirheumatic drugs relieves pain, swelling, and inflammation. Damage to cartilage and bone may be halted so that further deformity is minimized.

The joint in osteoarthritis

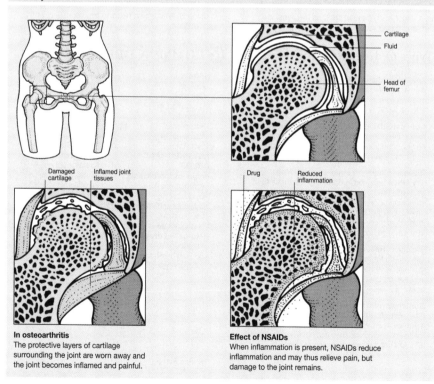

In osteoarthritis
The protective layers of cartilage surrounding the joint are worn away and the joint becomes inflamed and painful.

Effect of NSAIDs
When inflammation is present, NSAIDs reduce inflammation and may thus relieve pain, but damage to the joint remains.

OSTEOPOROSIS

What is it?
Osteoporosis is a common bone disorder in which the strength and density of the bone are reduced. When the loss of bone is significant, it increases the risk of fractures. In most people, bone density decreases very gradually from the age of 30. One in four women and one in eight men above the age of 50 have osteoporosis.

Most individuals with osteoporosis have no symptoms. Commonly, the vertebrae are affected and can become so weakened that they are not able to bear the body's weight and may collapse spontaneously or after a minor accident. Subsequently, the individual suffers from back pain, reduced height, and a round-shouldered appearance. Fractures usually tend to occur in the wrist or hip.

What causes it?
Bone is a living structure – minerals such as phosphorus and calcium are continually deposited and removed, and stored in a honeycombed protein framework called the matrix. Old bone is continually replaced with new bone. However, when the overall balance results in more bone being resorbed than deposited, loss of bone tissue occurs. In women, loss of the estrogen hormone at menopause increases the amount of bone loss. Any condition that accelerates the decline of sex hormones will increase the risk of osteoporosis, such as early menopause in women or untreated hypogonadism in men. Those who have had long-term treatment with a corticosteroid, or an overactive thyroid gland or chronic kidney failure are at an increased risk of developing the condition. Other risk factors include a family history of osteoporosis and a poor diet.

What can help?
Osteoporosis can be prevented by ensuring an adequate intake of protein, calcium, and vitamin D. Also, regular exercise throughout life is important for maintaining bone health. Quitting smoking and limiting alcohol consumption can also be of benefit. For people whose diet is deficient in calcium or vitamin D, supplements may be required. Drug treatment can

Types of drugs for osteoporosis

- **Bisphosphonates** bind to bone matrix, resulting in a decrease in bone loss. These drugs may be administered daily, weekly, or as a monthly dose. An injectable bisphosphonate, zoledronic acid, is administered once yearly. Other drugs that can be helpful include **raloxifene, calcitonin** and **teriparatide**.

- **Calcium supplements** (see p.180) may also be taken to prevent the body from obtaining the calcium it needs from the bones. Calcium carbonate is the most common form of calcium supplement. Adequate **vitamin D** is usually required for calcium to be absorbed well.

help prevent further deterioration and help fractures to heal. Drugs that inhibit removal of calcium from the bones are usually prescribed for osteoporosis, along with adequate calcium and vitamin D intake. Any treatment for osteoporosis should be monitored regularly. A bone mineral density (BMD) test is done periodically to see if the drug is effective.

🄺 COMMON DRUGS

Bisphosphonates	Other drugs
Alendronate ✳	Calcitonin
Etidronate ✳	Calcitriol (active
Risedronate ✳	Vitamin D)
Zoledronic acid	Conjugated estrogens
Supplements	Raloxifene ✳
Calcium carbonate ✳	Teriparatide
Calcium citrate	
Ergocalciferol	
(Vitamin D2)	
Vitamin D ✳	

> ✳ See Part 3

Action of drugs for osteoporosis

Normal bone
Regulated by hormones, bone cells constantly renew the hard mineralized tissue in the bone matrix with minerals from the blood.

In osteoporosis
Hormonal disturbance and other factors lead to wasting of active bone cells. The bones become less dense and more fragile. Most drug treatments and mineral supplements usually only prevent further bone loss.

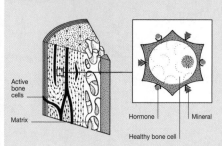

Active bone cells

Matrix

Hormone | Mineral

Healthy bone cell

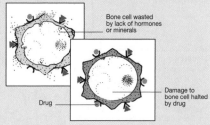

Bone cell wasted by lack of hormones or minerals

Damage to bone cell halted by drug

Drug

URINARY INCONTINENCE

What is it?

In normal bladder function, muscles in the bladder wall squeeze urine out of the bladder, while the ring of muscle (sphincter) around the bladder neck that normally keeps the bladder closed is consciously relaxed to allow the urine to pass out of the body. Urinary incontinence is characterized by complete or partial loss of voluntary control over the muscles of the bladder, causing leaking of urine. It is more common with increasing age and in women.

What causes it?

Urinary incontinence can occur for several reasons. A weak sphincter muscle allows the involuntary passage of urine when abdominal pressure is raised by coughing or physical exertion. This is known as stress incontinence and commonly affects women who have had children and post-menopausal women. Urgency – the sudden need to urinate – stems from oversensitivity of the bladder muscle; small quantities of urine stimulate the urge to urinate frequently. Incontinence can also occur due to loss of nerve control in neurological disorders such as multiple sclerosis. Some drugs can also worsen incontinence in a predisposed individual. In children, inability to control urination at night (nocturnal enuresis) is also a form of urinary incontinence.

What can help?

Drug treatment is not necessary or appropriate for all forms of incontinence. In stress incontinence, exercises to strengthen the pelvic floor muscles or surgery to tighten stretched ligaments may be effective. Intravaginal estrogen therapy may be tried in some women. In urgency, regular emptying of the bladder can often avoid the need for medical intervention. Frequency of urination in urgency may be reduced by anticholinergic drugs. Incontinence caused by loss of nerve control is unlikely to be helped by drug treatment.

🔅 COMMON DRUGS

Drugs used in incontinence
Darifenacin
Desipramine
Flavoxate
Imipramine
Oxybutynin
Solifenacin

Tolterodine ✱
Trospium
Other drugs
Estrogens

✱ See Part 3

Types of drugs for urinary incontinence

- **Anticholinergic drugs** reduce response of bladder muscles to nerve signals, allowing greater volumes of urine to accumulate without stimulating the urge to pass urine. Tricyclic antidepressants have a strong anticholinergic action, but also have other side effects and carry a high risk of overdose.

- **Topical estrogen** may be administered vaginally to post-menopausal women. This may help to slow the thinning of tissues lining the vagina and the urinary system; this may improve symptoms of stress incontinence.

Action of drugs on urination

Normal bladder action

Urination occurs when the sphincter keeping the exit from the bladder into the urethra closed is consciously relaxed in response to signals from the bladder indicating that it is full. As the sphincter opens, the bladder wall contracts and urine is expelled.

How drugs act to improve bladder control

Anticholinergic drugs relax the bladder muscle by interfering with the response of bladder muscles to nerve signals.

Sympathomimetics act directly on the sphincter muscle, causing it to contract.

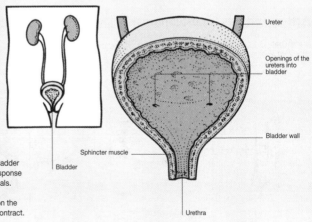

Ureter

Openings of the ureters into bladder

Bladder wall

Sphincter muscle

Bladder

Urethra

ORAL CONTRACEPTIVES

What are they?
Oral contraceptives provide an artificial method for controlling fertility in women, allowing people to choose whether and when to have children. There are many different methods of ensuring that conception and pregnancy do not follow sexual intercourse, but for most women the oral contraceptive is the most effective and convenient method, especially when combined with condoms to protect from sexually transmitted diseases. Oral contraceptives are available as a combined pill of estrogen and progestin or a progestin-only pill.

How do they work?
In a normal menstrual cycle, the ripening and release of an egg and the preparation of the uterus for implantation of the fertilized egg are the result of a complex interplay between the natural female sex hormones, estrogen and progesterone, and the pituitary hormones, follicle-stimulating hormone (FSH) and luteinizing hormone (LH). The estrogen and progestins contained in oral contraceptives disrupt the normal menstrual cycle in such a way that conception is less likely.

Types of oral contraceptives

- The **combined pill** is the most widely used form of oral contraceptive and has the lowest failure rate in terms of unwanted pregnancies. It is commonly referred to as the pill and is particularly suitable for those women who regularly experience exceptionally painful, heavy, or prolonged periods. The combined pill contains a fixed dose of an estrogen and a progestin drug. Different varieties contain either higher or lower amounts of estrogen; low-dose products are chosen when possible to minimize the risk of adverse effects.

- The combined pill is also available as **phased pills,** where each pack is divided into two or three groups or phases, each containing a different proportion of an estrogen and a progestin. This provides a hormonal balance that closely resembles the fluctuations of a normal menstrual cycle. Phased pills provide effective protection for many women who suffer side effects from other available forms of oral contraceptive.

With combined and phased pills, the increased levels of estrogen and progesterone produce similar effects to the hormonal changes of pregnancy. The actions of the hormones inhibit the production of FSH and LH, thereby preventing the egg from ripening in the ovary and from being released.

- The **progestin-only pill** is often prescribed for women who react adversely to the estrogen in the combined pill or for whom the combined pill is considered unsuitable due to their age or medical history (see Risks and special precautions, below). It is also prescribed for women who are breast-feeding since it does not reduce milk production. The progestin pill has a higher failure rate than the combined pill and must be taken at precisely the same time each day for maximum contraceptive effect. Progestin-only pills work mainly by thickening the mucus that lines the cervix, preventing sperm from crossing it.

🖐 Risks and special precautions
All oral contraceptives need to be taken regularly for maximum protection against pregnancy. Contraceptive protection can be reduced by missing a pill (see What to do if you miss a pill, p.68). Vomiting or diarrhea can affect the absorption of the pill. If you suffer from either of these symptoms, it is advisable to act as if you had missed your last pill. Many drugs may also affect the action of oral contraceptives; inform your doctor and pharmacist that you are taking oral contraceptives before taking additional prescribed medications.

One of the most serious potential adverse effects of estrogen-containing pills is development of a thrombus (blood clot) in a vein or artery, which may travel to the lungs or cause a stroke or heart attack. The risk of thrombus formation is increased with age, obesity, diabetes mellitus, high blood pressure, and smoking. Contraceptive pills containing the progestin desogestrel may carry a higher risk of thrombus formation than those containing other progestins. Please discuss with your doctor or pharmacist.

Oral contraceptives may cause high blood pressure in some women; blood pressure should be measured before the pill is prescribed and monitored regularly thereafter.

Some very rare liver cancers have occurred in contraceptive pill-users, and breast cancer may be slightly more common. However, cancers of the ovaries and uterus are less common in women who take the contraceptive pill.

Although there is no evidence that oral contraceptives reduce a woman's fertility or that they damage the babies conceived after they are discontinued, doctors recommend that you wait for at least one normal menstrual period after stopping the pill before you attempt to become pregnant.

🔵 COMMON DRUGS

Progestins	Estrogens
Desogestrel	Ethinyl estradiol
Drospirenone	
Ethynodiol diacetate	
Etonogestrel	
Levonorgestrel	
Norelgestromin	
Norethindrone	
Norgestimate	

ORAL CONTRACEPTIVES continued

Comparison of reliability of different methods of contraception

The table indicates the number of pregnancies that occur with each method of contraception among 100 women using that method in a year. The wide variation that occurs with some methods takes into account pregnancies that occur as a result of incorrect use of the method.

Methods	Pregnancies *
Combined and phased pills	2–3
Progestin-only pill	2.5–10
IUD (Intrauterine device)	up to 5
Condom	10–14
Diaphragm	10–14
Rhythm	25–30
Contraceptive sponge	10–14
Vaginal spermicide alone	2–30
Medroxyprogesterone depot	Less than 1
No contraception	80–85
"Morning after" pill	11–25

*Per 100 users per year.

What to do if you miss a pill

Contraceptive protection may be reduced as a result of missing a pill. It is particularly important to ensure that the progestin-only pills are taken punctually. If you miss a pill, the action you should take depends on the degree of lateness and the type of pill being used (see below).

	Combined and phased pills	Progestin-only pills
3–12 hours late	Take the missed pill now. No additional precautions necessary.	Take the missed pill now. Take additional precautions for contraception over the next 7 days.
Over 12 hours late	Take the missed pill now and take the next pill on time (even if on same day). If more than one pill has been missed, take the latest missed pill now and the next on time. Take additional precautions for contraception over the next 7 days. If the 7 days extends into the pill-free (or inactive pill) period, start the next pack without a break (or without taking inactive pills).	Take the missed pill now, and take the next on time. Take additional precautions for contraception over the next 7 days.

Postcoital contraception

Pregnancy following intercourse without contraception may be avoided by taking a short course of postcoital (morning after) pills. The preparation used for this purpose contains a progestin and is usually taken in one dose of two tablets, within 72 hours following intercourse. Depending on when during the menstrual cycle they are taken, these drugs may postpone ovulation or act on the lining of the uterus to prevent implantation of the egg. The high doses required make them unsuitable for regular use. This method has a higher failure rate than the usual oral contraceptives.

Risks and benefits of oral contraceptives

Oral contraceptives are safe for the vast majority of young women. However, every woman considering oral contraception should discuss with her doctor and pharmacist the risks and possible side effects of the drugs. Factors that must be taken into account include the woman's age, her own medical history and that of her close relatives, and whether she is a smoker. The table below gives the main advantages and disadvantages of estrogen-containing and progestin-only pills.

Type of oral contraceptive	Estrogen-containing combined and phased	Progestin-only

Advantages	● Very reliable
	● Convenient/unobtrusive
	● Regularizes menstruation
	● Reduced menstrual pain and blood loss
	● Reduced risk of:
	  ▼ benign breast disease
	  ▼ endometriosis
	  ▼ ectopic pregnancy
	  ▼ ovarian cysts
	  ▼ pelvic infection
	  ▼ ovarian and endometrial cancer
		● Reasonably reliable
		● Convenient/unobtrusive
		● Suitable during breast-feeding
		● Avoids estrogen-related side effects and risks
		● Allows rapid return to fertility

Side effects	● Weight gain ● Depression ● Breast swelling ● Reduced sex drive ● Headaches ● Increased vaginal discharge ● Nausea	● Irregular menstruation ● Breast tenderness
Risks	● Thrombosis/embolism ● Heart disease ● High blood pressure ● Jaundice ● Cancer of the liver (rare) ● Gallstones	● Ectopic pregnancy ● Ovarian cysts
Factors that may prohibit use	● Previous thrombosis* ● Heart disease or high levels of lipid in blood ● Breast cancer ● Liver disease ● Blood disorders ● High blood pressure ● Unexplained vaginal bleeding ● Migraine with aura ● Less than 6 weeks postpartum if breast-feeding ● Presence of several risk factors (below)	● Previous ectopic pregnancy ● Heart or circulatory disease ● Unexplained vaginal bleeding ● Breast cancer
Factors that increase risks	● Smoking* ● Obesity* ● Increasing age ● Diabetes mellitus ● Family history of heart or circulatory disease* ● Current treatment with other drugs	● As for estrogen-containing pills, but to a lesser degree

*Products containing desogestrel have a higher excess risk with these factors than other progestins.

How to minimize your health risks while taking the pill

▼ Give up smoking.
▼ Maintain a healthy weight and diet.
▼ Have regular blood pressure and blood lipid checks.
▼ Have regular cervical smear tests.
▼ Remind your doctor that you are taking oral contraceptives before taking other prescription drugs.

MENOPAUSE

What is it?

Menopause is the term given to the natural, permanent end of menstruation, signaling the end of the fertile phase of a woman's life. It usually occurs at about 51 years of age; one of the first signs is irregular menstruation. Although some women experience few or no symptoms, others suffer from mood swings, hot flashes, vaginal dryness, and night sweats. Menopause is also often associated with an increased risk of developing osteoporosis (see p.65).

What causes it?

The female sex hormones estrogen and progesterone are secreted by the ovaries starting at puberty, and are responsible for the development of female sexual characteristics and for preparing the lining of the uterus for the implantation of a fertilized egg. Estrogen is also needed to give bones strength. In menopause, the ovaries begin to produce less of these hormones, which brings an end to ovulation and menstruation. Menopause is defined as the cessation of menses for 12 months; the time leading up to menopause is called the perimenopausal period and may last between 1 and 5 years.

What can help?

Although menopause is part of a woman's natural aging process, it can often cause distressing symptoms. Various options are available for the management of these, including ovarian hormone replacement therapy (HRT). HRT, a combination of an estrogen and a progesterone, can also delay some of the long-term consequences of reduced estrogen levels, such as osteoporosis.

A balance between the benefits and risks of HRT for individual women must be considered, because there can be a slight increase in risk of breast cancer, high blood pressure, and thrombosis. It should be used with caution, especially in women with heart disease.

Another alternative for hot flashes is progestin therapy; venlafaxine and gabapentin have also been tried. For local symptoms such as vaginal dryness, vaginal estrogen therapy or lubricants can be helpful. Generally, for menopausal symptoms, maintaining a healthy diet and exercise program as well as managing stress levels or joining a menopause support group may be beneficial.

🔣 COMMON DRUGS

Estrogens
Conjugated estrogens
Estradiol
Estropipate
Progestins
Levonorgestrel
Medroxyprogesterone
acetate

Megestrol acetate
Norethindrone acetate
Progesterone
Other drugs
Venlafaxine ✳

✳ See Part 3

Types of Hormone Replacement Therapy

Hormone Replacement Therapy may be prescribed as pills, skin gel, patch, implants, vaginal cream, vaginal ring, or injection. It is usually given for the shortest period to alleviate menopausal symptoms, usually for less than 5 years.

Effects of HRT

Besides alleviating the symptoms of menopause, such as hot flashes and vaginal dryness, HRT has a beneficial effect in preventing osteoporosis (p.65). Benefits must, however, be weighed against a slightly increased risk of breast cancer and other side effects.

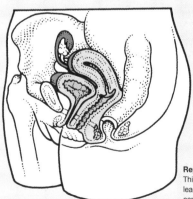

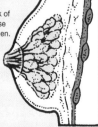

Bones
HRT reduces the thinning of bone that occurs in osteoporosis and thus protects against fractures.

Breasts
There is a slightly increased risk of breast cancer with long-term use of HRT, especially in older women.

Reproductive organs
Thinning of the vaginal tissues leading to painful intercourse can be prevented by HRT.

INDIGESTION AND OTHER STOMACH COMPLAINTS

What are they?
Indigestion is pain or discomfort in the upper abdomen that is brought on by eating. Usually indigestion occurs after a meal, especially one that included rich, fatty, or spicy food. If indigestion is recurrent and persistent, or occurs without an identifiable cause, it is called **dyspepsia.** If the symptoms increase in severity, and are accompanied by loss of appetite, weight loss, nausea, and sometimes vomiting, this may indicate a **peptic ulcer.** However, sometimes, peptic ulcers can occur with no specific symptoms. A peptic ulcer is an inflamed and eroded area of the tissue lining the stomach or the duodenum. **Gastroesophageal reflux disease** (commonly called GERD or acid reflux) refers to symptoms of heartburn and/or regurgitation due to excessive reflux of acidic juices from the stomach into the esophagus.

What causes them?
Digestive juices in the stomach contain acid and enzymes that break down food before it passes into the intestine. The wall of the stomach is normally protected from the action of digestive acid by a layer of mucous that is constantly secreted by the stomach lining. Problems arise when the stomach lining is damaged or too much acid is produced and eats away at the mucous layer, or when acid is regurgitated up into the esophagus, which may lead to irritation and inflammation.

Excess acid that leads to the pain of indigestion, dyspepsia, and GERD may result from anxiety and stress, overeating or eating certain foods, obesity, coffee, alcohol, or smoking. Peptic ulcers are most commonly associated with *Helicobacter pylori*, a bacterium that releases substances that reduce the effectiveness of the mucous layer protecting the wall of the stomach. Some drugs, notably ASA and non-steroidal anti-inflammatory drugs (NSAIDs), can irritate the stomach lining and cause ulcers to develop.

GERD may be caused by poor muscle tone in the esophageal sphincter, the muscular ring at the lower end of the esophagus that normally prevents the stomach acids from entering. The increased abdominal pressure due to pregnancy may also cause an attack of acid reflux.

What can help?
Often lifestyle changes can help to prevent indigestion and to reduce the frequency and severity of dyspepsia. Eat small portions of food at regular intervals without rushing, avoid eating three hours before going to bed, reduce or eliminate intake of coffee, alcohol, and tea, avoid rich, fatty, or spicy foods, lose excess weight, and learn coping strategies for stress.

Antacids and anti-ulcer drugs may be used to alleviate symptoms and promote healing of the stomach lining. Antibiotics may be combined with an anti-ulcer drug to eradicate the *Helicobacter pylori* infection that seems to cause many ulcers; this treatment may provide a cure in one to two weeks.

Ongoing symptoms of GERD may require longer-term treatment with a class of drugs called proton-pump inhibitors (PPI). The use of these drugs should be reevaluated periodically.

🔟 Risks and special precautions
Antacids and anti-ulcer drugs should not be taken to prevent abdominal pain on a regular basis except under medical supervision, as they may suppress the symptoms of stomach cancer. Antacids can interfere with the absorption of other drugs; check with your doctor or pharmacist before taking an antacid if you are on other medications. Aluminium compounds can interfere with the absorption of phosphate from the diet, causing weakness and bone damage if taken in high doses over a long period. Magnesium compounds can cause a high blood magnesium level to build up in people who have impaired kidney function, causing weakness, lethargy, and drowsiness.

Types of drugs for indigestion, ulcers, and GERD

- **Antacids** are used to neutralize stomach acid, and prevent inflammation, relieve pain and allow the mucous layer and lining to mend. Aluminum and magnesium compounds have a prolonged action and are used for the treatment of GERD.

- **Anti-ulcer drugs,** such as H₂ blockers and proton pump inhibitors, reduce the amount of acid released; they protect ulcers from the action of stomach acid, allowing the tissue to heal. They are used for dyspepsia or GERD.

- **Misoprostol** provides a mucosal protective effect and inhibits acid secretion; **sucralfate** forms a protective coating over the ulcer.

- **Alginates** form a protective barrier between the stomach and esophagus, which helps manage GERD symptoms

🥣 COMMON DRUGS

Antacids
Aluminum hydroxide
Calcium carbonate
Magnesium
 hydroxide ✳
Anti-ulcer
Proton pump inhibitors
Esomeprazole
Lansoprazole
Omeprazole
Pantoprazole ✳
Rabeprazole ✳
H₂-blockers
Cimetidine
Famotidine
Nizatidine
Ranitidine ✳

Other drugs
Alginic acid
Antibiotics (see p.62)
Misoprostol
Sucralfate

| ✳ See Part 3 |

INDIGESTION AND OTHER STOMACH COMPLAINTS continued

Action of antacids

Excess acid in the stomach may eat away at the layer of mucus that protects the stomach. When this occurs, or when the mucous lining is damaged, for example, by an ulcer, stomach acid comes into contact with the underlying tissues, causing pain and inflammation (right). Antacids combine with stomach acid to reduce the acidity of the digestive juices. This helps to prevent pain and inflammation, and can allow the mucous lining to repair itself (far right).

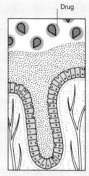

Mucus

Mucous lining

Stomach wall

Before drug
Acid damages mucous layer of stomach lining.

After drug
Acid is neutralized by antacid action.

Action of anti-ulcer drugs

Proton pump inhibitors
A cell membrane protein called the proton pump secretes acid into the stomach. Proton pump inhibitors work by blocking this system, which stops the secretion of stomach acid until a new supply of proton pumps can be made by the body.

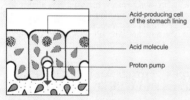

The proton pump
Acid secretion from the stomach lining is stimulated by the proton pump system.

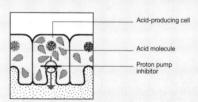

The action of proton pump inhibitors
Proton pump inhibitors block the proton pump system, stopping the secretion of acid.

H_2 blockers
Histamine, a chemical released by mast cells, can produce a number of effects in different parts of the body (see also Allergies, p.33). In the stomach, histamine stimulates H_2 receptors, causing acid production. A class of antihistamines called H_2 blockers work by blocking these receptors and stopping the production of stomach acid.

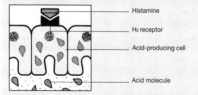

The action of histamine on the stomach
Histamine binds to specialized H_2 receptors and stimulates acid-producing cells in the stomach wall to release acid.

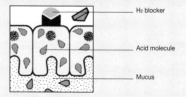

The action of H_2 blockers
H_2 blockers occupy H_2 receptors, preventing histamine from triggering the production of acid. This allows the mucous lining to heal.

NAUSEA AND VOMITING

What is it?

Nausea is a sensation of discomfort and unease in the stomach, and can lead to vomiting. Vomiting is a reflex action for getting rid of harmful substances from the stomach, but it may also be a symptom of disease. Nausea and vomiting occur when the vomiting centre in the brain is stimulated by signals from three places in the body: the digestive tract, the part of the inner ear controlling balance, and the brain itself via thoughts and emotions and via its chemoreceptor trigger zone, which responds to harmful substances in the blood.

What causes it?

Nausea and vomiting are often caused by a digestive tract infection, travel sickness, pregnancy, or vertigo (a balance disorder involving the inner ear). They can also occur as a side effect of some drugs, especially those used for cancer, radiation therapy, or general anesthesia.

Types of drugs for nausea and vomiting

There are three main types of anti-emetics, which act on the vomiting centre in the brain.

- **Antihistamines** are used to treat nausea caused by vertigo, Ménière's disease, and motion sickness.

- **Phenothiazines** may be used to treat severe vomiting in pregnancy, or vomiting caused by anesthetics.

- **5HT₃ antagonists** are prescribed mainly to relieve severe cases of vomiting caused by many anticancer drugs.

What can help?

Relief from nausea and vomiting will depend on the underlying cause. Many episodes of nausea and vomiting are short-lived and will not require medical treatment. Peppermint or ginger tea, dry toast, or crackers may help to settle an upset stomach. Doctors usually diagnose the cause of vomiting before prescribing an anti-emetic drug because vomiting may be due to another condition that may require further treatment. Anti-emetics may be taken to prevent travel sickness, vomiting resulting from anticancer and other drug treatments, to help the nausea in vertigo, and occasionally to relieve cases of severe vomiting during pregnancy.

🖐 Risks and special precautions

Always check with your doctor or pharmacist before taking an anti-emetic drug. These should not be taken for longer than a couple of days without consulting your doctor. As some antihistamines can make you drowsy, it may be advisable not to drive while taking them.

💊 COMMON DRUGS

Antihistamines	**Anti-vertigo**
Dimenhydrinate ✳	Betahistine
Diphenhydramine	**5HT₃ antagonists**
Promethazine	Dolasetron
Phenothiazines	Ondansetron
Chlorpromazine	**Butyrophenones**
Perphenazine	Haloperidol
Prochlorperazine	**Other drugs**
	Dexamethasone
✳ See Part 3	Dronabinol
	Scopolamine

Action of anti-emetics

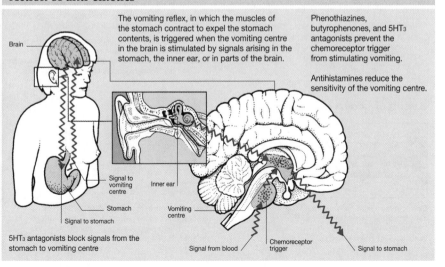

The vomiting reflex, in which the muscles of the stomach contract to expel the stomach contents, is triggered when the vomiting centre in the brain is stimulated by signals arising in the stomach, the inner ear, or in parts of the brain.

Phenothiazines, butyrophenones, and 5HT₃ antagonists prevent the chemoreceptor trigger from stimulating vomiting.

Antihistamines reduce the sensitivity of the vomiting centre.

Brain

Signal to vomiting centre

Inner ear

Stomach

Vomiting centre

Signal to stomach

5HT₃ antagonists block signals from the stomach to vomiting centre

Signal from blood

Chemoreceptor trigger

Signal to stomach

CONSTIPATION

What is it?
When your bowels do not move as frequently as usual and the feces are hard and difficult to pass, you are suffering from constipation.

What causes it?
The most common cause is lack of sufficient fiber in the diet; fiber supplies the bulk that makes the feces soft and easy to pass. Ignoring the urge to defecate can also cause constipation, because the feces become dry and too small to stimulate the intestinal muscles. Certain drugs may be constipating: for example, opioid analgesics and tricyclic antidepressants. Some diseases, such as hypothyroidism, can cause constipation. Injury to the spinal cord can also affect normal evacuation of the bowel. The onset of constipation in a middle-aged or elderly person may be an early symptom of bowel cancer. Consult your doctor about any persistent change in bowel habit.

What can help?
Increasing fluid intake, a high-fibre diet, and regular exercise can help with constipation. When these strategies alone don't work or if the constipation is due to medications, laxatives may be needed. Doctors may prescribe laxatives to prevent pain and straining after childbirth or abdominal surgery. Laxatives are also used to clear the bowel before investigative procedures such as colonoscopy. They may be prescribed for patients who are elderly or bedridden as lack of exercise can often lead to constipation.

✋ Risks and special precautions
Long-term use of some laxatives can be harmful. Discontinue use as soon as normal bowel movements have been re-established. Do not give children laxatives except on the advice of a doctor.

✪ COMMON DRUGS

Stimulant laxatives
  Bisacodyl ✲
  Cascara
  Sennosides
Bulk-forming agents
  Psyllium
Softening agents
  Docusate sodium ✲
  Glycerine suppositories

Osmotic laxatives
  Lactulose ✲
  Magnesium citrate
  Magnesium hydroxide
  Polyethylene glycol
  Sodium phosphate
Lubricant laxative
  Mineral oil

✲ See Part 3

Types of laxatives

- **Bulk-forming laxatives,** such as psyllium, absorb water in the bowel, thereby increasing the volume of feces, making them softer and easier to pass. They are relatively slow acting but are less likely than other laxatives to interfere with normal bowel action. Consult your doctor before taking laxatives if you have abdominal pain or discomfort.

- **Stimulant laxatives** cause the bowel muscles to contract, increasing the speed at which fecal matter goes through the intestine. These are suitable for occasional use when other treatments have failed or when rapid onset of action is needed. Constipation due to regular use of opioid medications for chronic pain management may be helped by this type of laxative. Stimulant laxatives should usually not be used for longer than a week.

- **Softening agents** make bowel movements easier to pass without increasing their bulk, and are often used when hard bowel movements cause pain on defecation – for example, when hemorrhoids are present, or after surgery when straining must be avoided.

- **Osmotic laxatives** act by keeping water in the bowel, and thereby make the bowel movements softer and easier to pass. Magnesium salts such as magnesium citrate may be used to evacuate the bowel before surgery or investigative procedures. They are not normally used for the long-term relief of constipation because they can cause chemical imbalances in the blood.

- **Lactulose** causes fluid to accumulate in the intestine, and is an alternative to bulk-forming laxatives for treatment of chronic constipation. It may cause stomach cramps and flatulence but is usually well tolerated.

Action of laxatives

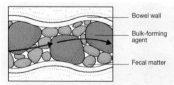

Bowel wall
Bulk-forming agent
Fecal matter

Bulk-forming agents contain particles that absorb many times their own volume of water. By doing so, they increase the bulk of the bowel movements and thus encourage bowel action.

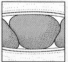
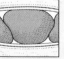

Increased contractions

Before drug   **After drug**

Stimulant laxatives trigger contraction of the intestinal muscles, speeding the passage of fecal matter through the large intestine and allowing less time for water to be absorbed. Thus feces become more liquid and are passed more frequently.

DIARRHEA

What is it?

Diarrhea is an increase in the fluidity, frequency, and sometimes volume of bowel movements. In some cases, diarrhea is accompanied by abdominal pain, cramping, bloating, loss of appetite, and vomiting. Severe diarrhea can lead to dehydration that may be life-threatening, particularly in babies or the elderly.

What causes it?

In some cases diarrhea protects the body from harmful substances in the intestine by hastening their removal. The most common causes are viral infection, food poisoning, and parasites. Traveller's diarrhea is usually associated with contaminated food or water and can be caused by bacteria, viruses, or parasites. Diarrhea can also occur as a symptom of other illnesses, such as Crohn's disease or ulcerative colitis. It can be a side effect of some drugs and may follow radiation therapy for cancer. Mild diarrhea may also be caused by anxiety. A doctor should be consulted with any changes in bowel function such as diarrhea or constipation, especially in those over 40.

What can help?

An attack of diarrhea related to a viral infection or food poisoning usually clears up quickly without medical attention. Traveller's diarrhea may resolve itself in 3–4 days. The best treatment is to drink plenty of clear fluids, such as apple juice. Rehydration solutions containing sugar as well as potassium and sodium salts are widely recommended for preventing dehydration and chemical imbalances, particularly in children. You should consult your doctor if: the condition does not improve within 48 hours; the diarrhea contains blood; severe abdominal pain and vomiting are present; you have just returned from a foreign country; or if the diarrhea occurs in a small child or an elderly person. Severe diarrhea can impair absorption of drugs; seek advice from a doctor or pharmacist. A woman taking oral contraceptives may need additional contraceptive measures.

An antidiarrheal drug may be prescribed to provide relief when simple remedies are not effective, and once it is confirmed that the diarrhea is neither infectious nor toxic. Sometimes, antispasmodic drugs may also be used to relieve accompanying pain. Antibacterials may also be prescribed, especially for traveller's diarrhea.

🖑 Risks and special precautions

Opioid drugs should be used under medical supervision when diarrhea is caused by an infection, since they may slow the elimination of microorganisms from the intestine, causing serious complications. Do not take a bulk-forming agent together with an opioid or antispasmodic drug, because a bulky mass could form and obstruct the bowel.

🖎 COMMON DRUGS

Antispasmodics	Bulk-forming agents
Dicyclomine	and adsorbents
Scopolamine	Attapulgite
Opioids	Bismuth subsalicylate
Codeine ✳	Psyllium
Diphenoxylate	**Antibacterials**
Loperamide ✳	Azithromycin
	Ciprofloxacin ✳

✳ See Part 3

Action of antidiarrheal drugs

Opioid antidiarrheals

These drugs reduce contractions in the intestinal muscles. This allows more time for water to be absorbed from the food residue and therefore reduces the fluidity as well as the frequency of bowel movements.

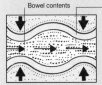

Bowel contents — Bowel wall

Before drug
Rapid bowel contraction prevents water from being absorbed.

After drug
Slowed bowel action allows more water to be absorbed.

Bulk-forming agents

These preparations contain particles that swell up as they absorb water from the large intestine. This makes the feces firmer and less fluid. It is thought that bulk-forming agents may absorb irritants and harmful chemicals along with excess water.

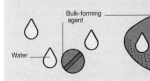

Bulk-forming agent

Water

Water is attracted by bulk-forming agent.

Bulk-forming agent swells as water is absorbed.

Types of antidiarrheal drugs

- **Bulk-forming agents and adsorbents** absorb water and irritants from the bowel, thereby producing larger, firmer stools at less frequent intervals. They have a milder effect and are often used when it is necessary to regulate bowel action over a prolonged period – for example, in people with colostomies or ileostomies.

- **Opioid drugs** decrease contractions in the intestinal muscles so that fecal matter passes more slowly through the bowel. They are the most effective antidiarrheals and are used when the diarrhea is severe and debilitating.

DIABETES MELLITUS

What is it?

The body obtains most of its energy from glucose, a simple form of sugar made in the intestine from the breakdown of starch and other sugars and absorbed into the blood. Insulin, one of the hormones produced in the pancreas, enables body tissues to take up glucose from the blood, either to use it for energy or to store it. In diabetes mellitus, insulin production is defective. This results in reduced uptake of glucose by the tissues, and thus the glucose level in the blood rises abnormally. A high blood glucose level is medically known as hyperglycemia.

There are two main types of diabetes mellitus. **Type 1** occurs when the pancreas produces too little insulin or none at all, and usually develops suddenly in childhood or adolescence. Symptoms of Type 1 diabetes include extreme thirst, increased urination, lethargy, blurred vision, and weight loss. This type of diabetes is fatal if it is left untreated. **Type 2** occurs either when the pancreas is secreting sufficient insulin but the cells in the body become resistant to it, or there is not enough insulin produced. This type of diabetes mainly affects people over 40 and is more common in overweight people.

What causes it?

In Type 1 diabetes, the insulin-secreting cells in the pancreas are gradually destroyed. An autoimmune reaction, where the body recognizes its own insulin-producing cells as foreign and tries to eliminate them, is the likely cause. Although it is not clear what causes this, a trigger may be a childhood viral infection. The causes of Type 2 diabetes are less well understood, but genetics and obesity are important factors. Diabetes can also be caused by corticosteroid drugs or excess levels of natural corticosteroid hormones (such as Cushing syndrome). Other drugs, such as some types of antipsychotics, can also cause a diabetes-like condition.

What can help?

It is important to treat diabetes, as continuous high blood glucose levels will damage various parts of the body. The major problems are caused by the build-up of fatty deposits in arteries (atherosclerosis, see p.47), which narrows the vessels, reducing the flow of blood. This can result in heart attacks, blindness, kidney failure, reduced circulation in the legs, and decreased nerve sensation, especially in the legs and hands.

In Type 1 diabetes, insulin treatment is the only option. It has to be continued for life and will be tailored to each person's particular needs. A regular record of home blood glucose monitoring should be kept. Several types of insulin are available, which are broadly classified by their duration of action (short-, medium-, and long-acting). Short-acting insulin is generally taken 15–30 minutes before eating to deal with the increased amount of glucose generated through digestion. Longer-acting insulin is usually taken once or twice a day to maintain a constant low background level of the hormone.

In both types of diabetes, management of the diet is vital. A healthy diet consisting of a low-fat, high-fibre, low simple sugar (cakes, sweets) and high complex sugar (pasta, rice, potatoes) intake is advised. In Type 2 diabetes, a reduction in weight alone, through diet and exercise, may be sufficient to lower the body's energy requirements and restore blood glucose to normal.

If an alteration in diet fails, oral antidiabetic drugs are prescribed. Insulin may need to be given to people with Type 2 diabetes if the above treatments fail, or in pregnancy, during severe illness, and before the patient undergoes any surgery requiring a general anesthetic. Other changes in lifestyle, such as quitting smoking, drinking alcohol only in moderation, and exercising regularly, can also help.

It is advisable for diabetics to carry a card or bracelet detailing their condition and treatment in case of a medical emergency.

🛈 Risks and special precautions

Insulin injection sites should be regularly rotated to avoid disturbing the fat layer beneath the skin, which alters the rate of insulin absorption.

Insulin requirements increase during illness and pregnancy. During an illness, check the urine for high levels of ketones, which indicate that insulin levels are too low. The combination of high blood sugars, high urinary ketones, and vomiting is a diabetic emergency and the person should be taken to an Emergency department without delay. Too much insulin can cause a condition called hypoglycemia, which should be corrected quickly with intake of a sugar/glucose source. Hypoglycemia, left untreated, can be life threatening.

The sulfonylureas may lower the blood glucose too much, causing a condition called hypoglycemia. Avoid this by starting with low doses of these drugs and ensuring regular food intake. Interactions may occur with other drugs; consult with your doctor before taking any other medications.

Exercise increases the body's need for glucose; extra calories should be taken prior to exertion. The effects of vigorous exercise on blood sugar levels may last up to 18 hours, and the post-exercise doses of insulin may need to be reduced by 10–25 percent to avoid hypoglycemia.

Types of drugs for diabetes

- **Insulin** treatment directly replaces the natural insulin hormone that is deficient in Type 1 diabetes. Animal-sourced (commonly pork) and biosynthetic human insulins are available. Insulin is usually self-administered by injection.

- **Sulfonylurea** oral antidiabetic drugs encourage the pancreas to secrete insulin. They are effective only when some insulin-secreting cells remain active, and are used in the treatment of Type 2 diabetes.

- **Other antidiabetic drugs** slow the increase in blood sugar that occurs after a meal and reduce the body's resistance to insulin, and can be used in combination to treat Type 2 diabetes.

Monitoring blood glucose

Diabetics need to check their blood glucose level at home. There are a variety of devices, called glucometers, that can measure the blood sugar level in a drop of blood obtained from a finger prick.

Glucometers can be purchased at most pharmacies. Ask your doctor or pharmacist which meter would be best for you. You should also ask for training on how to use the chosen meter properly.

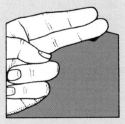

1 Prick your finger to give a large drop of blood.

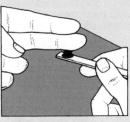

2 Touch the blood on to the test pads of the testing strip.

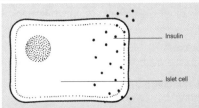

3 Within the specified time, insert the strip into the meter. Your reading (e.g. 6.8) will appear within the specified time on the meter (usually within 2 minutes).

Action of sulfonylurea drugs

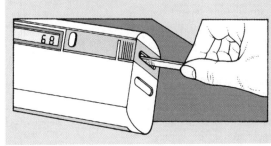

Insulin

Islet cell

Before drug treatment
In Type 2 diabetes, the islet cells of the pancreas secrete insufficient insulin to meet the body's needs.

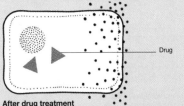

Drug

After drug treatment
The drug stimulates the islet cells to release increased amounts of insulin.

✪ COMMON DRUGS

Sulfonylurea drugs
  Chlorpropamide
  Gliclazide
  Glimepiride
  Glyburide ✳
  Tolbutamide
Antiobesity agent
  Orlistat
Other drugs
  Acarbose
  Glucagon
  Insulins ✳
    Aspart
    Detemir
    Glargine
    Lente (pork)
    Lispro
    NPH (human
      biosynthetic, pork)
    Regular (human
      biosynthetic)

Metformin ✳
Nateglinide
Pioglitazone
Repaglinide
Rosiglitazone ✳
Sitagliptin ✳

✳ See Part 3

COMMON MEDICAL DRUGS

The drug profiles in this section provide information and practical advice on 100 individual drugs commonly taken by Canadians. The profiles are intended to provide reference and guidance for non-medical readers taking drug treatment. However, it is impossible for this kind of book to take into account every variation in individual circumstances; readers should always follow their doctor's or pharmacist's instructions in instances where these differ from the advice in this section.

The drugs have been selected in order to provide representative coverage of the principal classes of drugs in medical use today. For disorders for which a number of drugs are available, the most commonly used drugs have been selected.

At the end of this section, there are additional profiles on common vitamins, minerals, and natural health product supplements (pp.179–186).

HOW TO UNDERSTAND THE PROFILES

For ease of reference, each drug profile is organized in the same way, using standard headings.

Drug name
Tells you the drug's generic name, common brand names under which the drug is marketed, and combined preparations that contain the drug.

Information for users
Practical information on how and when to take the drug, the usual recommended dosage, how soon it takes effect, how long it is active, and advice on diet, storage, missed doses, and prolonged use.

Special precautions
Describes circumstances in which the drug should be taken with special caution or in which it might not be suitable.

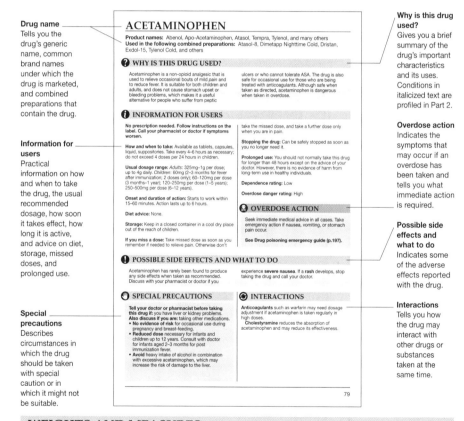

Why is this drug used?
Gives you a brief summary of the drug's important characteristics and its uses. Conditions in italicized text are profiled in Part 2.

Overdose action
Indicates the symptoms that may occur if an overdose has been taken and tells you what immediate action is required.

Possible side effects and what to do
Indicates some of the adverse effects reported with the drug.

Interactions
Tells you how the drug may interact with other drugs or substances taken at the same time.

WEIGHTS AND MEASURES

Metric equivalents of measurements used in this book:

1,000mcg (microgram) = 1mg (milligram)
1,000mg = 1g (gram)
1,000ml (millilitre) = 1l (litre)

Units or international units
Units (u) and international units (IU) are also used to express drug dosages. They represent the biological activity of a drug (its effect on the body) and are calculated in a laboratory.

ACETAMINOPHEN

Product names: Abenol, Apo-Acetaminophen, Atasol, Tempra, Tylenol, and many others
Used in the following combined preparations: Atasol-8, Dimetapp Nighttime Cold, Dristan, Exdol-15, Tylenol Cold, and others

❓ WHY IS THIS DRUG USED?

Acetaminophen is a non-opioid analgesic that is used to relieve occasional bouts of mild *pain* and to reduce fever. It is suitable for both children and adults, and does not cause stomach upset or bleeding problems, which makes it a useful alternative for people who suffer from peptic ulcers or who cannot tolerate ASA. The drug is also safe for occasional use for those who are being treated with anticoagulants. Although safe when taken as directed, acetaminophen is dangerous when taken in overdose.

ℹ️ INFORMATION FOR USERS

No prescription needed. Follow instructions on the label. Call your pharmacist or doctor if symptoms worsen.

How and when to take: Available as tablets, capsules, liquid, suppositories. Take every 4–6 hours as necessary; do not exceed 4 doses per 24 hours in children.

Usual dosage range: *Adults*: 325mg–1g per dose; up to 4g daily. *Children*: 60mg (2–3 months for fever after immunization; 2 doses only); 60–120mg per dose (3 months–1 year); 120–250mg per dose (1–5 years); 250–500mg per dose (6–12 years).

Onset and duration of action: Starts to work within 15–60 minutes. Action lasts up to 6 hours.

Diet advice: None.

Storage: Keep in a closed container in a cool dry place out of the reach of children.

If you miss a dose: Take missed dose as soon as you remember if needed to relieve pain. Otherwise don't take the missed dose, and take a further dose only when you are in pain.

Stopping the drug: Can be safely stopped as soon as you no longer need it.

Prolonged use: You should not normally take this drug for longer than 48 hours except on the advice of your doctor. However, there is no evidence of harm from long-term use in healthy individuals.

Dependence rating: Low

Overdose danger rating: High

☠️ OVERDOSE ACTION

Seek immediate medical advice in all cases. Take emergency action if nausea, vomiting, or stomach pain occur.

See Drug poisoning emergency guide (p.197).

❗ POSSIBLE SIDE EFFECTS AND WHAT TO DO

Acetaminophen has rarely been found to produce any side effects when taken as recommended. Discuss with your pharmacist or doctor if you experience **severe nausea**. If a **rash** develops, stop taking the drug and call your doctor.

✋ SPECIAL PRECAUTIONS

Tell your doctor or pharmacist before taking this drug if: you have liver or kidney problems.
Also discuss if you are: taking other medications.
• **No evidence of risk** for occasional use during pregnancy and breast-feeding.
• **Reduced dose** necessary for infants and children up to 12 years. Consult with doctor for infants aged 2–3 months for post immunization fever.
• **Avoid** heavy intake of alcohol in combination with excessive acetaminophen, which may increase the risk of damage to the liver.

🔄 INTERACTIONS

Anticoagulants such as warfarin may need dosage adjustment if acetaminophen is taken regularly in high doses.
    Cholestyramine reduces the absorption of acetaminophen and may reduce its effectiveness.

ALENDRONATE

Product names: Apo-Alendronate, Fosamax, PMS-Alendronate, and other generics
Used in the following combined preparation: Fosavance

❓ WHY IS THIS DRUG USED?

Alendronate is used to treat *osteoporosis* in men and post-menopausal women. It is also used to treat Paget's disease. Take tablets first thing in the morning on an empty stomach, and swallow them whole with a glass of water (do not take them with mineral water or other drinks as these could affect the absorption of the drug). Remain upright for at least 30 minutes to prevent the drug from staying in the esophagus, where it could cause irritation. Wait for at least 30 minutes (preferably longer) before taking other medications and food.

ℹ INFORMATION FOR USERS

Prescription needed. Do not alter dosage without checking with your doctor.

How and when to take: Available as tablets and liquid. Take once daily, first thing in the morning. Once weekly, first thing in the morning (post-menopausal women).

Usual adult dosage range: *Treatment*: men and postmenopausal women, 10mg; postmenopausal women may also use 70mg once weekly. *Prevention*: 5mg (postmenopausal women). *Prevention and treatment of corticosteroid-induced osteoporosis*: 5mg; postmenopausal women not taking HRT, 10mg.

Onset and duration of effect: It may take months to notice an improvement. Some effects may persist for months or years.

Diet advice: Absorption of alendronate is reduced by foods, especially those containing calcium (e.g. dairy products), so the drug should be taken on an empty stomach. The diet must contain adequate calcium and vitamin D; supplements may be given.

Storage: Keep in a closed container in a cool, dry place out of the reach of children.

If you miss or exceed a dose: Take the next dose at the usual time next morning. An occasional unintentional extra dose is unlikely to cause problems. Large overdoses may cause stomach problems including heartburn, irritation, and ulcers. Notify your doctor at once, and try to remain upright.

Stopping the drug: Do not stop the drug without consulting your doctor, as it may lead to worsening of the underlying condition.

Prolonged use: Alendronate is usually prescribed indefinitely for osteoporosis without causing any problems. Blood and urine tests may be carried out at intervals.

Dependence rating: Low

Overdose danger rating: Medium

❗ POSSIBLE SIDE EFFECTS AND WHAT TO DO

The most common side effect caused by alendronate is **abdominal pain** as a result of irritation to the esophagus, stomach, or the small intestine – discuss with your doctor if bothersome. Other possible side effects are **diarrhea, constipation, headache, nausea** and **vomiting** – discuss with doctor if bothersome. If you develop **muscle or bone pain, a rash** or **photosensitivity,** or **eye inflammation,** call your doctor now. If you experience **jaw pain,** stop taking the drug and call your doctor now.

🛑 SPECIAL PRECAUTIONS

Tell your doctor if you have: abnormality of the esophagus; unusual bone pain; stomach problems or a history of ulcers; hypocalcemia; kidney impairment. **Also discuss if you are:** unable to stand or sit upright for at least 30 minutes; taking any other medications.
• **Not recommended** in pregnancy, breast-feeding, or for infants and children.
• **Avoid** alcohol as it may cause further stomach irritation.

🔄 INTERACTIONS

Antacids, calcium, iron salts, and other medications reduce the absorption of alendronate. Separate dosing times are required.

ALLOPURINOL

Product names: Apo-Allopurinol, Teva-Allopurinol
Used in the following combined preparations: None

❓ WHY IS THIS DRUG USED?

Allopurinol is used to prevent gout, which is caused by deposits of uric acid crystals in joints, by blocking an enzyme called xanthine oxidase that is involved in forming uric acid. It is also used to lower high uric acid levels (hyperuricemia) caused by other drugs, such as anticancer drugs.

At the start of treatment, the drug may cause an acute attack of gout, and an anti-inflammatory drug may also be given to reduce uric acid levels. Also, allopurinol should never be started until an acute attack is over because it may cause a further episode. Treatment with the drug should be continued indefinitely to prevent further attacks.

ℹ️ INFORMATION FOR USERS

Prescription needed. Do not alter dosage without checking with your doctor.

How and when to take: Available as tablets. Take 1–3 x daily after food.

Usual adult dosage range: 100–300mg daily.

Onset and duration of effect: Starts to work within 24–48 hours. Full effect may take several weeks. Action lasts up to 30 hours. Some effects may last for 1–2 weeks after the drug has been stopped.

Diet advice: A high fluid intake (2 litres of fluid daily) is recommended.

Storage: Keep in a closed container in a cool, dry place out of the reach of children.

If you miss or exceed a dose: If your next dose is not due for another 12 hours or more, take a dose as soon as you remember and take the next one as usual. Otherwise skip the missed dose and take your next dose on schedule. An occasional unintentional extra dose is unlikely to cause problems. Large overdoses may cause nausea, vomiting, abdominal pain, diarrhea, and dizziness; notify your doctor.

Stopping the drug: Do not stop the drug without consulting your doctor; symptoms may recur.

Prolonged use: Apart from an increased risk of gout in the first weeks or months, the drug is usually well tolerated. Periodic checks on uric acid levels in the blood, and liver and kidney function tests are usually performed, and the dose of allopurinol adjusted if necessary.

Dependence rating: Low

Overdose danger rating: Medium

❗ POSSIBLE SIDE EFFECTS AND WHAT TO DO

The most serious side effect is an allergic rash; nausea can be avoided by taking allopurinol after food. If you experience **nausea, drowsiness,** or **dizziness,** discuss with your doctor if bothersome. If you develop **headache, metallic taste,** or **visual disturbances,** discuss with your doctor in all cases. Stop taking the drug now and see your doctor if you experience a **rash/itching, sore throat,** or **fever and chills.**

👐 SPECIAL PRECAUTIONS

Tell your doctor if you have: long-term liver or kidney problems; a history of sensitivity reaction to allopurinol; a current attack of gout. **Also discuss if you are:** taking large amounts of vitamin C; taking other medications.
- **Safety not established** in pregnancy. The drug passes into the breast milk and may affect the baby. Discuss with your doctor in both cases.
- **Reduced dose necessary** for infants and children, and possibly for those over 60.
- **Avoid** driving and hazardous work until you have learned how allopurinol affects you because the drug can cause drowsiness.
- **Avoid** alcohol as it may worsen gout.

⚙️ INTERACTIONS

Allopurinol may increase the effects of **ACE inhibitors, anticoagulant drugs,** and **cyclosporine.**
  Large doses of **ASA** may reduce the effects of allopurinol.
  Allopurinol may increase levels of **theophylline.**
  Allopurinol blocks the breakdown of **mercaptopurine** and **azathioprine,** requiring a reduction in their dosage.
  Thiazide diuretics may increase the level of allopurinol.
  The risk of rash may be increased when taken with **amoxicillin** or **ampicillin.**
  The hypoglycemic effects of **chlorpropamide** may be increased.

ALPRAZOLAM

Product names: Apo-Alpraz, Nu-Alpraz, Teva-Alprazolam, Xanax, and others
Used in the following combined preparations: None

❓ WHY IS THIS DRUG USED?

Alprazolam is used for the short-term symptomatic relief of excessive *anxiety*. It is also used in the treatment of panic disorders and agoraphobia (fear of open spaces), other phobias, and anxiety disorders of a general nature. Panic disorders are characterized by recurrent panic attacks, which may present as periods of intense fear or discomfort.

Alprazolam can be habit-forming if taken regularly over a long period, and its effects may grow weaker over time. For these reasons, your doctor will review your treatment regularly.

ℹ️ INFORMATION FOR USERS

Prescription needed. Do not alter dosage without checking with your doctor.

How and when to take: Available as tablets. Take 2–3 x daily.

Usual dosage range: 0.75–1.5mg daily. Occasionally, larger doses may be prescribed.

Onset and duration of effect: Starts to work within 1–2 hours. Action lasts for up to 24 hours.

Diet advice: None.

Storage: Keep in a tightly closed container in a cool, dry place away from reach of children. Protect from light.

If you miss or exceed a dose: Take missed dose when you remember. If your next dose is due within 2 hours, take a single dose now and skip the next one.

An occasional unintentional extra dose is unlikely to cause problems. Larger overdoses may cause unusual drowsiness, unsteadiness, or coma – notify your doctor.

Stopping the drug: If you have been taking the drug continuously for less than 2 weeks, it can be safely stopped as soon as you feel you no longer need it. However, if you have been taking it for longer, stopping abruptly may lead to withdrawal symptoms – consult your doctor.

Prolonged use: Regular use over several weeks can lead to a reduction in its effect as the body adapts. It may also be habit-forming when taken for extended periods, especially if larger-than-average doses are taken.

Dependence rating: High

Overdose danger rating: Medium

❗ POSSIBLE SIDE EFFECTS AND WHAT TO DO

The principal side effects of this drug are related to its sedative and tranquilizing properties, and can often be reduced by adjustment of dosage. If you experience **drowsiness** or **headache**, discuss with your doctor if bothersome. Discuss with your doctor in all cases if you experience **dizziness** or **unsteadiness, forgetfulness** or **confusion, blurred vision, rash,** or **jaundice**.

✋ SPECIAL PRECAUTIONS

Tell your doctor or pharmacist before taking this drug if you have: impaired liver or kidney function; myasthenia gravis; glaucoma; problems with alcohol or drug abuse. **Also discuss if you are:** taking other medications; pregnant; breast-feeding.
- **Not recommended** for children under 18 years.
- **Reduced dose** likely for those over 60 due to increased likelihood of adverse effects.
- **Avoid** driving and hazardous work until you have learned how the drug affects you: it can cause reduced alertness, blurred vision, and slowed reactions.
- **Avoid** alcohol as it may increase the sedative effects of this drug.

⚙️ INTERACTIONS

All drugs that have a sedative effect on the central nervous system are likely to increase the sedative properties of alprazolam. Such drugs include **alcohol, sleeping drugs, antihistamines, antidepressants, opioid analgesics,** and **antipsychotics**.

AMLODIPINE

Product names: Apo-Amlodipine, Norvasc, PMS-Amlodipine, and others
Used in the following combined preparation: Caduet

❓ WHY IS THIS DRUG USED?

Amlodipine, a calcium channel blocker, is used in the treatment of *angina* to help prevent attacks of chest pain. Unlike some other anti-angina drugs, it can be used safely by individuals with asthma and noninsulin-dependent diabetes. Amlodipine is also used to reduce *high blood pressure* (hypertension).

Amlodipine may cause blood pressure to fall too low at the start of treatment. In rare cases, angina may become worse at the start of amlodipine treatment. The drug may sometimes cause mild to moderate leg and ankle swelling.

ℹ INFORMATION FOR USERS

Prescription needed. Do not alter dosage without checking with your doctor.

How and when to take: Available as tablets. Take once daily.

Usual adult dosage range: 5–10mg daily.

Onset and duration of effect: Starts to work within 6–12 hours. Action lasts 24 hours.

Diet advice: None.

Storage: Keep in a closed container in a cool, dry place out of the reach of children.

If you miss or exceed a dose: If you remember a missed dose within 12 hours, take it as soon as you remember. If you do not remember until later, do not take the missed dose and do not double up the next one. Instead, go back to your regular schedule. An occasional unintentional extra dose is unlikely to cause problems. Large overdoses may cause a marked lowering of blood pressure – notify your doctor immediately.

Stopping the drug: Consult your doctor, as stopping the drug may lead to worsening of the underlying condition.

Prolonged use: No problems expected.

Dependence rating: Low

Overdose danger rating: Medium

❗ POSSIBLE SIDE EFFECTS AND WHAT TO DO

Amlodipine can cause a variety of minor side effects, including **leg and ankle swelling, headache, dizziness, fatigue,** and **flushing** – discuss with your doctor if bothersome. If you experience **nausea** or **palpitations,** discuss with your doctor in all cases. Stop taking the drug now and discuss with your doctor if you develop a **worsening of angina, skin rash,** or **breathing difficulties**.

🖐 SPECIAL PRECAUTIONS

Tell your doctor if you have: long-term liver or kidney problems; heart failure; diabetes. **Also discuss if you are:** taking other medications; pregnant; breast-feeding.
• **Not recommended** for infants and children.
• **Avoid** driving and hazardous work until you have learned how amlodipine affects you as the drug can cause dizziness owing to lowered blood pressure.
• **Avoid** alcohol as it may further reduce blood pressure, causing dizziness or other symptoms.

⊙ INTERACTIONS

Amlodipine may increase the effect of **beta blockers** and other blood pressure lowering drugs.
  Fluconazole, ketoconazole, clarithromycin, and **erythromycin** can increase the effect of amlodipine.
  Amlodipine may decrease the effect of **clopidogrel**; monitor therapy.
  Grapefruit juice may increase the effect of amlodipine.
  Amlodipine may increase the effect of **phenytoin**.

AMOXICILLIN

Product names: Apo-Amoxi, Mylan-Amoxicillin, and others
Used in the following combined preparations: Apo-Amoxi Clav, Clavulin, Hp-PAC

❓ WHY IS THIS DRUG USED?

Amoxicillin is a penicillin antibiotic. It is prescribed to treat a variety of *infections*, but is particularly useful for treating ear, nose, and throat infections, respiratory tract infections, cystitis, and uncomplicated gonorrhea. Amoxicillin can cause minor stomach upsets and a skin rash. It can also provoke a severe allergic reaction, which suggests that the patient is allergic to penicillin antibiotics.

ℹ INFORMATION FOR USERS

Prescription needed. Do not alter dosage without checking with your doctor.

How and when to take: Available as tablets, capsules, powder (dissolved in water). Taken normally 3 x daily.

Usual dosage range: *Adults* 750mg–1.5g daily. In some cases a short course of up to 6g daily is given. A single dose of 3g may be given as a preventative. *Children* Reduced dose according to age and weight.

Onset and duration of effect: Starts to work in 1–2 hours. Action lasts up to 8 hours.

Diet advice: None.

Storage: Keep in a closed container in a cool, dry place out of the reach of children.

If you miss or exceed a dose: Take missed dose as soon as you remember. Take your next dose at the scheduled time. An occasional unintentional extra dose is unlikely to be a cause for concern. If you notice any unusual symptoms, or if a large overdose has been taken, notify your doctor.

Stopping the drug: Take the full course. The original infection may recur if treatment is stopped too soon.

Prolonged use: Amoxicillin is usually given only for short courses of treatment.

Dependence rating: Low

Overdose danger rating: Low

❗ POSSIBLE SIDE EFFECTS AND WHAT TO DO

If you develop a **rash, wheezing, itching, fever, joint swelling,** or **swollen mouth or tongue,** this may indicate an allergy. Stop taking the drug and call your doctor, who may prescribe a different antibiotic. You may also experience **diarrhea** or **nausea** and **vomiting** – discuss with your doctor if bothersome.

SPECIAL PRECAUTIONS

Tell your doctor if you have: long-term kidney problems; allergies (for example, asthma, hay fever, or eczema); ulcerative colitis; glandular fever; chronic leukemia; had a previous allergic reaction to a penicillin or cephalosporin antibiotic. **Also discuss if you are:** taking other medications; breast-feeding.
- **Reduced dose** necessary for infants and children.

🗘 INTERACTIONS

Amoxicillin may reduce the effectiveness of the **oral contraceptive pill** and also increase the risk of breakthrough bleeding. Discuss with your pharmacist or doctor.
  Amoxicillin may alter the effect of **anticoagulant drugs** so patients may have to be monitored more closely.

ASA (ACETYLSALICYLIC ACID)

Product names: Aspirin, Entrophen, Novasen, and others
Used in the following combined preparations: Fiorinal, Midol, 222 Tablets, Robaxisal, and others

❓ WHY IS THIS DRUG USED?

ASA relieves *pain*, reduces fever, and alleviates the symptoms of *arthritis*. In low doses, it helps to prevent blood clots, particularly in those with *atherosclerosis* or *angina* due to coronary artery disease, and it reduces the risk of *heart attacks* and *strokes*. Many medicines for *colds, flu,* headaches, menstrual period pains, and joint or muscular aches contain ASA.

ASA can provoke asthma attacks, and, in children, can cause Reye's syndrome, a rare but serious brain and liver disorder.

ℹ️ INFORMATION FOR USERS

Prescription not needed. Follow instructions on the label. Call your pharmacist or doctor if symptoms worsen.

How and when to take: Available as tablets, chewable tablets, enteric coated tablets, and suppositories. Take every 4–6 hours for relief of pain or fever. For prevention of blood clots, take once daily.

Usual adult dosage range: *Relief of pain or fever* 300–900mg per dose. *Prevention of blood clots* 75–300mg daily.

Onset and duration of effect: Starts to work in 30–60 minutes (regular aspirin); 1½–8 hours (enteric coated or sustained-release). Action lasts up to 12 hours; effect on blood clotting lasts several days.

Diet advice: Take with or immediately after food or milk.

Storage: Keep in a closed container in a cool, dry place out of the reach of children.

If you miss a dose: Take missed dose as soon as you remember. If your next dose is due within 2 hours, take a single dose now and skip the next.

Stopping the drug: If prescribed for a long-term condition, seek medical advice before stopping the drug. Otherwise it can be safely stopped.

Prolonged use: Do not take for longer than 2 days except on your doctor's advice. Prolonged use of ASA may lead to bleeding in the stomach and stomach ulcers.

Dependence rating: Low

Overdose danger rating: High

☠️ OVERDOSE ACTION

Seek immediate medical advice in all cases. Take emergency action if there is restlessness, stomach pain, ringing noises in the ears, blurred vision, or vomiting.

See Drug poisoning emergency guide (p.197).

❗ POSSIBLE SIDE EFFECTS AND WHAT TO DO

An **upset stomach** may be helped by taking the drug with food or in buffered or enteric coated forms. If you experience **nausea and vomiting,** discuss with your doctor in all cases. If you develop a **rash, breathlessness, wheezing, blood in vomit, black feces, ringing in the ears, dizziness,** or **severe indigestion** stop taking the drug and call your doctor now.

✋ SPECIAL PRECAUTIONS

Tell your doctor or pharmacist if you have: long-term liver or kidney problems; asthma; a blood clotting disorder; a stomach ulcer. **Also discuss if you are:** allergic to ASA; taking any other medications.
- **Not usually recommended** in pregnancy or during breast-feeding.
- **Do not give** to children under 16 years, except on a doctor's advice.
- **Adverse effects** more likely for those over 60.
- **Avoid** alcohol; it can cause stomach irritation.
- **Discuss** with your doctor or dentist before surgery; ASA may need to be stopped.

🔄 INTERACTIONS

Anticoagulants may have their effects increased by ASA, leading to an increased risk of abnormal bleeding.

Drugs for gout may have their effects reduced by ASA.

Corticosteroids may increase the risk of stomach bleeding with ASA.

NSAIDs may increase the likelihood of stomach irritation with ASA.

Methotrexate may have its toxicity increased by ASA.

Oral antidiabetic drugs may have their effects increased by ASA.

ATENOLOL

Product names: Apo-Atenol, Tenormin, Teva-Atenolol, and others
Used in the following combined preparations: Novo-Atenolthalidone, Tenoretic

❓ WHY IS THIS DRUG USED?

Atenolol is a beta blocker. It prevents the heart from beating too quickly and is used mainly to treat chest pain (*angina*), and *high blood pressure* (hypertension). Atenolol is sometimes prescribed with a diuretic for high blood pressure, and may also be given after a *heart attack* to protect the heart from further damage.

Atenolol should be used with caution by people with asthma, bronchitis, or other forms of respiratory disease.

ℹ️ INFORMATION FOR USERS

Prescription needed. Do not alter dosage without checking with your doctor.

How and when to take: Available as tablets. Take once daily.

Usual adult dosage range: 25–100mg daily.

Onset and duration of effect: Starts to work in 2–4 hours. Action lasts for 20–30 hours.

Diet advice: None.

Storage: Keep in a tightly closed container in a cool, dry place out of the reach of children. Protect from light.

If you miss or exceed a dose: Take missed dose as soon as you remember. If your next dose is due within 6 hours, do not take the missed dose but take the next scheduled dose as usual. An occasional unintentional extra dose is unlikely to be a cause for concern. Notify your doctor if you notice any unusual symptoms, or if a large overdose has been taken.

Stopping the drug: Do not stop taking the drug without consulting your doctor; sudden withdrawal may lead to dangerous worsening of the underlying condition.

Prolonged use: No special problems expected.

Dependence rating: Low

Overdose danger rating: Medium

❗ POSSIBLE SIDE EFFECTS AND WHAT TO DO

Side effects are usually temporary and tend to diminish with long-term use. If you experience **muscle ache, cold hands and feet, nightmares/sleeplessness,** or **dizziness,** discuss with your doctor if bothersome. If you experience **fatigue, dry eyes,** or **headache,** discuss with your doctor in all cases. If you develop a **rash** or **breathing difficulties,** stop taking the drug and call your doctor now.

🖐️ SPECIAL PRECAUTIONS

Tell your doctor if you have: any other heart condition; a long-term kidney problem; diabetes; a lung disorder such as asthma or bronchitis.
Also discuss if you are: taking other medications.
* **Safety not established** in pregnancy and breast-feeding; discuss with your doctor.
* **Not recommended** for infants and children.
* **Reduced dose** may be necessary for those over 60 if there is impaired kidney function.
* **Avoid** driving and hazardous work until you have learned how atenolol affects you because the drug can cause dizziness.
* **Limit** alcohol consumption.
* **Discuss** with your doctor or dentist before any operation; atenolol may need to be stopped before you have surgery.

🔄 INTERACTIONS

Anti-arrhythmic drugs used with atenolol may increase the risk of adverse effects on the heart.

Antidiabetic drugs, including insulin, used with atenolol may increase the risk and/or mask many symptoms of low blood sugar.

Decongestants used with atenolol may increase blood pressure and heart rate.

Calcium channel blockers used with atenolol may further decrease blood pressure, heart rate, and/or the force of the heart's pumping action.

Non-steroidal anti-inflammatory drugs (NSAIDs) may reduce the antihypertensive effect of atenolol.

ATORVASTATIN

Product names: Apo-Atorvastatin, GD-Atorvastatin, Lipitor, and others
Used in the following combined preparation: Caduet

❓ WHY IS THIS DRUG USED?

Atorvastatin is used to treat hypercholesterolemia (*high blood cholesterol* levels) in patients who have not responded to other treatments, such as a special diet, and are at risk of developing heart disease. It blocks the action, in the liver, of an enzyme that is needed for the manufacture of cholesterol. As a result, blood levels of cholesterol are lowered, which can help to prevent coronary heart disease.

ℹ️ INFORMATION FOR USERS

Prescription needed. Do not alter dosage without checking with your doctor.

How and when to take: Available as tablets. Take once daily.

Usual adult dosage range: 10–40mg; up to 80mg in some cases.

Onset and duration of effect: Starts to work within 2 weeks. Full beneficial effects may not be seen for 4–6 weeks. Action lasts 20–30 hours.

Diet advice: A low-fat diet is usually recommended.

Storage: Keep in a closed container in a cool, dry place out of the reach of children.

If you miss or exceed a dose: Take missed dose as soon as you remember. If your next dose is due within 8 hours, do not take the missed dose, but take the next one on schedule. An occasional unintentional extra dose is unlikely to cause problems. Large overdoses may cause liver problems; notify your doctor.

Stopping the drug: Do not stop taking the drug without consulting your doctor, as it may lead to a recurrence of the original condition.

Prolonged use: Long-term use of atorvastatin can affect liver function. Regular blood tests to check liver function are needed. Tests of muscle function may be carried out if problems are suspected.

Dependence rating: Low

Overdose danger rating: Medium

❗ POSSIBLE SIDE EFFECTS AND WHAT TO DO

Most side effects are mild and usually disappear with time. If you experience **headache, nausea,** or **fatigue,** discuss with your doctor if bothersome. If you experience **chest or abdominal pain, muscle pain,** or **jaundice,** discuss with your doctor in all cases. Stop taking the drug now and call your doctor if you develop a **rash, muscle weakness,** or **change in cognition.**

🖐️ SPECIAL PRECAUTIONS

Tell your doctor if you have: liver or kidney problems; thyroid problems; a family history of muscular disorders. **Also discuss if you are:** a heavy drinker; taking other medications; allergic to statins or atorvastatin; diabetic.
- **Not usually prescribed** in pregnancy and safety not established in breast-feeding; discuss with your doctor.
- **Not recommended** for infants and children.
- **Avoid** excessive amounts of alcohol, which may increase the risk of developing liver problems with atorvastatin.

🔄 INTERACTIONS

Anticoagulant drugs may have their effects increased by atorvastatin.
   Itraconazole, ketoconazole, and possibly other **antifungals,** may increase the risk of muscle damage with atorvastatin.
   Clarithromycin and **erythromycin** may also increase the level of atorvastatin.
   Grapefruit juice may increase the level of atorvastatin in the blood.
   Other lipid-lowering drugs taken with atorvastatin may increase the risk of muscle damage.
   Cyclosporine and other immunosuppressant drugs are not usually prescribed with atorvastatin because of the increased risk of muscle damage. However, if using the drugs together is unavoidable, close monitoring is advised.
   Atorvastatin may decrease the effect of **clopidogrel.**

AZITHROMYCIN

Product names: Apo-Azithromycin, CO Azithromycin, Novo-Azithromycin, PMS-Azithromycin, Teva-Azithromycin, Zithromax, Z-PAK
Used in the following combined preparations: None

WHY IS THIS DRUG USED?

Azithromycin is an antibiotic used for upper respiratory tract infections, such as *middle ear infections*, pharyngitis and tonsilitis, and lower respiratory tract infections, such as bacterial exacerbation of chronic obstructive lung disease, *bronchitis*, and *pneumonia*. It is also used for skin and soft tissue infections, including gonorrhea.

INFORMATION FOR USERS

Prescription needed. Do not alter dosage without checking with your doctor.

How and when to take: Available as tablets, liquid (reconstituted from powder), injection. Take once daily.

Usual dosage range: 250mg–1.5g daily.

Onset and duration of effect: Starts to work in 1–3 hours. Action lasts up to 24 hours.

Diet advice: None.

Storage: Keep in a closed container in a cool, dry place out of the reach of children. Store the reconstituted solution between 5 and 30°C and discard any unused portion after 10 days.

If you miss or exceed a dose: Take missed dose as soon as you remember. If it is near the time of the next dose, skip the missed dose and resume your usual dosing schedule. Do not double up to catch up on a missed dose. An occasional unintentional extra dose is unlikely to be a cause for concern. Notify your doctor if you notice any unusual symptoms, or if a large overdose has been taken.

Stopping the drug: Take the full course. The original infection may recur if treatment is stopped too soon.

Prolonged use: Usually not used for prolonged periods. During prolonged therapy, periodic liver function tests may be done.

Dependence rating: Low

Overdose danger rating: Low

POSSIBLE SIDE EFFECTS AND WHAT TO DO

Azithromycin is usually well tolerated. If you experience **abdominal pain, nausea, diarrhea, headache,** or **dizziness,** discuss with your doctor if bothersome. If you develop a **rash, edema of the skin,** or **jaundice,** stop taking the drug and call your doctor now.

SPECIAL PRECAUTIONS

Tell your doctor if you have: liver or kidney problems; a heart problem; porphyria. **Also discuss if you are:** taking other medications, or if you have had an allergic reaction to erythromycin, clarithromycin, or azithromycin.
• **Safety not established** in pregnancy or breast-feeding; discuss with your doctor.
• **Reduced dose** necessary for infants and children.

INTERACTIONS

Aluminum- and magnesium-containing **antacids** can affect azithromycin's peak effect. Do not take at the same time as azithromycin.
   Azithromycin may increase the effect of **cyclosporine, digoxin, triazolam,** and **disopyramide**.

BACLOFEN

Product names: Apo-Baclofen, Lioresal Intrathecal, Lioresal Oral, Mylan-Baclofen, PMS-Baclofen, ratio-Baclofen, and others
Used in the following combined preparations: None

❓ WHY IS THIS DRUG USED?

Baclofen is a muscle-relaxant drug that acts on the central nervous system, including the spinal cord. The drug relieves the spasms, cramping, and rigidity of muscles caused by a variety of disorders, including multiple sclerosis and spinal cord injury. Baclofen is also used to treat the spasticity that results from brain injury, cerebral palsy, or *stroke*. Although this drug does not cure any of these disorders, it increases mobility, allowing other treatment, such as physiotherapy, to be carried out. It is less likely to cause muscle weakness than similar drugs, and its side effects are usually temporary.

ℹ INFORMATION FOR USERS

Prescription needed. Do not alter dosage without checking with your doctor.

How and when to take: Available as tablets, intrathecal injection (specialist use). Take 3 x daily with food or milk.

Usual adult dosage range: 15mg daily (starting dose). Daily dose may be increased by 15mg every 3 days as necessary. Maximum daily dose: 80mg.

Onset and duration of effect: Some benefits may appear after 1–3 hours, but full beneficial effects may not be felt for several weeks. A dose 1 hour before a specific task will improve mobility. Action lasts up to 8 hours.

Diet advice: None.

Storage: Keep in a closed container in a cool, dry place out of the reach of children. Protect liquid from light.

If you miss or exceed a dose: Take missed dose as soon as you remember. If your next dose is due within 2 hours, take a single dose now and skip the next. An occasional unintentional extra dose is unlikely to cause problems. Large overdoses may cause weakness, vomiting, and severe drowsiness; notify your doctor.

Stopping the drug: Do not stop taking the drug without consulting your doctor who will supervise a gradual reduction in dosage. Abrupt cessation may cause hallucinations, seizures, and worsening spasticity.

Prolonged use: No problems expected.

Dependence rating: Low

Overdose danger rating: Medium

⚠ POSSIBLE SIDE EFFECTS AND WHAT TO DO

Common side effects are related to the sedative effects of the drug, and can be minimized by starting with a low dose that is gradually increased. If you experience **dizziness, drowsiness, nausea, muscle fatigue/weakness,** or **difficulty in passing urine,** discuss with your doctor if bothersome. If you develop **constipation, diarrhea,** or **headache**, discuss with your doctor in all cases. See your doctor in all cases if you experience **confusion**.

✋ SPECIAL PRECAUTIONS

Tell your doctor if you have: long-term liver or kidney problems; difficulty in passing urine; a history of peptic ulcers or epileptic seizures; diabetes; breathing problems. **Also discuss if you are:** taking other medications.
- **Safety not established** in pregnancy. The drug passes into the breast milk. Discuss with your doctor.
- **Reduced dose necessary** for infants and children, and possibly for those over 60; the elderly may be more sensitive to side effects.
- **Avoid** driving and hazardous work until you have learned how baclofen affects you.
- **Avoid** alcohol as it may increase the sedative effects of this drug.
- **Inform** your doctor or dentist that you are taking baclofen before you have a general anesthetic.

🔄 INTERACTIONS

The effect of **antihypertensive** and **diuretic drugs** may be increased.
Some **drugs for parkinsonism** may cause confusion or hallucinations if taken with baclofen.
Dosage of **antidiabetic drugs** or **insulin** may need adjusting, as baclofen may increase blood glucose levels.
Sedatives may increase the sedative properties of baclofen.
Tricyclic antidepressants may increase baclofen's effects, causing muscle weakness.

BISACODYL

Product names: Apo-Bisacodyl, Correctol, Dulcolax, PMS-Bisacodyl, Soflax Ex
Used in the following combined preparations: Royvac Bowel Evacuant Kit

❓ WHY IS THIS DRUG USED?

Bisacodyl is a stimulant laxative and is recommended for the treatment of occasional *constipation*. It may also be given in preparation for diagnostic procedures. It is thought to work by acting on the nerve endings on the wall of the bowel, which triggers contraction of the intestinal muscles and speeds up the process of fecal matter moving through the bowel.

Bisacodyl tablets should be swallowed whole and not taken with milk or antacids.

ℹ️ INFORMATION FOR USERS

No prescription needed. Follow instructions on the label. Call your pharmacist or doctor if symptoms worsen.

How and when to take: Available as tablets, enteric coated tablets, suppositories. Take once daily on an occasional basis.

Usual adult dosage range: *Oral tablets* 5–15mg. *Suppository* 10mg.

Onset and duration of effect: *Tablets* start to work within 6–8 hours; *suppository* within 30 minutes. Action lasts up to 24 hours.

Diet advice: Maintain adequate fluid and fibre intake to prevent constipation.

Storage: Keep in a closed container in a cool, dry place out of the reach of children.

If you miss or exceed a dose: Take missed dose as soon as you remember. Resume normal dose thereafter. Do not double up on a dose. An occasional unintentional extra dose is unlikely to be a cause for concern. Large doses can cause watery stools, abdominal cramps, and loss of electrolytes; notify your doctor.

Stopping the drug: Can be safely stopped as soon as you no longer need it.

Prolonged use: Prolonged use of the oral preparation can make the bowel dependent on laxatives. For regular use, consult your doctor or pharmacist.

Dependence rating: Low

Overdose danger rating: Medium

❗ POSSIBLE SIDE EFFECTS AND WHAT TO DO

Bisacodyl is generally well tolerated. If you experience **local irritation** with suppositories, discuss with your doctor if bothersome. If you develop **abdominal pain or discomfort, dizziness, diarrhea, muscle weakness,** or **painful sensation,** discuss with your doctor in all cases.

✋ SPECIAL PRECAUTIONS

Tell your doctor or pharmacist if you have: severe constipation, and/or nausea, vomiting, or abdominal pain; unexplained rectal bleeding; difficulty swallowing; a known narrowing of the bowel; any obstruction of the bowel; an acute appendicitis or inflammatory bowel disease. **Also discuss if you are:** sensitive or allergic to triarylmethane products; taking other medications.
* **Safety not established** in pregnancy; discuss with your doctor.
* **No evidence of risk** in breast-feeding; discuss with your doctor.
* **Not recommended** in children under 6 years of age without medical advice.

⟳ INTERACTIONS

Prolonged use of bisacodyl can affect electrolyte balance, which can be potentiated further with **diuretic** use.

Changes in electrolytes with bisacodyl could increase the effect of **digoxin**.

BUPROPION

Product names: PMS-bupropion SR, ratio-Bupropion SR, Wellbutrin SR, Wellbutrin XL, Zyban, and others
Used in the following combined preparations: None

WHY IS THIS DRUG USED?

Bupropion is an antidepressant. It is also used as an aid for people who are trying to give up *tobacco smoking*. Treatment is started while the patient is still smoking. The target stop date is decided on within the first two weeks of treatment. Bupropion will be stopped after 7 weeks if the smoker has not made significant progress in giving up smoking by then. This drug is not recommended in those with a seizure or eating disorder, or in those with manic depression or psychosis.

INFORMATION FOR USERS

Prescription needed. Do not alter dosage without checking with your doctor.

How and when to take: Available as SR and XL tablets. Take 1–2 x daily.

Usual adult dosage range: Single maximum dose 150mg; maximum daily dose 300mg.

Onset and duration of effect: Up to 4 weeks for full effect. Action lasts for 12 hours.

Diet advice: None.

Storage: Keep in original closed container in a cool, dry place out of the reach of children.

If you miss a dose: Take missed dose as soon as you remember. If your next dose is due within 2 hours, take a single dose now and skip the next dose.

Stopping the drug: Do not stop the drug without consulting your doctor, who may want to taper the dose.

Prolonged use: For smoking cessation, bupropion is used for up to 9 weeks. Progress will be reviewed after 3–4 weeks, and the drug continued only if useful.

Dependence rating: Low

Overdose danger rating: High

OVERDOSE ACTION

Seek immediate medical advice in all cases. Take emergency action if consciousness is lost.

See Drug poisoning emergency guide (p.197)

POSSIBLE SIDE EFFECTS AND WHAT TO DO

Some effects, such as agitation, tremor, sweating, and insomnia, may be due to the withdrawal of nicotine rather than to the effects of bupropion itself. If you experience **insomnia, poor concentration, headache, dizziness, tremor, nausea, vomiting,** or **dry mouth**, discuss with your doctor if bothersome. If you develop a **rash, fever, depression, palpitations, fainting, confusion** or **anxiety**, discuss with your doctor in all cases. Stop taking drug now and call your doctor if you have a **seizure**.

SPECIAL PRECAUTIONS

Tell your doctor if you have: a head injury or history of seizures; an eating disorder; cancer of the nervous system; diabetes; manic depression or a psychosis; kidney or liver problems. **Also discuss if you are:** withdrawing from alcohol or benzodiazepine dependence; taking other medications.
* **Safety not established** in pregnancy and breast-feeding; discuss with your doctor.
* **Not recommended** for infants and children.
* **Reduced dose** may be necessary for those over 60 due to increased sensitivity to drug's effects.
* **Avoid** driving and hazardous work until you have learned how bupropion affects you.
* **Avoid** alcohol; it will increase any sedative effects.

INTERACTIONS

A wide range of drugs increases the likelihood of seizures when taken with bupropion. Check with your doctor if you are on other medications.
   Ritonavir, amantadine, and **levodopa** may all increase the risk of side effects with bupropion.
   The antiepileptics **phenytoin** and **carbamazepine** may reduce the blood levels and effects of bupropion.
   Valproate may increase bupropion's blood levels and effects.

CANDESARTAN

Product name: Atacand
Used in the following combined preparation: Atacand Plus

❓ WHY IS THIS DRUG USED?

Candesartan is a member of the group of vasodilator drugs called angiotensin-II receptor blockers. Used to treat *hypertension*, the drug works by blocking the action of angiotensin-II (a naturally occurring substance that constricts blood vessels). This action causes the blood vessel walls to relax, thereby easing blood pressure. Candesartan is also used in the treatment of *heart failure* when someone is intolerant to ACE inhibitors.

ℹ️ INFORMATION FOR USERS

Prescription needed. Do not alter dosage without checking with your doctor.

How and when to take: Available as tablets. Take once daily.

Usual adult dosage range: 8–32mg. People over 75 years, and other groups that are especially sensitive to the drug's effects, and those with liver dysfunction, may start on 25mg.

Onset and duration of effect: *Blood pressure* Starts to work in 1–2 weeks, with maximum effect in 4 weeks from start of treatment. *Other conditions* Within 3–4 hours. Action lasts for 24 hours.

Diet advice: None.

Storage: Keep in a closed container in a cool, dry place out of the reach of children.

If you miss or exceed a dose: Take missed dose as soon as you remember. If your next dose is due within 12 hours, take a single dose now and skip the next. An occasional unintentional extra dose is unlikely to cause problems. Large overdoses may cause dizziness and fainting; notify your doctor.

Stopping the drug: Do not stop the drug without consulting your doctor as it may lead to worsening of the underlying condition.

Prolonged use: No special problems. Periodic checks on blood potassium levels may be performed.

Dependence rating: Low

Overdose danger rating: Medium

❗ POSSIBLE SIDE EFFECTS AND WHAT TO DO

Side effects are usually mild. If you experience **dizziness, fatigue, headache** or **cold symptoms**, discuss with your doctor. If you experience **muscle weakness or muscle pain,** a **rash/itching** or **jaundice**, discuss with your doctor in all cases. Stop taking the drug now and call your doctor if you develop **wheezing** or **facial swelling**.

✋ SPECIAL PRECAUTIONS

Tell your doctor if you have: stenosis (narrowing) of the kidney arteries; liver or kidney problems; congestive heart failure; primary aldosteronism; previously experienced angioedema. **Also discuss if you are:** taking other medications, especially diuretics.
- **Not prescribed** in pregnancy (may cause fetus abnormalities) or while breast-feeding.
- **Safety not established** for infants and children.
- **Avoid** driving and hazardous work until you have learned how candesartan affects you because the drug can cause dizziness and fatigue.
- **Avoid** alcohol; it may raise blood pressure, reducing the effectiveness of candesartan, or cause blood vessels to dilate, increasing the likelihood of an excessive fall in blood pressure.

⊘ INTERACTIONS

There is a risk of a sudden fall in blood pressure when candesartan is taken with **diuretics.**

Candesartan increases the effect of **potassium supplements, potassium-sparing diuretics,** and **cyclosporine,** leading to raised levels of potassium in the blood.

Candesartan may increase the levels and toxicity of **lithium.**

Candesartan may have an additive effect of a decrease in blood pressure, when used with **rituximab.**

Certain **non-steroidal anti-inflammatory drugs (NSAIDs)** may reduce the blood-pressure lowering effect of candesartan.

CARBAMAZEPINE

Product names: Apo-Carbamazepine, Teva-Carbamazapine, Tegretol, and others
Used in the following combined preparations: None

❓ WHY IS THIS DRUG USED?

Carbamazepine is used to treat some forms of epilepsy; it reduces the likelihood of seizures caused by abnormal nerve signals in the brain. It is also prescribed to relieve the intermittent severe pain caused by damage to the cranial nerves in trigeminal neuralgia. Carbamazepine is also occasionally prescribed to treat manic depression and diabetes insipidus and is used for pain relief in diabetic neuropathy.

ℹ INFORMATION FOR USERS

Prescription needed. Do not alter dosage without checking with your doctor.

How and when to take: Available as CR (controlled release) tablets, tablets, chewable tablets, and liquid. Take 1–2 x daily.

Usual adult dosage range: *Epilepsy* 100–2,000mg daily (low starting dose that is slowly increased every 2 weeks). *Pain relief* 100–1,600mg daily. *Psychiatric disorders* 400–1,600mg daily.

Onset and duration of effect: Starts to work within 4 hours. Action lasts for 12–24 hours.

Diet advice: None.

Storage: Keep in a closed container in a cool, dry place out of the reach of children.

If you miss or exceed a dose: Take missed dose as soon as you remember. If your next dose is due within 2 hours, take a single dose now and skip the next. An occasional unintentional extra dose is unlikely to cause problems. Large overdoses may cause tremor, convulsions, and coma; notify your doctor.

Stopping the drug: Do not stop the drug without consulting your doctor; symptoms may recur.

Prolonged use: There is a slight risk of changes in liver function or of skin or blood abnormalities occurring during prolonged use. Periodic blood tests are usually performed to monitor levels of the drug, blood cell counts, and liver and kidney function.

Dependence rating: Low

Overdose danger rating: Medium

❗ POSSIBLE SIDE EFFECTS AND WHAT TO DO

If blood levels of the drug get too high, side effects are common and the dose may need to be reduced. If you experience **dizziness/unsteadiness, drowsiness, nausea,** or **loss of appetite,** discuss with your doctor if bothersome.

If you develop **blurred vision, jaundice,** or **ankle swelling,** discuss with your doctor in all cases. Stop taking drug now and call your doctor if you develop a **rash,** or **sore throat/hoarseness**.

🖐 SPECIAL PRECAUTIONS

Tell your doctor if you have: long-term liver or kidney problems; heart problems; blood problems with other drugs or porphyria. **Also discuss if you are:** taking other medications.

- **Discuss** with your doctor if you are pregnant or breast-feeding; drug may cause abnormalities in an unborn baby; drug passes into breast milk.
- **Reduced dose** necessary for infants and children, and possibly for those over 60, as it may cause side effects in the elderly.
- **Discuss** with your doctor regarding driving and hazardous work; such activities may be inadvisable due to your underlying condition and the possibility of reduced alertness while taking carbamazepine.
- **Avoid** alcohol, as it may increase the sedative effects of this drug.

⊘ INTERACTIONS

Carbamazepine interacts with many drugs; discuss with your doctor or pharmacist before taking other medications.

Complex and variable interactions can occur between other **antiepileptic drugs** and carbamazepine.

Grapefruit juice may increase carbamazepine blood levels; avoid.

Carbamazepine may affect the blood level of **oral contraceptives**.

CELECOXIB

Product name: Celebrex
Used in the following combined preparations: None

❓ WHY IS THIS DRUG USED?

Celecoxib belongs to a sub-group of non-steroidal anti-inflammatory drugs (NSAIDs), called COX-2 selective inhibitors. This analgesic reduces the pain, stiffness, and inflammation of both rheumatoid *arthritis* and osteoarthritis. It has a lower risk of causing irritation and ulceration to the upper gastrointestinal tract than other NSAIDs, and is therefore useful for people who have had problems, such as stomach ulcers, with other drugs. It is also given to groups at high risk of developing gastrointestinal problems, such as the elderly.

ℹ INFORMATION FOR USERS

Prescription needed. Do not alter dosage without checking with your doctor.

How and when to take: Available as capsules. Take 1–2 x daily.

Usual adult dosage range: 200–400mg daily.

Onset and duration of effect: Starts to work in 1 hour. Action lasts 8–12 hours.

Diet advice: None.

Storage: Keep in a cool, dry place out of the reach of children.

If you miss or exceed a dose: Take missed dose as soon as you remember. If your next dose is due within 4 hours, take a single dose now and skip the next. An occasional unintentional extra dose is unlikely to cause problems. Large overdoses can cause stomach and intestinal pain and damage; notify your doctor.

Stopping the drug: The drug can safely be stopped if being used short term. If prescribed for long-term use, consult with your doctor first.

Prolonged use: There is a smaller risk of peptic ulcers compared to other similar drugs when used long-term. Periodic tests of kidney function may be performed.

Dependence rating: Low

Overdose danger rating: Medium

❗ POSSIBLE SIDE EFFECTS AND WHAT TO DO

If you experience **indigestion, abdominal pain, diarrhea, flatulence, dizziness,** or **insomnia**, discuss with your doctor if bothersome. If you develop a **rash** or **swollen ankles,** discuss with your doctor in all cases. Call your doctor now if you experience **palpitations** or **difficulty breathing,** and stop taking the drug now and call your doctor if you have **black/bloody vomit** or **feces**.

SPECIAL PRECAUTIONS

Tell your doctor if you have: asthma; angina/coronary heart disease or kidney disease; a peptic ulcer or gastrointestinal bleeding; inflammatory bowel disease; congestive heart failure. **Also discuss if you are:** allergic to ASA, celecoxib, or sulfonamides; taking other medicines.
- **Not prescribed** in pregnancy or while breast-feeding.
- **Not recommended** for infants and children.
- **Lower doses** may be necessary for those over 60; elderly people may be more sensitive to the drug's effects.
- **Avoid** driving and hazardous work until you learn how the drug affects you. It can cause dizziness, vertigo, and sleepiness. Alcohol may increase drowsiness and the risk of stomach irritation.

⊘ INTERACTIONS

Many potential interactions can occur; discuss with your doctor or pharmacist.
   Celecoxib can increase the effects of the anticoagulant **warfarin**.
   ACE inhibitors, cyclosporine, and tacrolimus increase the risk of kidney problems when taken with celecoxib.
   Blood pressure-lowering effects of **antihypertensives** and **diuretics** may be reduced by celecoxib.
   Lithium levels and effects are increased when taken with celecoxib.
   Excretion of **methotrexate** may be slowed by celecoxib, causing increased toxicity.
   Carbamazepine, fluconazole, rifampin, and **barbiturates** reduce the effects of celecoxib.

CEPHALEXIN

Product names: Apo-Cephalex, Teva-Cephalexin, and others
Used in the following combined preparations: None

❓ WHY IS THIS DRUG USED?

Cephalexin is a cephalosporin antibiotic that is prescribed for a variety of mild to moderate *infections*. It is helpful in treating *bronchitis*, cystitis, and certain skin and soft tissue infections.

In some cases it is prescribed as follow-up treatment for severe infections after a more powerful cephalosporin has been given by injection. People sensitive to penicillin may be allergic to cephalexin.

ℹ️ INFORMATION FOR USERS

Prescription needed. Do not alter dosage without checking with your doctor.

How and when to take: Available as tablets, capsules, liquid. Usually taken 4 x daily. May take with food.

Usual dosage range: *Adults* 1–2g daily, up to a maximum of 4g. *Children* Reduced dose according to age and weight.

Onset and duration of effect: Starts to work within 1 hour. Action lasts 6–12 hours.

Diet advice: None.

Storage: Keep tablets and capsules in a closed container in a cool, dry place out of the reach of children. Refrigerate liquid, but do not freeze, and keep for no longer than 10 days. Protect from light.

If you miss or exceed a dose: Take missed dose as soon as you remember. If your next dose is due at this time, take both doses now. An occasional unintentional extra dose is unlikely to be a cause for concern. If you notice any unusual symptoms, or if a large overdose has been taken, notify your doctor.

Stopping the drug: Take the full course. The original infection may recur if treatment is stopped too soon.

Prolonged use: Cephalexin is usually given only for short courses of treatment. Use of large doses or prolonged therapy requires close monitoring.

Dependence rating: Low

Overdose danger rating: Low

❗ POSSIBLE SIDE EFFECTS AND WHAT TO DO

Most people do not suffer serious side effects while taking cephalexin. If you experience **diarrhea** or **nausea/vomiting**, discuss with your doctor if bothersome. If you experience **abdominal pain,** discuss with your doctor in all cases. If you develop a **rash** or **itching, swelling,** or **wheezing,** stop taking the drug now and call your doctor – you may be allergic to the drug.

🖐️ SPECIAL PRECAUTIONS

Tell your doctor if you have: a long-term kidney problem; a previous allergic reaction to a penicillin or cephalosporin antibiotic; a history of blood disorders. **Also discuss if you are:** taking other medications.
- **No evidence of risk** to the baby during pregnancy.
- **Adverse effects unlikely** during breast-feeding at normal doses, even though the drug passes into the breast milk; discuss use with your doctor.
- **Reduced dose** necessary for infants and children.

⊘ INTERACTIONS

Probenecid increases the level of cephalexin in the blood. The dosage of cephalexin may need to be adjusted accordingly.
   Cephalexin may reduce the contraceptive effect of **oral contraceptives**. Discuss with your pharmacist or doctor.

CETIRIZINE

Product names: Apo-Cetrizine, Reactine, and others
Used in the following combined preparation: Reactine Allergy and Sinus

❓ WHY IS THIS DRUG USED?

Cetirizine is a long-acting antihistamine. Its main use is in the treatment of *allergic rhinitis*, particularly hay fever. It is also used to treat a number of allergic skin conditions, such as urticaria (hives). Cetrizine tends to cause less drowsiness than some other antihistamines and may be suitable for people who need to avoid sleepiness. But it can have a sedative effect on some people, so caution should be exercised until you learn how cetirizine affects you.

ℹ️ INFORMATION FOR USERS

Prescription needed for some preparations. Do not alter dosage without checking with your doctor.

How and when to take: Available as tablets, liquid. Take 1–2 x daily.

Usual adult dosage range: 5–10mg daily. Maximum dose: 20mg.

Onset and duration of effect: Starts to work in 1–3 hours. Some effects may not be felt for 1–2 days. Action lasts for up to 24 hours.

Diet advice: None.

Storage: Keep in a closed container in a cool, dry place out of the reach of children.

If you miss or exceed a dose: Take missed dose as soon as you remember. If your next dose is due within 8 hours, take a single dose now and skip the next. An occasional unintentional extra dose is unlikely to cause problems. Large overdoses may cause nausea or drowsiness and have adverse effects on the heart; notify your doctor.

Stopping the drug: Can be safely stopped as soon as you no longer need it.

Prolonged use: No problems expected.

Dependence rating: Low

Overdose danger rating: Medium

❗ POSSIBLE SIDE EFFECTS AND WHAT TO DO

The most common adverse effects are **drowsiness, dry mouth,** and **fatigue** – contact your doctor if bothersome. Side effects may be reduced if the dose of cetirizine is taken as 5mg twice a day.

🖐️ SPECIAL PRECAUTIONS

Tell your doctor if you have: long-term liver or kidney problems; glaucoma. **Also discuss if you are:** allergic to hydroxyzine; taking other medications.
* **Safety not established** in pregnancy or breast-feeding. Discuss with your doctor.
* **Not recommended** for children under 2 years, but may be prescribed for special use under 6 years.
* **Avoid** driving and hazardous work until you have learned how cetirizine affects you because the drug can cause drowsiness in some people.
* **Limit** alcohol consumption.

⊙ INTERACTIONS

The anticholinergic effects of cetirizine may be increased by all drugs that have anticholinergic effects, including **anti-psychotics** and **tricyclic antidepressants**.

Cetirizine may increase the sedative effects of **anti-anxiety drugs, sleeping drugs, antidepressants,** and **antipsychotic drugs**.

Antihistamines should be discontinued approximately 3 days before **allergy skin testing**.

CIPROFLOXACIN

Product names: Apo-Ciproflox, Ciloxan, Cipro, Cipro XL, CO-ciprofloxacin, and others
Used in the following combined preparation: Ciprodex

❓ WHY IS THIS DRUG USED?

Ciprofloxacin, a quinolone antibacterial, is used to treat several types of bacteria resistant to other commonly used antibiotics. It is especially useful for some types of chest infections, and *skin, intestinal*, and *urinary tract infections*. It can also be used to treat gonorrhea. When taken by mouth, ciprofloxacin is well absorbed by the body and works quickly and effectively. In more severe systemic bacterial infections the drug may need to be administered by injection.

❗ INFORMATION FOR USERS

Prescription needed. Do not alter dosage without checking with your doctor.

How and when to take: Available as tablets, liquid, injection, eye ointment and drops, ear drops. Take 2 x daily with plenty of fluids.

Usual adult dosage range: 500mg–1.5g daily (tablets); 200–400mg daily (injection).

Onset and duration of effect: Starts to work within a few hours, although full beneficial effect may not be felt for several days. Action lasts about 12 hours.

Diet advice: Do not get dehydrated; ensure that you drink fluids regularly.

Storage: Keep in a closed container in a cool, dry place out of the reach of children. The injection must be protected from light.

If you miss or exceed a dose: Take missed dose as soon as you remember, and take your next dose as usual. An occasional unintentional extra dose is unlikely to cause problems. Large overdoses may cause mental disturbance and seizures; notify your doctor.

Stopping the drug: Take the full course. The original infection may recur if treatment is stopped too soon.

Prolonged use: No problems expected. Blood tests may be necessary to monitor kidney and liver function.

Dependence rating: Low

Overdose danger rating: Medium

❗ POSSIBLE SIDE EFFECTS AND WHAT TO DO

Ciprofloxacin may commonly cause nausea and vomiting; other side effects are less common, except when very high doses are given. If you experience **nausea/vomiting, abdominal pain, diarrhea, dizziness, headache, joint pain,** or **sleep disturbance,** discuss with your doctor if bothersome. If you develop a **rash/itching, photosensitivity,** or **jaundice,** discuss with your doctor in all cases. Stop taking the drug now and call your doctor if you experience **confusion, convulsions,** or **painful, inflamed tendons**.

✋ SPECIAL PRECAUTIONS

Tell your doctor if you have: long-term liver or kidney problems; epileptic fits; glucose-6-phosphate dehydrogenase (G6PD) deficiency. **Also discuss if you are:** taking other medications.
* **Safety not established** in pregnancy or breast-feeding; discuss with your doctor.
* **Not usually recommended** for infants and children.
* **Discuss** with your doctor if you are over 60; ciprofloxacin may make you more susceptible to tendinitis.
* **Avoid** driving and hazardous work until you have learned how ciprofloxacin affects you as the drug can cause dizziness.
* **Avoid** alcohol and excessive exposure to sunlight.

⚙ INTERACTIONS

Oral iron preparations and **antacids** containing magnesium or aluminum hydroxide interfere with absorption of ciprofloxacin. Do not take antacids within 2 hours of taking ciprofloxacin tablets.
   Blood levels of **anticoagulants, oral antidiabetics, theophylline**, and **phenytoin** may be increased; their dosage may need adjusting.
   Non-steroidal anti-inflammatory drugs increase the risk of epileptic seizures.

CLARITHROMYCIN

Product names: Apo-Clarithromycin, Biaxin, Biaxin BID, Biaxin XL, Mylan-Clarithromycin, PMS-Clarithromycin, ratio-Clarithromycin, and others
Used in the following combined preparation: Hp-PAC

❓ WHY IS THIS DRUG USED?

Clarithromycin is a macrolide antibiotic. It is used for upper respiratory tract infections, such as *middle ear infections*, *sinusitis*, and pharyngitis, and lower respiratory tract infections, including whooping cough, *bronchitis*, and *pneumonia*, as well as for skin and soft tissue infections, including gonorrhoea. Given with anti-ulcer drugs and other antibiotics, clarithromycin is used to eradicate Helicobacter pylori, the bacterium that causes many peptic ulcers.

ℹ️ INFORMATION FOR USERS

Prescription needed. Do not alter dosage without checking with your doctor.

How and when to take: Available as tablets, suspension (made from granules), extended release tablets. Take 2 x daily, up to 14 days.

Usual adult dosage range: 500mg–1g daily.

Onset and duration of effect: Starts to work in 1–4 hours. Action lasts up to 12 hours.

Diet advice: None.

Storage: Keep in a closed container in a cool, dry place out of the reach of children. Protect from light.

If you miss or exceed a dose: Take missed dose as soon as you remember. If your next dose is due within 2 hours, take a single dose now and skip the next. An occasional unintentional extra dose is unlikely to be a cause for concern. If you notice any unusual symptoms, or if a large overdose has been taken, notify your doctor.

Stopping the drug: Take the full course. The original infection may recur if treatment is stopped too soon.

Prolonged use: Prolonged use is usually not necessary. In courses of over 14 days, there is a risk of developing antibiotic-resistant infections.

Dependence rating: Low

Overdose danger rating: Low

❗ POSSIBLE SIDE EFFECTS AND WHAT TO DO

Clarithromycin is generally well tolerated. If you experience **nausea, vomiting, diarrhea, indigestion, headache, or joint/muscle pain,** discuss with your doctor if bothersome. If you experience a **rash, altered sense of taste/smell,** **anxiety, insomnia, confusion, hallucinations,** or **hearing loss,** discuss with your doctor in all cases. Stop taking the drug now and call your doctor if you develop **jaundice.**

✋ SPECIAL PRECAUTIONS

Tell your doctor if you have: liver or kidney problems; a history of allergic reaction to erythromycin or clarithromycin; a heart problem; porphyria. **Also discuss if you are:** taking other medications.
* **Safety not established** in pregnancy. Clarithromycin passes into the breast milk and may affect the baby. Discuss with your doctor in both cases.
* **Reduced dose necessary** for infants and children.

🔄 INTERACTIONS

Blood levels and effects of **digoxin, warfarin, triazolam, midazolam, disopyramide, lovastatin, rifabutin, phenytoin, cyclosporine,** and **tacrolimus** are increased by clarithromycin.
Blood levels and toxicity of **carbamazepine, theophylline,** and **digoxin** are increased by clarithromycin.
Blood levels are reduced if **zidovudine** is taken at the same time as clarithromycin.
There is an increased risk of ergot toxicity if **ergot derivatives,** such as ergotamine or dihydroergotamine, are taken with clarithromycin.
Pimozide may cause cardiac arrhythmias if taken with clarithromycin.
If **lipid-lowering drugs whose names end in 'statin'** are taken with clarithromycin, there is a risk of rhabdomyolysis (muscle and kidney damage).

CLOPIDOGREL

Product name: Plavix
Used in the following combined preparations: None

❓ WHY IS THIS DRUG USED?

Clopidogrel is an antiplatelet drug that is used to prevent blood clots from forming. It is prescribed to patients who have a tendency to form clots in the fast-flowing blood of the arteries and heart, or those who have had a *stroke* or a *heart attack*. The drug may be suitable for people who cannot take

ASA for its antiplatelet effects. However, it can cause abnormal bleeding. You should report any unusual bleeding to your doctor at once, and, if you require dental treatment, you should tell your dentist that you are taking the drug.

ℹ️ INFORMATION FOR USERS

Prescription needed. Do not alter dosage without checking with your doctor.

How and when to take: Available as tablets. Take once daily.

Usual dosage range: 75mg.

Onset and duration of effect: Starts to work in 1 hour. Action lasts for 24 hours.

Diet advice: None.

Storage: Keep in a closed container in a cool, dry place out of the reach of children.

If you miss or exceed a dose: Take missed dose as soon as you remember. If your next dose is due within 4 hours, take a single dose now and skip the next. An

occasional unintentional extra dose is unlikely to be a cause for concern. If you notice any unusual symptoms, or if a large overdose has been taken, notify your doctor.

Stopping the drug: Do not stop taking the drug without consulting your doctor. Stopping the drug may lead to a recurrence of the original condition.

Prolonged use: No special problems.

Dependence rating: Low

Overdose danger rating: Medium

⚠️ POSSIBLE SIDE EFFECTS AND WHAT TO DO

The most frequent side effects of clopidogrel are bleeding and bruising. If you experience **nausea, vomiting, diarrhea, abdominal pain, headache,** or **dizziness,** discuss with your doctor if bothersome. If you experience **bruising,**

nosebleeds, gastrointestinal bleeding/ulcers, blood in urine, or a **rash/itching,** discuss with your doctor in all cases. Call your doctor now if you develop a **sore throat.**

✋ SPECIAL PRECAUTIONS

Tell your doctor if you have: liver or kidney problems; a condition, such as a peptic ulcer or recent surgery, that makes you more likely to bleed. **Also discuss if you are:** taking other medications, especially proton pump inhibitors.
- **Safety not established** in pregnancy or breast-feeding; discuss with your doctor.
- **Not recommended** for infants and children.
- **Avoid** excessive intake of alcohol, which may irritate the stomach and increase the risk of bleeding.
- **Discuss** with your doctor or dentist if you require surgery; clopidogrel may need to be stopped a week before surgery.

🔄 INTERACTIONS

Clopidogrel increases the effect of **ASA** and other **non-steroidal anti-inflammatory drugs** (NSAIDs) on platelets. The risk of gastrointestinal bleeding is increased when clopidogrel is used with these drugs.
   The effect of **anticoagulant drugs** (e.g., warfarin) is increased if they are taken with clopidogrel.
   Proton pump inhibitors may decrease the therapeutic effect of clopidogrel and should be used cautiously; discuss with your doctor.
   Atorvastatin and other drugs like erythromycin, which affect the enzyme CYP3A4, may decrease the effect of clopidogrel.
   Fluvoxamine, fluoxetine, sertraline, moclobemide, fluconazole, and **ketoconazole** may decrease the effectiveness of clopidogrel.

CODEINE

Product names: Codeine, Codeine Contin
Used in the following combined preparations: Atasol-8, CoActifed, Covan, Fiorinal-C¼, and many others

❓ WHY IS THIS DRUG USED?

Codeine is an opioid analgesic used to relieve mild to moderate *pain*, and is often combined with a non-opioid analgesic such as acetaminophen. It is also an effective cough suppressant and is included as an ingredient in many non-prescription cough and cold relief preparations. There is variability in how an individual may metabolize codeine, which in some can result in either too much or too little effect. Although codeine is habit-forming, addiction is rare if the drug is used as directed for a limited period of time.

ℹ️ INFORMATION FOR USERS

Prescription needed for some preparations. Do not alter dosage without checking with your doctor.

How and when to take: Available as tablets, controlled release tablets, liquid, injection. Take 4–6 x daily (pain); 3–4 x daily when necessary (cough); every 4–6 hours when necessary (diarrhea).

Usual adult dosage range: 120–240mg daily (pain); 45–120mg daily (cough); 30–180mg daily (diarrhea).

Onset and duration of effect: Starts to work in 30–60 minutes. Action lasts for 4–6 hours.

Diet advice: None.

Storage: Keep in a closed container in a cool, dry place out of the reach of children. Protect from light.

If you miss a dose: Take missed dose as soon as you remember if needed for relief of symptoms. If not needed, do not take the missed dose, and return to your normal dose schedule when necessary.

Stopping the drug: Can be safely stopped as soon as you no longer need it. However, if taken for a prolonged period, stopping should be discussed with your doctor and pharmacist.

Prolonged use: Codeine is normally used only for short-term relief of symptoms. It can be habit-forming if taken for extended periods, especially if higher-than-average doses are taken.

Dependence rating: Medium

Overdose danger rating: High

☠️ OVERDOSE ACTION

Seek immediate medical advice in all cases. Take emergency action if there are symptoms such as slow or irregular breathing, severe drowsiness, or loss of consciousness.

See Drug poisoning emergency guide (p.197).

❗ POSSIBLE SIDE EFFECTS AND WHAT TO DO

If you experience severe **constipation**, discuss with your doctor. If you experience **nausea/vomiting, drowsiness,** or **dizziness,** discuss with your doctor in all cases. Stop taking the drug now and call your doctor if you develop a **rash/hives, agitation/ restlessness,** or **wheezing/breathlessness**. Rarely, some may experience extreme **sedation** and **shallow breathing;** see your doctor right away.

✋ SPECIAL PRECAUTIONS

Tell your doctor if you have: long-term liver or kidney problems; a lung disorder such as asthma or bronchitis. **Also discuss if you are:** taking other medications.
- **Discuss** with your doctor if pregnant or breast-feeding; may adversely affect the baby's breathing if taken during labour, or may cause sedation or difficulty breathing in your nursing baby; seek help right away.
- **Reduced dose necessary** for infants and children, and possibly for those over 60.
- **Avoid** driving and hazardous work until you have learned how codeine affects you.
- **Avoid** alcohol; it may increase sedation.

🔄 INTERACTIONS

All **sedatives**, including alcohol, are likely to increase sedation with codeine. Such drugs include **sleeping drugs, antidepressant drugs,** and **antihistamines**.

DABIGATRAN ETEXILATE

Product name: Pradax
Used in the following combined preparations: None

❓ WHY IS THIS DRUG USED?

Dabigatran is an anticoagulant used to prevent blood clots, particularly in the leg and pelvic veins. It works by blocking the activity of a protein called thrombin. The drug is used to reduce the risk of clot formation after elective orthopedic surgery of the hip and knee (replacements). Dabigatran etexilate, once absorbed, releases the active drug dagibatran, which starts to work much sooner than other anticoagulants such as warfarin. Dabigatran is not recommended for those who have had a recent stroke or any conditions that may increase the risk of bleeding.

ℹ️ INFORMATION FOR USERS

Prescription needed. Do not alter dosage without checking with your doctor.

How and when to take: Available as capsules. Take once daily, at the same time each day.

Usual dosage range: 110–220mg daily.

Onset and duration of effect: Starts to work within 30 mins to 2 hours. Action lasts for 24 hours or longer.

Diet advice: None.

Storage: Keep in a closed container in a cool, dry place out of the reach of children. Protect from light.

If you miss a dose: Take as soon as you remember. Take the following dose on your original schedule. Do not double up on your doses. Discuss any missed doses with your doctor.

Stopping the drug: Do not stop taking the drug without consulting your doctor as it may lead to worsening of the underlying condition.

Prolonged use: Usually used for a specific number of days following surgery; not used long-term.

Dependence rating: Low

Overdose danger rating: High

☠️ OVERDOSE ACTION

Seek immediate medical advice in all cases. Take emergency action if severe bleeding or loss of consciousness occur.

See Drug poisoning emergency guide (p.197).

❗ POSSIBLE SIDE EFFECTS AND WHAT TO DO

Bleeding is the most common and serious side effect with dabigatran. If you experience any **signs of bruising or bleeding**, such as a nose bleed, discuss with your doctor and pharmacist. Call your doctor now if you notice **blood in your stools or urine**. If you develop symptoms such as **red and lumpy skin, rash, hives, swelling** or have **trouble breathing,** call your doctor now.
    If you experience anything else which is unusual for you, discuss with your doctor.

🖐️ SPECIAL PRECAUTIONS

Tell your doctor if you have: liver disease or kidney problems; previous stroke; any problems with bleeding; peptic ulcers. **Also discuss** if you are taking other medications including over-the-counter or natural health products.
- **Not recommended** in women who are pregnant or breast-feeding, or for use in children. Discuss with your doctor.
- **Reduced dose** may be needed for those over 75 due to changes in kidney function.
- **Use caution** with driving and hazardous work; even minor bumps can cause bad bruises and excessive bleeding.
- **Avoid** excessive amounts of alcohol as it may increase the effects of this drug.
- **Consult** with your doctor or dentist before surgery; dabigatran may need to be stopped.

🔄 INTERACTIONS

Amiodarone, atorvastatin, clarithromycin, itraconazole, verapamil, amiodarone and **clarithromycin** may increase the level of dabigatran.
    Quinidine can increase the level of dabigatrin and the two are not recommended to be used together.
    Rifampin and **St. John's wort** may decrease the effectiveness of dabigatrin.
    Avoid **grapefruit juice**, which may increase blood levels of dabigatrin.
    Warfarin, heparin, LMWH, clopidogrel, and **other drugs** that act as anticoagulants should not be used with dabigatrin as the risk of bleeding is increased.
    ASA and **NSAIDs** should be used cautiously with dabigatran. Discuss with your doctor.

DEXTROMETHORPHAN

Product names: Balminil DM, Benylin DM, Koffex DM, Robitussin Children's, and many others
Used in the following combined preparations: Neocitran DM, Triaminic Cold, Cough and Fever, Tylenol Cough, and others

❓ WHY IS THIS DRUG USED?

Dextromethorphan is a cough suppressant available over-the-counter in a large number of cough and *cold* remedies. It is useful for suppressing persistent, dry coughing, especially if the cough is causing disturbed sleep.

Dextromethorphan should not be used to treat phlegm-producing coughs. It has little general sedative effect, and its use is unlikely to lead to dependence when it is taken as recommended.

ℹ INFORMATION FOR USERS

Prescription not needed. Follow instructions on the label. Call your doctor if symptoms worsen.

How and when to take: Available as tablets, chewable tablets, oral strips, capsules, liquid, controlled release syrup, powder for solution. Take up to 4 x daily as required; controlled release products 1–2 x daily.

Usual dosage range: *Adults* 12 years and older, 15–30mg per dose, up to a maximum of 120mg/24 hours. *Children* 6–11 years, 15mg per dose up to a maximum of 60mg/24 hours; 2–5 years, 7.5mg per dose up to a maximum of 30mg/24 hours.

Onset and duration of effect: Starts to work within 30 minutes. Action lasts for 4–8 hours.

Diet advice: None.

Storage: Keep in a closed container in a cool, dry place out of the reach of children.

If you miss or exceed a dose: Take missed dose as soon as you remember if needed to relieve coughing. If you are using a sustained release product, and if your next dose is less than 4 hours away, take a dose now and skip the next dose. An occasional unintentional extra dose is unlikely to cause problems. Larger overdoses may cause nausea, vomiting, stomach pain, dizziness, drowsiness, and breathing problems; notify your doctor.

Stopping the drug: Can be safely stopped as soon as you no longer need it.

Prolonged use: Should not be taken for longer than 1 week except on the advice of a doctor.

Dependence rating: Medium

Overdose danger rating: Medium

⚠ POSSIBLE SIDE EFFECTS AND WHAT TO DO

Most side effects normally diminish after a few days and can often be reduced by adjustment of dosage. If you experience **dizziness, drowsiness,** **constipation, nausea, vomiting,** or **abdominal pain,** discuss with your doctor only if bothersome.

✋ SPECIAL PRECAUTIONS

Tell your doctor or pharmacist if you have: a liver disorder; asthma or another serious respiratory problem. **Also discuss if you are:** taking other medications.
- **No evidence of risk** during pregnancy when normal doses are used for short periods. The drug passes into the breast milk, but at normal doses adverse effects on the baby are unlikely. Discuss with your doctor in both cases.
- **Not recommended** for children under 2 years of age; consult with your doctor or pharmacist before using this medication in children.
- **Reduced dose** necessary for those over 60.
- **Avoid** driving and hazardous work until you have learned how the drug affects you; it may reduce alertness.
- **Avoid** alcohol as it may increase the sedative effects of this drug.

⊕ INTERACTIONS

All **sedative drugs**, including alcohol, can increase the sedative properties of dextromethorphan. Such drugs include **anti-anxiety and sleeping drugs, antihistamines, opioid analgesics, antidepressants, and antipsychotics.**
   Monoamine oxidase inhibitors (MAOIs) may interact dangerously with dextromethorphan to cause excitation and fever.
   Fluoxetine, quinidine, paroxetine, rizatriptan and similar drugs can increase dextromethorphan levels.

DICLOFENAC

Product names: Apo-Diclo, Nu-Diclo, Teva-Diclofenac, Teva-Diclofenac SR, Voltaren, Voltaren Emulgel, Voltaren Rapide, and others
Used in the following combined preparation: Arthrotec

❓ WHY IS THIS DRUG USED?

Taken as a single dose, diclofenac acts as an analgesic and is taken to relieve mild to moderate headache, menstrual *pain*, and pain following minor surgery. When diclofenac is given regularly over a long period, it acts as an anti-inflammatory and is used to relieve the pain and stiffness of *rheumatoid arthritis* and advanced *osteoarthritis*. Diclofenac may also be prescribed to treat acute attacks of gout.

ℹ️ INFORMATION FOR USERS

Prescription needed. Do not alter dosage without checking with your doctor.

How and when to take: Available as tablets, extended-release tablets, enteric coated tablets, topical solution, ophthalmic solution, rectal suppository, topical gel. Take or use 1–3 x daily.

Usual adult dosage range: 75–150mg daily.

Onset and duration of effect: Starts to work in about 1 hour (pain relief); full anti-inflammatory effect may take 2 weeks. Action lasts up to 12 hours; up to 24 hours (SR-preparations).

Diet advice: Take oral tablets with food.

Storage: Keep in a closed container in a cool, dry place out of the reach of children.

If you miss or exceed a dose: Take missed dose as soon as you remember. If your next dose is due within 2 hours, take a single dose now and skip the next. An occasional unintentional extra dose is unlikely to be a cause for concern. If you notice any unusual symptoms or if a large overdose has been taken, notify your doctor.

Stopping the drug: The drug can safely be stopped if being used short term. If prescribed for long-term use (e.g., for arthritis), consult with your doctor first.

Prolonged use: There is an increased risk of bleeding from peptic ulcers and in the gastrointestinal tract with prolonged use of diclofenac.

Dependence rating: Low

Overdose danger rating: Low

❗ POSSIBLE SIDE EFFECTS AND WHAT TO DO

If you experience **gastrointestinal disorders, headache, dizziness,** or **drowsiness,** discuss with your doctor if bothersome. If you develop **swollen feet/ankles,** discuss with your doctor in all cases. Stop taking the drug now and call your doctor if you develop a **rash, wheezing/ breathlessness,** or **black or bloodstained feces/vomit**.

SPECIAL PRECAUTIONS

Tell your doctor if you have: long-term liver or kidney problems; a bleeding disorder; a peptic ulcer or esophagitis; porphyria; indigestion; asthma; heart problems or high blood pressure. **Also discuss if you are:** allergic to ASA; taking other medications.
- **Not usually prescribed** in the last 3 months of pregnancy as it may increase the risk of adverse effects on the baby's heart and may prolong labour. Small amounts of the drug pass into the breast milk during breast-feeding, but adverse effects on the baby are unlikely.
- **Reduced dose** necessary for infants and children, and possibly for those over 60.
- **Avoid** driving and hazardous work until you know how the drug affects you. **Alcohol** may increase the risk of stomach irritation.
- **Discuss** with your doctor or dentist before any surgery.

⚙️ INTERACTIONS

Diclofenac interacts with other **NSAIDs, oral anticoagulants,** and **corticosteroids** to increase the risk of bleeding and/or ulcers.
  The beneficial effects of **antihypertensive drugs** and **diuretics** may be reduced with diclofenac.
  Diclofenac may increase the risk of kidney problems with **cyclosporine**.
  Diclofenac may increase the blood levels of **lithium, digoxin,** and **methotrexate** to an undesirable extent.
  Antacids and other medications used for indigestion should not be taken at the same time of day as enteric coated diclofenac preparations as they disrupt this coating.

DILTIAZEM

Product names: Apo-Diltiaz, Cardizem CD, Tiazac, and others
Used in the following combined preparations: None

❓ WHY IS THIS DRUG USED?

Diltiazem is a calcium channel blocker used in the treatment of *angina*; longer acting formulations are used to treat *high blood pressure*. When this drug is taken regularly, it reduces the frequency of angina attacks but does not work quickly enough to reduce the pain of an angina attack that is already in progress. Diltiazem does not adversely affect breathing and is valuable for people who suffer from asthma. Some brands of diltiazem are not interchangeable; check with your pharmacist to make sure that you are taking the right product for you. Do not chew or crush SR or CD formulations; swallow whole. The contents of Tiazac capsules may be sprinkled on a spoonful of applesauce, and swallowed.

ℹ️ INFORMATION FOR USERS

Prescription needed. Do not alter dosage without checking with your doctor.

How and when to take: Available as tablets, SR-capsules, CD-capsules, injection. Take 3 x daily (tablets); 2 x daily (SR-capsules), 1 x daily (CD capsules).

Usual adult dosage range: 180–360mg daily.

Onset and duration of effect: Starts to work in 1 hour and action lasts 6–8 hours.

Diet advice: None.

Storage: Keep in a closed container in a cool, dry place out of the reach of children.

If you miss or exceed a dose: Take missed dose as soon as you remember. If your next dose is due within 2 hours, take a single dose now and skip the next. An occasional unintentional extra dose is unlikely to cause problems. Large overdoses may cause dizziness or collapse; notify your doctor urgently.

Stopping the drug: Do not stop taking the drug without consulting your doctor as symptoms may recur. Stopping suddenly may worsen angina.

Prolonged use: No problems expected.

Dependence rating: Low

Overdose danger rating: Medium

⚠️ POSSIBLE SIDE EFFECTS AND WHAT TO DO

Diltiazem can cause minor symptoms that are common to other calcium channel blockers. These effects can sometimes be controlled by an adjustment in dosage. If you experience **headache, nausea,** or **dry mouth,** discuss with your doctor if bothersome. If you develop **leg and ankle swelling, tiredness,** or **dizziness,** discuss with your doctor in all cases. If you develop a **rash,** stop taking the drug now and call the doctor.

✋ SPECIAL PRECAUTIONS

Tell your doctor if you have: long-term liver or kidney problems; heart failure. **Also discuss if you are:** taking other medications.
• **Not usually prescribed** in pregnancy. The drug passes into the breast milk and may affect the baby. Discuss with your doctor in both cases.
• **Not recommended** for infants and children.
• **Reduced dose** may be necessary for those over 60 due to increased likelihood of adverse effects.
• **Avoid** driving and hazardous work until you have learned how diltiazem affects you because the drug can cause dizziness.
• **Avoid** alcohol.

🔄 INTERACTIONS

Diltiazem increases the effects of **antihypertensive drugs**, leading to a further reduction in blood pressure.
  Levels of **anticonvulsant drugs** may be altered by diltiazem.
  There is a risk of side effects on the heart if **anti-arrhythmic drugs** are taken with diltiazem.
  Blood levels and adverse effects of **digoxin** may be increased if it is taken with diltiazem. The dose of digoxin may need to be reduced.
  Diltiazem may increase the levels of theophylline/aminophylline and cyclosporine.
  Beta blockers increase the risk of the heart slowing.

DIMENHYDRINATE

Product names: Apo-Dimenhydrinate, Gravol, Novo-Dimenate, PMS Dimenhydrinate, Travel Tabs, and others
Used in the following combined preparation: Gravergol

❓ WHY IS THIS DRUG USED?

Dimenhydrinate is an antihistamine that is mainly used as an anti-emetic drug. It is especially effective for treating the *nausea and vomiting* that occur with vertigo. It is also prescribed to relieve the symptoms of inner ear disorders such as Meniere's disease and to prevent and treat motion sickness. Dimenhydrinate is often effective in treating other forms of nausea and vomiting, including those caused by drugs and radiation treatments for cancer.

ℹ️ INFORMATION FOR USERS

Prescription not needed, except for the combination product. Follow instructions on the label. Call your doctor if symptoms worsen.

How and when to take: Available as tablets, capsule, oral liquid, injection, rectal suppositories, quick dissolve chewable tablets. Take as follows: *Adults* Every 4 hours *Children* Every 6–8 hours. To prevent motion sickness the first dose should be taken 30 minutes before travel.

Usual oral dosage range: *Adults* 50–100mg per dose (maximum 400mg/24 hours) *Children* 2–6 years, 15–25mg per dose (maximum 75mg/24 hours); 6–12 years, 25–50mg per dose (maximum 150mg/24 hours); 12 years and over, 50mg per dose (maximum 300mg/24 hours).

Onset and duration of effect: Starts to work within 30 minutes. Action lasts 6–8 hours.

Diet advice: None.

Storage: Keep in a closed container in a cool, dry place away from reach of children.

If you miss or exceed a dose: Take missed dose when you remember. Adjust the timing of your next dose accordingly. An occasional unintentional extra dose is unlikely to cause problems. Larger overdoses may cause unusual drowsiness; notify your doctor.

Stopping the drug: Can be safely stopped as soon as you no longer need it.

Prolonged use: No special problems, but this drug should not be used for more than a few days except on medical advice.

Dependence rating: Low

Overdose danger rating: Medium

❗ POSSIBLE SIDE EFFECTS AND WHAT TO DO

Side effects can sometimes be reduced by adjustment of dosage. If you experience **drowsiness** or **dry mouth,** discuss with your doctor if bothersome. If you develop **blurred vision, confusion,** or **nervousness,** discuss with your doctor in all cases.

🖐️ SPECIAL PRECAUTIONS

Tell your doctor or pharmacist if you have: impaired liver or kidney function; chronic lung disease; a history of glaucoma or seizures; prostate trouble. **Also discuss if you are:** taking other medications.
• **Safety not established** in pregnancy. The drug passes into the breast milk, and the effects on the baby are not clearly known.
• **Only as prescribed** by your doctor in children under 2 years. Reduced dose necessary in older children.
• **Reduced dose** recommended for those over 60 due to possible increased sensitivity to side effects.
• **Avoid** driving and hazardous work until you have learned how the drug affects you.
• **Avoid** alcohol as it may increase the sedative effects of this drug.

🔄 INTERACTIONS

Anti-emetics may mask the presence of underlying organic abnormalities or the toxic effects of other drugs.
    Antihistamines should be discontinued approximately 48 hours prior to allergy skin testing.
    Sedatives are likely to increase the sedative properties of dimenhydrinate. Such drugs include alcohol, anti-anxiety and sleeping drugs, antidepressants, opioid analgesics, and antipsychotics.

DIPHENHYDRAMINE

Product names: Allerdryl, Benadryl, Nytol, Simply Sleep, Unisom, and others
Used in the following combined preparations: Balminil Night-Time, Sinutab Nighttime, and others

❓ WHY IS THIS DRUG USED?

Diphenhydramine is an antihistamine used for treating *allergies* such as allergic rhinitis and urticaria (hives). Injected diphenhydramine is also used in the treatment of anaphylaxis and hypersensitivity reactions to food, drugs, or insect stings. It can also be used to treat involuntary muscle movements of parkinsonism and other movement disorders caused by antipsychotic drugs, and in the treatment and prevention of vertigo and motion sickness. It is included in several over-the-counter sleeping preparations because of its sedative effect.

ℹ️ INFORMATION FOR USERS

No prescription needed. Follow instructions on the label. Call your doctor if symptoms worsen.

How and when to take: Available as tablets, chewable tablets, capsules, oral liquid, injection, cream, spray. Take *by mouth* 3–4 x daily (allergic conditions); 30 minutes before travelling and before meals (motion sickness); 30 minutes before bedtime (insomnia). *Injection* Every 2–3 hours (adults). *Cream* As directed.

Usual dosage range: *Adults* 25–200mg daily (by mouth); up to 400mg daily (by injection). *Children* Reduced dose necessary according to age and weight.

Onset and duration of effect: Starts to work within 1 hour (by mouth); within 20 minutes (injection). Action lasts for 4–6 hours.

Diet advice: None.

Storage: Keep in a closed container in a cool, dry place away from reach of children. Do not freeze.

If you miss or exceed a dose: Take missed dose as soon as you remember. If your next dose is due within 2 hours, take a single dose now and skip the next. An occasional, unintentional extra dose is unlikely to cause problems. Large overdoses may cause drowsiness or agitation; notify your doctor.

Stopping the drug: Can be safely stopped as soon as you no longer need it.

Prolonged use: The effect of this drug may become weaker with prolonged use as the body adapts. Transfer to a different antihistamine may be recommended. Antihistamines should be discontinued approximately 48 hours prior to allergy skin testing.

Dependence rating: Low

Overdose danger rating: Medium

❗ POSSIBLE SIDE EFFECTS AND WHAT TO DO

If you experience drowsiness, **dry mouth, nausea,** or **abdominal pain,** discuss with your doctor if bothersome. If you develop **blurred vision,** **urinary difficulties, disorientation,** or **excitation,** discuss with your doctor in all cases.

SPECIAL PRECAUTIONS

Tell your doctor or pharmacist if you have: impaired liver function; chronic lung disease; epileptic seizures; glaucoma; urinary difficulties.
Also discuss if you are: taking other medications.
- **No evidence of risk** in pregnancy for normal doses.
- **Discuss** with your doctor if breast-feeding as the drug passes into the breast milk and may make the baby drowsy or irritable. It may also inhibit milk secretion.
- **Not recommended** for newborn/premature infants.
- **Reduced dose** necessary for older children, and possibly for those over 60.
- **Avoid** driving and hazardous work until you have learned how the drug affects you.
- **Avoid** alcohol; it may increase sedation.

⊙ INTERACTIONS

All **sedatives,** including alcohol, are likely to enhance the sedative effect of this drug.
    Anticholinergic drugs are likely to increase the anticholinergic effects of diphenhydramine.
    Antihistamines should be discontinued approximately 3 days before **allergy skin testing**.

DOCUSATE SODIUM

Product names: Colace, Correctol Stool Softener, Novo-Docusate Sodium, Selax, Soflax
Used in the following combined preparations: Senna-S Tablets, Senokot-S

WHY IS THIS DRUG USED?

Docusate is a stool softener and is used in the management of *constipation* due to hard stools. Taking it regularly makes the stools softer and easier to pass. Docusate may be recommended for those with heart conditions to ease the passage of stools and to avoid straining on defecation. Laxatives, including docusate, should not be used in those experiencing vomiting, abdominal pain, or fever.

INFORMATION FOR USERS

Prescription not needed. Follow instructions on the label. Call your doctor if symptoms worsen.

How and when to take: Available as tablets, capsules, liquid, drops. Take once or twice daily.

Usual adult dosage range: 100–200mg.

Onset and duration of effect: Starts to work within 1–2 days. Action lasts up to 24 hours.

Diet advice: In general, increasing fluid intake can help constipation.

Storage: Keep in a closed container in a cool, dry place out of the reach of children.

If you miss or exceed a dose: Take missed dose as soon as you remember, and resume normal dose thereafter. An occasional unintentional extra dose is unlikely to be a cause for concern. If you notice unusual symptoms, or if a large overdose has been taken, notify your doctor. Large overdoses may cause constipation and cramping.

Stopping the drug: Can be safely stopped as soon as you no longer need it.

Prolonged use: No problems expected.

Dependence rating: Low

Overdose danger rating: Low

POSSIBLE SIDE EFFECTS AND WHAT TO DO

Generally well tolerated. If you experience **abdominal pain, cramping,** or **rash,** discuss with your doctor in all cases.

SPECIAL PRECAUTIONS

Tell your doctor or pharmacist if you have: severe constipation, and/or nausea, vomiting, or abdominal pain; unexplained rectal bleeding; difficulty swallowing; a known narrowing of the bowel. **Also discuss if you are:** taking other medications.
• **Safety not established** in pregnancy or breast-feeding; discuss with your doctor.
• **Reduced dose** recommended in children.

INTERACTIONS

Docusate should not be administered with **mineral oil** as this may increase the absorption of the oil.

DONEPEZIL

Product name: Aricept
Used in the following combined preparations: None

 ## WHY IS THIS DRUG USED?

Donepezil is an inhibitor of the enzyme acetylcholinesterase; blocking this enzyme causes increased alertness in the brain. Donepezil has been found to improve the symptoms of dementia in Alzheimer's disease and is used to diminish deterioration in that disease. It is not currently recommended for dementia due to other causes. It is usual to assess anyone being treated with donepezil after about three months to decide whether the drug is helping and whether it is worth continuing treatment.

ℹ INFORMATION FOR USERS

Prescription needed. Do not alter dosage without checking with your doctor.

How and when to take: Available as tablets, and orally disintegrating tablets. Take once daily in the evening.

Usual adult dosage range: 5–10mg.

Onset and duration of effect: Starts to work in 1 hour. Full effects might take up to 3 months. Action lasts for 1–2 days.

Diet advice: None.

Storage: Keep in a closed container in a cool, dry place out of the reach of children.

Missed dose: Take missed dose as soon as you remember. A caregiver should ensure that the maximum dose taken in 24 hours does not exceed 10mg. An occasional unintentional extra dose is unlikely to be a cause for concern. If you notice any unusual symptoms, or if a large overdose has been taken, notify your doctor.

Stopping the drug: Do not stop taking the drug without consulting your doctor; symptoms may recur.

Prolonged use: May be continued for as long as there is benefit. Stopping the drug leads to a gradual loss of the improvements. Periodic checks may be performed to test whether the drug is still providing some benefit.

Dependence Rating: Low

Overdose danger rating: Medium

 ## POSSIBLE SIDE EFFECTS AND WHAT TO DO

Side effects include such problems as accidents, which are common in this group of people even when not treated. If you experience **nausea/vomiting, diarrhea, fatigue, insomnia, muscle cramps,** or **headache,** discuss with your doctor if bothersome. If you experience **fainting, dizziness, palpitations,** or **difficulty in passing urine,** discuss with your doctor in all cases.

 ## SPECIAL PRECAUTIONS

Tell your doctor if you have: a heart problem; asthma or respiratory problems; a gastric or duodenal ulcer. **Also discuss if you are:** taking an NSAID regularly; taking other medications.
* **Safety not established** in pregnancy.
* **Not recommended** while breast-feeding, or for infants and children.
* **Discuss** with your doctor before driving and performing hazardous work; such activities may be inadvisable due to your underlying condition.
* **Avoid** alcohol as it may reduce the effect of donepezil.
* **Discuss** with your doctor or dentist before any surgery; treatment with donepezil may need to be stopped before you have a general anesthetic.

 ## INTERACTIONS

Drugs with **anticholinergic** effects may diminish the effects of donepezil.
 Donepezil may enhance the effects of **antipsychotics, cholinergic drugs** and some effects of **beta-blockers**.
 Paroxetine, erythromycin, and **grapefruit juice** could increase donepezil levels in the blood and possibly its side effects.
 Donepezil may increase the effect of some **muscle relaxants used in surgery**, but it may also block some others.
 Carbamazepine, phenytoin, and **rifampin** can all decrease the effectiveness of donepezil.
 St. John's wort may decrease donepezil levels.
 Ginkgo biloba may increase adverse effects of acetylcholinesterase inhibitors.

ENALAPRIL/ENALAPRILAT

Product names: Apo-enalapril, CO enalapril, Teva-enalapril, Vasotec, and others
Used in the following combined preparations: Teva-enalapril HCTZ, Vaseretic

WHY IS THIS DRUG USED?

Enalapril is used to treat hypertension (*high blood pressure*) and *heart failure* (inability of the heart to cope with its workload). It is also given to patients following a *heart attack*. The first dose of enalapril may cause a sudden drop in blood pressure. For this reason, you should be resting at the time and be able to lie down for 2 to 3 hours afterwards.

INFORMATION FOR USERS

Prescription needed. Do not alter dosage without checking with your doctor.

How and when to take: Available as tablets, injection. Take 1–2 x daily.

Usual adult dosage range: 2.5–5mg daily (starting dose), increased to 10–40mg daily (maintenance dose).

Onset and duration of effect: Starts to work within 1 hour. Action lasts for 24 hours.

Diet advice: None.

Storage: Keep in a closed container in a dry place below 25°C out of the reach of children. Protect from light.

If you miss or exceed a dose: Take missed dose as soon as you remember. If your next dose is due within 8 hours, take a single dose now and skip the next. An occasional unintentional extra dose is unlikely to be a cause for concern. Large overdoses may cause dizziness or fainting; notify your doctor.

Stopping the drug: Do not stop the drug without consulting your doctor as it may lead to worsening of the underlying condition.

Prolonged use: No problems expected. Periodic tests on blood and urine should be performed.

Dependence rating: Low

Overdose danger rating: Medium

POSSIBLE SIDE EFFECTS AND WHAT TO DO

Common side effects usually diminish with long-term treatment, but dose adjustment may be necessary. The drug can increase the level of potassium in the blood or affect kidney function; both require periodic monitoring. If you experience **dizziness, headache, nausea, loss of appetite,** or **diarrhea,** discuss with you doctor if bothersome. If you experience a **persistent dry cough, fainting, rash/uticaria,** or **muscle cramps,** discuss with your doctor in all cases. Stop taking the drug now and call your doctor if you develop **wheezing** or **swelling**.

SPECIAL PRECAUTIONS

Tell your doctor if you have: a long-term kidney problem; a heart problem; angioedema; a previous allergic reaction to an ACE inhibitor drug; porphyria. **Also discuss if you are:** taking other medications.
• **Not normally prescribed** in pregnancy.
• **Discuss** with your doctor if you are breast-feeding as the drug passes into the breast milk.
• **Not recommended** for infants and children.
• **Reduced dose** may be necessary for those over 60.
• **Avoid** driving and hazardous work until you have learned how enalapril affects you as the drug can cause dizziness and fainting.
• **Avoid** alcohol as it increases the likelihood of an excessive drop in blood pressure that may cause dizziness.
• **Discuss** with your doctor or dentist before any surgery.

INTERACTIONS

Antihypertensive drugs and NSAIDs are likely to enhance the blood pressure-lowering effect of enalapril.
Enalapril increases the levels of **lithium** in the blood, and serious adverse effects from lithium excess may occur.
Taken with enalapril, **cyclosporine** may increase blood levels of potassium.
Enalapril may enhance the effect of **potassium supplements** and **potassium-sparing diuretics,** leading to raised levels of potassium in the blood.
Some **non-steroidal anti-inflammatory drugs (NSAIDs)** may reduce the effectiveness of enalapril, and may increase the risk of kidney damage when taken with enalapril.

ETIDRONATE

Product names: CO etidronate, Didronel, and others
Used in the following combined preparations: CO etidrocal, Didrocal, and others

❓ WHY IS THIS DRUG USED?

Etidronate is used to treat bone disorders such as Paget's disease. It acts only on the bones, stopping the progress of the disease and the releasing of calcium from the bones into the bloodstream. Etidronate is also packaged together with calcium tablets to treat *osteoporosis* in post-menopausal women and to prevent corticosteroid-induced osteoporosis. If taken at high doses, the drug can lead to thinning of the bones and fractures. The effect is reversed on stopping the drug. Your doctor will tailor your treatment to deal with this effect.

ℹ️ INFORMATION FOR USERS

Prescription needed. Do not alter dosage without checking with your doctor.

How and when to take: Available as tablets. Take once daily on an empty stomach, 2 hours before or after food.

Usual dosage range: *Paget's disease* 5–20mg/kg body weight daily for a maximum of 3–6 months. Courses may be repeated after a break of at least 3 months. *Osteoporosis* 400mg daily for 2 weeks, repeated every 3 months. Package contains a daily calcium dose for remaining 76 days.

Onset and duration of effect: *Paget's disease/osteoporosis* Beneficial effects may take several months. Some effects may persist for several weeks or months.

Diet advice: Absorption of etidronate is reduced by foods, especially those containing calcium (e.g., dairy products), so the drug should be taken on an empty stomach. For prevention of osteoporosis, the daily diet must contain adequate calcium, and vitamin D; supplements may be given.

Storage: Keep in a closed container in a dry place below 30°C out of the reach of children. Protect from light.

If you miss or exceed a dose: Take missed dose as soon as you remember on an empty stomach. If your next dose is due within 6 hours, take a single dose now and skip the next. An occasional unintentional extra dose is unlikely to cause problems. Large overdoses may cause numbness and muscle spasm; notify your doctor.

Stopping the drug: Do not stop the drug without consulting your doctor as it may lead to worsening of the underlying condition.

Prolonged use: When used in bone disorders such as Paget's disease, courses of treatment longer than 3 to 6 months are not usually prescribed, but repeat courses may be required. This drug can be used long term for osteoporosis. Blood and urine tests may be carried out.

Dependence rating: Low

Overdose danger rating: Medium

❗ POSSIBLE SIDE EFFECTS AND WHAT TO DO

The most common side effect, diarrhea, is more likely if the dose is increased above 5mg/kg daily. If you experience **diarrhea, nausea, constipation, abdominal pain,** or **headache,** discuss with your doctor only if bothersome. If you develop a **rash/itching, eye inflammation,** or **vision changes,** discuss with your doctor in all cases. If you experience **bone pain, bruising, fever,** or **sore throat,** call your doctor now.

🖐 SPECIAL PRECAUTIONS

Tell your doctor if you have: a long-term kidney problem; osteomalacia; unusual bone pain; a previous allergic reaction to etidronate or other bisphosphonates; an overactive parathyroid gland; a high concentration of calcium in your blood or urine; colitis. **Also discuss if you are:** taking other medications.
- **Safety not established** in pregnancy or in breast-feeding; discuss with your doctor.
- **Not recommended** for infants and children.

⚙️ INTERACTIONS

Antacids and products containing calcium, magnesium, or iron should be given at least 2 hours before or after etidronate to minimize the risk of reduced absorption of etidronate.

EZETIMIBE

Product name: Ezetrol
Used in the following combined preparations: None

❓ WHY IS THIS DRUG USED?

Ezetimibe is a lipid-lowering drug used in the treatment of *high cholesterol*. It works by blocking the absorption of cholesterol, including dietary cholesterol, from the intestines. It is usually used in addition to another lipid-lowering medication, a statin. Ezetimibe can be taken at any time, once daily, and preferably taken at the same time every day.

ℹ️ INFORMATION FOR USERS

Prescription needed. Do not alter dosage without checking with your doctor.

How and when to take: Available as tablets. Take once daily.

Usual adult dosage range: 10mg daily.

Onset and duration of effect: Starts to work in 1–4 hours. Action lasts up to 24 hours.

Diet advice: Patients should be on a low saturated fat diet.

Storage: Keep in a closed container in a cool, dry place out of the reach of children.

If you miss or exceed a dose: Take missed dose as soon as you remember. If it is near the time of the next dose, skip the missed dose and resume your usual dosing schedule. An occasional unintentional extra dose is unlikely to cause problems. If you notice any unusual symptoms, or if a large overdose has been taken, notify your doctor.

Stopping the drug: Do not stop the drug without consulting your doctor as it may lead to worsening of the underlying condition.

Prolonged use: No known problems. If administered with a statin, certain blood tests will be done periodically.

Dependence rating: Low

Overdose danger rating: Low

❗ POSSIBLE SIDE EFFECTS AND WHAT TO DO

Ezetimibe is usually well tolerated and serious side effects are rare. If you experience **diarrhea, headache, abdominal pain,** or **dizziness,** discuss with your doctor if bothersome. If you develop **sinusitis, muscle ache, excessive tiredness,** or **dark urine,** discuss with your doctor in all cases.

🔺 SPECIAL PRECAUTIONS

Tell your doctor if you have: an allergic reaction to ezetimibe; liver problems or liver disease; kidney problems or kidney disease. **Also discuss if you are:** on any other medications.
- **Safety not established** in pregnancy or in breast-feeding; discuss with your doctor.
- **Not recommended** in children less than 10 years of age.

🔄 INTERACTIONS

Antacids may decrease the rate of absorption of ezetimibe, although these do not significantly affect the total amount of ezetimibe absorbed.
Cholestyramine may decrease absorption of ezetimibe, when taken at the same time.
Ezetimibe is not recommended to be used with **fibrates,** which also decrease cholesterol.
Cyclosporine may increase levels of ezetimibe; close monitoring recommended.

FENTANYL

Product names: Duragesic MAT, Fentanyl citrate, Ratio-Fentanyl, Teva-Fentanyl, and others
Used in the following combined preparations: None

❓ WHY IS THIS DRUG USED?

Fentanyl is an opioid analgesic. It is used in the management of persistent, moderate to severe, chronic *pain* in people already requiring continuous opioid medication. It is available as a patch or an injection. The patch provides a more constant management of pain and should be applied to non-irritated skin on a flat surface such as the chest, back, flank, or upper arm. Dispose of an old patch safely by folding it so that the adhesive side sticks to itself and flushing it down the toilet. Patches should not be cut or divided as this may lead to uncontrolled release of the drug.

ℹ️ INFORMATION FOR USERS

Prescription needed. Do not alter dosage without checking with your doctor.

How and when to take: Available as injection, patch. Apply one patch every 72 hours (3 days).

Usual adult dosage range: Variable and based on previous opioid dose. Patch available in 4 different strengths.

Onset and duration of effect: The peak effect from a patch usually occurs around 12 hours. Action lasts up to 72 hours.

Diet advice: To relieve constipation, increase intake of fluids and high fibre foods.

Storage: Keep in a closed container in a cool, dry place out of the reach of children before and after use.

If you miss a dose: Apply the missed patch when you remember; the next patch should be used at the appropriate interval of 72 hours. Do not double up on a dose.

Stopping the drug: Always discuss with your doctor. When stopping opioid medications, a gradual reduction is recommended.

Prolonged use: The effects of fentanyl usually become weaker during prolonged use as the body adapts. Other effects of long-term use include physical and psychological dependence.

Dependence rating: High

Overdose danger rating: High

☠️ OVERDOSE ACTION

Seek immediate medical advice. Take emergency action in cases of slow, shallow, or irregular breathing, severe drowsiness, inability to think, or slow pulse.

See Drug poisoning emergency guide (p.197).

❗ POSSIBLE SIDE EFFECTS AND WHAT TO DO

Individuals at risk of serious side effects include those with a fever, those whose patch area is exposed to sources of heat such as heating pads and hot water bottles, and those using drugs that may interact with this medication. If you experience **sedation** or **constipation,** discuss with your doctor if bothersome. If you experience **nausea/vomiting, dizziness/light headedness, confusion,** or **vivid dreams,** discuss with your doctor in all cases. Stop taking the drug now and call your doctor if you develop **wheezing** or **difficulty breathing**.

🖐️ SPECIAL PRECAUTIONS

Tell your doctor if you have: impaired liver or kidney function; heart or circulatory problems; a lung disorder such as asthma, bronchitis, or emphysema; sleep apnea; thyroid disease. **Also discuss if you are:** taking other medications.
- **Safety not established** in pregnancy or breast-feeding. Discuss with your doctor.
- **Not recommended** for infants and children.
- **Reduced dose necessary** for those over 60.
- Driving and hazardous work **not recommended.**
- **Avoid** alcohol; it increases sedation.

⚙️ INTERACTIONS

Fentanyl increases the sedative properties of **central nervous system depressants.**
  Ritonavir, ketoconazole, itraconazole, troleandomycin, clarithromycin, nelfinavir verapamil, diltiazem, and **amiodarone** may increase the effect of fentanyl, leading to serious effects on breathing. If any of these drugs is used with fentanyl, very close monitoring is required.
  Grapefruit juice may also increase the effect of fentanyl.
  Monoamine oxidase inhibitors may produce a severe rise in blood pressure when taken with fentanyl.

FLUOXETINE

Product names: Apo-Fluoxetine, PMS-Fluoxetine, Prozac, Teva-Fluoxetine, and others
Used in the following combined preparations: None

❓ WHY IS THIS DRUG USED?

Fluoxetine is an antidepressant that elevates mood, increases physical activity, and restores interest in everyday pursuits. It is used to treat *depression*, to reduce binge eating and purging activity (bulimia nervosa), and to treat obsessive-compulsive disorder. Fluoxetine belongs to the group of antidepressants called selective serotonin re-uptake inhibitors (SSRIs) – these drugs tend to cause less sedation and have different side effects to older antidepressants.

ℹ️ INFORMATION FOR USERS

Prescription needed. Do not alter dosage without checking with your doctor.

How and when to take: Available as capsules, liquid. Take once daily in the morning.

Usual adult dosage range: 20–60mg daily.

Onset and duration of effect: The full benefits may not be felt for 4 weeks or more. Beneficial effects may last for up to 6 weeks following prolonged treatment. Side effects may wear off within a few days.

Diet advice: None.

Storage: Keep in a closed container in a cool, dry place out of the reach of children.

If you miss or exceed a dose: Take missed dose as soon as you remember. If your next dose is due within 8 hours, take a single dose now and skip the next. An occasional unintentional extra dose is unlikely to cause problems. Large overdoses may cause adverse effects; notify your doctor.

Stopping the drug: Do not stop the drug without consulting your doctor, who may supervise a gradual reduction in dosage.

Prolonged use: No problems expected. Side effects tend to decrease with time.

Dependence rating: Low

Overdose danger rating: Medium

❗ POSSIBLE SIDE EFFECTS AND WHAT TO DO

The most common side effects of this drug are restlessness, insomnia, and intestinal irregularities. If you experience **headache, nervousness, drowsiness,** or **sexual dysfunction,** discuss with your doctor if bothersome. If you develop **insomnia, anxiety, nausea, diarrhea,** or **weight loss,** discuss with your doctor in all cases. Stop taking the drug now and call your doctor if you develop a **rash.**

✋ SPECIAL PRECAUTIONS

Tell your doctor if you have: long-term liver or kidney problems; heart problems; diabetes; epileptic seizures; bleeding problems; previously had an allergic reaction to fluoxetine or other SSRIs. **Also discuss if you are:** taking other medications.
- **Safety not established** in pregnancy. The drug passes into the breast milk while breast-feeding. Discuss with your doctor in both cases.
- **Safety and effectiveness not established** with infants and children; discuss with your doctor.
- **Reduced dose** may be necessary for those over 60.
- **Avoid** driving and hazardous work until you have learned how fluoxetine affects you because the drug can cause drowsiness and can affect your judgment and coordination.

🔄 INTERACTIONS

Any drug that affects the breakdown of other drugs in the liver may alter blood levels of fluoxetine.
    Sedatives may increase the sedative effects of fluoxetine.
    Fluoxetine should not be started less than 14 days after stopping a **monoamine oxidase inhibitor (MAOI)** – except moclobemide – as serious adverse effects can occur. An MAOI should not be started less than 5 weeks after stopping fluoxetine.
    Fluoxetine reduces the breakdown and may increase the toxicity of **tricyclic antidepressants**.
    Fluoxetine increases blood levels and toxicity of **lithium**.
    Taken together, **tryptophan** and fluoxetine may produce agitation, restlessness, and gastric distress.
    Fluoxetine can increase the effect of **warfarin** so dose may need adjustment.

FLUTICASONE

Product names: Apo-Fluticasone, Avamys, Flonase, Flovent Diskus, Flovent HFA, ratio-Flucatisone
Used in the following combined preparation: Advair

❓ WHY IS THIS DRUG USED?

Fluticasone is a corticosteroid drug used to control inflammation and relieve restricted breathing in *asthma* and *allergic rhinitis*. Fluticasone does not produce relief immediately: for allergic rhinitis, treatment with the nasal spray needs to begin two to three weeks before the hay fever season commences. People who suffer from asthma should take fluticasone regularly by inhaler in order to prevent attacks. Proper instruction is essential to ensure that the inhaler is used correctly.

ℹ️ INFORMATION FOR USERS

Prescription needed. Do not alter dosage without checking with your doctor.

How and when to take: Available as inhaler, nasal spray. *Allergic rhinitis* take 1–2 x daily; *asthma* take 2 x daily.

Usual adult dosage range: *Allergic rhinitis* 2 sprays into each nostril; *asthma* 200–500mcg per day.

Onset and duration of effect: 4–7 days (asthma); 3–4 days (allergic rhinitis). The effects can last for several days after stopping the drug.

Diet advice: None.

Storage: Keep in a cool, dry place out of the reach of children.

If you miss or exceed a dose: Take missed dose as soon as you remember. An occasional unintentional extra dose is unlikely to be a cause for concern. Adverse effects may occur if the recommended dose is regularly exceeded over a prolonged period.

Stopping the drug: Do not stop the drug without consulting your doctor as symptoms may recur.

Prolonged use: Long-term use of high doses may, rarely, lead to suppression of adrenal gland function. Patients on long-term fluticasone should carry a steroid card or wear a Medic-alert bracelet, and may have their adrenal gland function checked periodically.

Dependence rating: Low

Overdose danger rating: Low

❗ POSSIBLE SIDE EFFECTS AND WHAT TO DO

Fungal infection of the throat and mouth is a main side effect of the inhaled form but can be minimized by thoroughly rinsing the mouth and gargling with water after each inhalation If you experience **nasal irritation,** or **taste/smell disturbances,** discuss with your doctor if bothersome. If you develop a **sore throat/mouth, hoarseness,** or **nosebleeds,** discuss with your doctor in all cases. Call your doctor now if you develop **breathing difficulties,** a **rash,** or **facial swelling**.

🖐️ SPECIAL PRECAUTIONS

Tell your doctor if you have: chronic sinusitis; previous nasal ulcers or surgery; tuberculosis or another respiratory infection. **Also discuss if you are:** taking other medications.
- **Safety not established** in pregnancy or breast-feeding. Discuss with your doctor in both cases.
- **Not recommended** for children under 2 years.
- **Reduced dose necessary** in older children. For use in children, discuss with their doctor.

🔄 INTERACTIONS

No significant interactions with inhaled corticosteroid.

FLUVOXAMINE

Product names: Apo-Fluvoxamine, Dom-Fluvoxamine, Luvox, and others
Used in the following combined preparations: None

❓ WHY IS THIS DRUG USED?

Fluvoxamine is an antidepressant that elevates mood and restores interest in usual activities. It is used to treat *depression* and obsessive-compulsive disorder. Fluvoxamine belongs to the group of antidepressants called selective serotonin re-uptake inhibitors (SSRIs) – these drugs tend to cause less sedation than older antidepressants such as amitriptyline (tricyclic antidepressants).

ℹ️ INFORMATION FOR USERS

Prescription needed. Do not alter dosage without checking with your doctor.

How and when to take: Available as tablets. Take once daily.

Usual adult dosage range: *Initial dose:* 50mg at bedtime; may increase gradually as appropriate; maximum 300mg/day.

Onset and duration of effect: The full benefits may not be felt for 4 weeks or more. Action lasts up to 24 hours.

Diet advice: None.

Storage: Keep in a closed container in a cool, dry place out of the reach of children.

If you miss or exceed a dose: Take missed dose as soon as you remember. If it is near the time of the next dose, skip the missed dose and resume your usual dosing schedule. Do not exceed the total daily prescribed dose in a day. An occasional unintentional extra dose is unlikely to cause problems. For overdoses seek immediate medical advice and contact your doctor right away. Take emergency action if seizures or loss of consciousness occur. See **Drug poisoning emergency guide** (p.197).

Stopping the drug: Do not stop the drug without consulting your doctor. This drug needs to be withdrawn gradually over several weeks to minimize the potential for withdrawal effects.

Prolonged use: No problems expected.

Dependence rating: Low

Overdose danger rating: Medium

❗ POSSIBLE SIDE EFFECTS AND WHAT TO DO

If you experience **tiredness/drowsiness, nausea, constipation, headache,** or **insomnia,** discuss with your doctor if bothersome. If you develop **diarrhea, tremor, agitation,** or **changes in sexual performance,** discuss with your doctor in all cases. Call your doctor now if you experience **mental or mood changes.**

✋ SPECIAL PRECAUTIONS

Tell your doctor if you have: diabetes; seizure disorders or epilepsy; a history of mania or hypomania, or seizures; liver or kidney disease; high blood pressure. **Also discuss if:** you or anyone else in your family has depression or obsessive compulsive disorder; you are taking any other medications, especially those that can affect bleeding.
• **Safety not established** in pregnancy, breast-feeding, or for use with infants and children; discuss with your doctor.
• **Reduced dose** may be necessary for those over 60.
• **Avoid** driving and hazardous work until you have learned how fluvoxamine affects you; the drug can cause drowsiness and impair judgment and coordination.

🔄 INTERACTIONS

Grapefruit juice can increase the level of fluvoxamine.
  Fluvoxamine should not be used with **tizanidine** and **monoamine oxidase inhibitors (MAOIs)**. Fluvoxamine and **MAOIs** should not be used within 2 weeks of each other.
  Use **St. John's wort, lithium,** or **tryptophan** cautiously with fluvoxamine as there is a potential for interaction.
  Fluvoxamine can increase the effect of **warfarin**; may require dose adjustment.

FORMOTEROL

Product names: Foradil, Oxeze Turbuhaler
Used in the following combined preparation: Symbicort Turbuhaler

❓ WHY IS THIS DRUG USED?

Formoterol is a long-acting sympathomimetic bronchodilator used to treat conditions, such as *asthma* and bronchospasm, in which the airways become constricted. For these conditions, it is usually added to an inhaled corticosteroid. Formoterol may also be used in *chronic obstructive*

pulmonary disease such as bronchitis and emphysema. Its advantage over salbutamol (p.163) is that it is longer acting. It is not used for immediate relief of asthma because of its slow onset of effect. It is prescribed to prevent attacks, however, and can be helpful in preventing night-time asthma.

ℹ️ INFORMATION FOR USERS

Prescription needed. Do not alter dosage without checking with your doctor.

How and when to take: Available as powder in capsules for inhalation, metered dose inhaler. Take 2 x daily.

Usual dosage range: *Adult* 1 puff or inhaled capsule (6 or 12mcg) once or twice daily. Daily maximum: 48mcg. *Children* 6–16 years: 1 puff or inhaled capsule (6 or 12mcg). Daily maximum: 24mcg. Not recommended in children less than 6 years. Combination product (Symbicort): one to two inhalations once or twice daily. Maximum 4 inhalations daily.

Onset and duration of effect: Peaks at about 15 minutes. Action lasts for 12 hours.

Diet advice: None.

Storage: Keep in a cool, dry place out of the reach of children.

If you miss or exceed a dose: If a dose of twice daily schedule is missed, take the missed dose as soon as you remember if this is within 6 hours of the missed dose. If more than 6 hours has elapsed, should not take the missed dose and take your next scheduled dose on time. An occasional unintentional extra dose is unlikely to cause problems. If you notice any unusual symptoms, or if a large overdose has been taken, notify your doctor.

Stopping the drug: Do not stop the drug without consulting your doctor; symptoms may recur.

Prolonged use: Formoterol is intended to be used long term. The main problem comes from using combinations of anti-asthma drugs, leading to low blood potassium levels. Periodic blood tests are usually carried out to monitor potassium levels.

Dependence rating: Low

Overdose danger rating: Low

❗ POSSIBLE SIDE EFFECTS AND WHAT TO DO

Side effects are usually mild. If you experience **tremor**, discuss with your doctor if bothersome. If you experience **palpitations, a fast heart rate,**

or **headache,** discuss with your doctor in all cases. Stop taking the drug now and call your doctor if you develop **sudden breathlessness**.

🖐️ SPECIAL PRECAUTIONS

Tell your doctor if you have: heart problems including rhythm problems; high blood pressure; an overactive thyroid; diabetes; allergy to milk or lactose. **Also discuss if you are:** taking other medications.
* **Safety not established** in pregnancy. Discuss with your doctor.
* **Not recommended** while breast-feeding. Discuss with your doctor.
* **Not recommended** for children under 6 years. Combination product not recommended in children under 12 years of age.
* **Avoid** driving and hazardous work until you have learned how formoterol affects you because the drug can cause tremors.

⚙️ INTERACTIONS

There is an increased risk of low blood potassium levels when high doses of formoterol are taken with **corticosteroids, theophylline,** and **diuretics.**
    Beta blockers may decrease the action of formoterol.
    Monoamine oxidase inhibitiors can interact with formoterol, causing a rise in blood pressure.

FUROSEMIDE

Product names: Lasix, Lasix Special, Teva-Furosemide, and others
Used in the following combined preparations: None

❓ WHY IS THIS DRUG USED?

Furosemide is a diuretic that is used to treat edema (accumulation of fluid in tissue spaces) caused by *heart failure*, and certain lung, liver, and kidney disorders. Because it is fast acting, furosemide is often used in emergencies to relieve pulmonary edema (fluid in the lungs). Furosemide is particularly useful for people who have impaired kidney function because they do not respond well to thiazide diuretics. Furosemide increases potassium loss and for this reason, potassium supplements are often given with it.

ℹ️ INFORMATION FOR USERS

Prescription needed. Do not alter dosage without checking with your doctor.

How and when to take: Available as tablets, liquid, injection. Take once daily, usually in the morning; 4–6 x hourly (high dose therapy).

Usual adult dosage range: 20–80mg daily. Dose may be increased to a maximum of 2g daily if kidney function is impaired.

Onset and duration of effect: Starts to work within 1 hour (by mouth); within 5 minutes (by injection). Action lasts up to 6 hours.

Diet advice: Use of this drug may reduce potassium in the body. Eat plenty of potassium-rich fresh fruits and vegetables, such as bananas and tomatoes.

Storage: Keep in a closed container in a cool, dry place out of the reach of children. Protect from light.

If you miss or exceed a dose: Take missed dose as soon as you remember. However, if it is late in the day do not take the missed dose, or you may need to get up during the night to pass urine. Take the next scheduled dose as usual. An occasional unintentional extra dose is unlikely to be a cause for concern. If you notice any unusual symptoms, or if a large overdose has been taken, notify your doctor.

Stopping the drug: Do not stop the drug without consulting your doctor; symptoms may recur.

Prolonged use: Levels of salts, such as potassium, sodium, and calcium, may become depleted; periodic monitoring may be required. Low blood pressure, palpitations, headaches, problems passing urine, or muscle cramps may develop, particularly in the elderly.

❗ POSSIBLE SIDE EFFECTS AND WHAT TO DO

Side effects tend to diminish as the body adjusts to taking the drug. If you experience **dizziness** or **nausea**, discuss with your doctor if bothersome. If you develop **noise in ears, lethargy,** or **muscle cramps,** discuss with your doctor in all cases. Stop taking the drug now and call your doctor if you develop a **rash, photosensitivity,** or **palpitations**. Excessive use may lead to fluid and electrolyte loss; dose adjustments require medical follow-up.

⚠️ SPECIAL PRECAUTIONS

Tell your doctor if you have: long-term liver problems; gout; diabetes; previously had an allergic reaction to furosemide or sulfonamides; prostate trouble. **Also discuss if you are:** taking laxatives; taking other medications.
- **Safety not established** in pregnancy. The drug may reduce milk supply in breast-feeding. Discuss with your doctor.
- **Reduced dose necessary** for infants and children, and possibly for those over 60.
- **Avoid** driving and hazardous work until you have learned how furosemide affects you; it may reduce mental alertness and cause dizziness.
- **Avoid** excessive intake of alcohol; furosemide increases the likelihood of dehydration and hangovers.

🔄 INTERACTIONS

Non-steroidal anti-inflammatory drugs (NSAIDs) may reduce the diuretic effect of furosemide.

Furosemide may increase blood levels of **lithium**, leading to an increased risk of lithium poisoning.

Loss of potassium may lead to digoxin toxicity when furosemide is taken with **digoxin**.

The risk of hearing and kidney problems may be increased when **aminoglycoside antibiotics** are taken with furosemide.

There is a risk of low blood pressure when **angiotensin-converting enzyme inhibitors** are taken with furosemide.

GEMFIBROZIL

Product names: Apo-Gemfibrozil, Lopid, Nu-Gemfibrozil, Teva-Gemfibrozil, and others
Used in the following combined preparations: None

❓ WHY IS THIS DRUG USED?

Gemfibrozil belongs to a group of drugs called fibrates, which lower lipid (fat) levels in the blood, particularly triglycerides and total cholesterol. Saturated fats are associated with *atherosclerosis* (deposition of fat in blood vessel walls). When gemfibrozil is combined with a diet low in saturated fats, there is some evidence that the risk of coronary heart disease (such as *angina* and *heart attack*) is reduced.

ℹ️ INFORMATION FOR USERS

Prescription needed. Do not alter dosage without checking with your doctor.

How and when to take: Available as tablets, capsules. Take twice daily, 30 minutes before morning and evening meals.

Usual adult dosage range: 1,200mg.

Onset and duration of effect: Starts to work in 2–5 days; may take up to 4 weeks to see maximum benefit. Action lasts for 3–6 hours.

Diet advice: A low-fat diet is usually recommended.

Storage: Keep in a closed container in a cool, dry place out of the reach of children.

If you miss or exceed a dose: Take missed dose as soon as you remember. If it is near the time of the next dose, skip the missed dose and resume your usual dosing schedule. Do not double up on a dose. An occasional unintentional extra dose is unlikely to cause problems. Large overdoses may cause liver problems. Notify your doctor and seek medical assistance right away.

Stopping the drug: Do not stop the drug without consulting your doctor as it may lead to worsening of the underlying condition.

Prolonged use: No problems expected, but patients with kidney disease will need special care as there is a high risk of developing muscle problems. Blood tests will be performed occasionally to monitor the effect of the drug on lipids in the blood, and to periodically measure kidney and liver function.

Dependence rating: Low

Overdose danger rating: Medium

❗ POSSIBLE SIDE EFFECTS AND WHAT TO DO

The common side effects are loss of appetite and nausea, and normally diminish as treatment continues. If you experience **nausea, loss of appetite, abdominal pain,** or **epigastric pain,** discuss with your doctor if bothersome. If you experience **vomiting, headache, skin rash, muscle pain/cramp, dizziness,** or **fatigue,** discuss with your doctor in all cases.

✋ SPECIAL PRECAUTIONS

Tell your doctor if you have: liver or kidney problems; muscle weakness; angina or other heart disease; high blood pressure. **Also discuss if you are:** taking other medications.
• **Safety not established** in pregnancy or breast-feeding; discuss with your doctor.
• **Not usually prescribed** for infants and children.

🔄 INTERACTIONS

Gemfibrozil may increase the effect of anticoagulants such as **warfarin**. Dosage adjustment may be needed.
   Pravastatin, atorvastatin, simvastatin, and other lipid-lowering drugs belonging to 'statins' will increase the risk of muscle damage when taken with gemfibrozil.
   Cholestyramine and **colestipol** may decrease absorption of gemfibrozil. Take two hours apart.
   Gemfibrozil can increase the effect of **repaglinide**.
   Gemfibrozil may increase the effect of **amlodipine, verapamil, carvedilol, losartan, phenytoin, diazepam,** and **tolbutamide.**

GLYBURIDE

Product names: Diabeta, Euglucon, Med-Glybe, Mylan-Glybe, Rhoxal-Glyburide, and others
Used in the following combined preparations: None

❓ WHY IS THIS DRUG USED?

Glyburide is an oral antidiabetic drug used in the treatment of Type II *diabetes mellitus* (usually diagnosed in adults), in conjunction with a diet low in carbohydrates and fats. It stimulates the production and secretion of insulin, which lowers blood sugar levels. In conditions of severe illness, injury, or stress, glyburide may lose its effectiveness, making insulin injections necessary.

ℹ️ INFORMATION FOR USERS

Prescription needed. Do not alter dosage without checking with your doctor.

How and when to take: Available as tablets. Take once daily in the morning with breakfast.

Usual adult dosage range: 5–15mg daily.

Onset and duration of effect: Starts to work within 3 hours. Action lasts for 10–15 hours.

Diet advice: A low-carbohydrate, low-fat diet must be maintained in order for the drug to be fully effective.

Storage: Keep in a closed container in a cool, dry place out of the reach of children. Protect from light.

If you miss a dose: Take missed dose with next meal; do not double the dose to account for missed dose.

Stopping the drug: Consult your doctor; stopping may lead to worsening of your diabetes.

Prolonged use: No problems expected. Regular monitoring of levels of sugar in the blood and urine is needed. Periodic assessment of the eyes, heart, and kidneys may also be advised.

Dependence rating: Low

Overdose danger rating: High

☠️ OVERDOSE ACTION

Seek immediate medical advice in all cases. If any early warning symptoms of excessively low blood sugar (such as fainting, sweating, trembling, confusion, or headache) occur, eat or drink something sugary. Take emergency action if seizures or loss of consciousness occur.

See Drug poisoning emergency guide (p.197).

❗ POSSIBLE SIDE EFFECTS AND WHAT TO DO

Common symptoms, often accompanied by hunger, may be signs of low blood sugar due to lack of food or too high a dose of the drug. If you experience **constipation** or **diarrhea**, discuss with your doctor if bothersome. If you experience **weakness, tremor, sweating, nausea, vomiting, rash/itching,** or **weight changes,** discuss with your doctor in all cases. Call your doctor now if you experience **faintness, confusion,** or **jaundice.**

✋ SPECIAL PRECAUTIONS

Tell your doctor if you have: long-term liver or kidney problems; thyroid problems; porphyria; problems with adrenal glands. **Also discuss if you are:** allergic to sulfonylurea drugs; taking other medications.
- **Not usually prescribed** in pregnancy; insulin is generally substituted. The drug passes into the breast milk while breast-feeding.
- **Not prescribed** for infants and children.
- **Reduced dose** may be necessary for those over 60 due to a greater likelihood of low blood sugar.
- **Avoid** driving and hazardous work if you have warning signs of low blood sugar.
- **Avoid** alcohol as it may upset diabetic control.
- **Notify** your doctor or dentist that you are diabetic before undergoing any type of surgery.

⊘ INTERACTIONS

Many drugs reduce glyburide's effect and raise blood sugar. These include **corticosteroids, estrogens, diuretics,** and **rifampin.**
    Warfarin, sulfonamides and other antibacterials, antifungals, ASA, beta blockers, and **ACE inhibitors** may increase the risk of low blood sugar.

HEPARIN/LMWH

Product names: [Heparin] Hepalean, Heparin-LEO; [LMWH] Fragmin, Fraxiparine, Fraxiparine Forte, Innohep, Lovenox, Lovenox HP
Used in the following combined preparations: None

❷ WHY IS THIS DRUG USED?

Heparin is an anticoagulant drug used to prevent the formation of, and aid in the dispersion of, blood clots. It acts quickly and is useful in emergencies, for instance, to prevent further clotting when a clot has already reached the lungs or the brain. It can be prescribed before or after surgery, before kidney dialysis, or to treat unstable *angina*. Low molecular weight heparins (LMWH), such as dalteparin, enoxaparin, nadroparin, and tinzaparin, act longer and do not require close blood monitoring as heparin does.

❶ INFORMATION FOR USERS

Generally prescribed by a medical practitioner. Do not alter dosage without checking with your doctor.

How and when to take: Available as solution for injection (IV and SC). Take every 8–12 hours or continuous intravenous infusion; LMWH usually once daily.

Usual dosage range: Dosage is determined by the nature of the condition being treated or prevented.

Onset and duration of effect: Starts to work within 15 minutes. Action lasts for 4–12 hours after treatment is stopped; LMWH usually lasts 24 hours after end of treatment.

Diet advice: None.

Storage: Keep in a cool, dry place out of the reach of children.

If you miss a dose: Notify your doctor.

Stopping the drug: Do not stop taking the drug without consulting your doctor. Stopping the drug may lead to clotting of blood.

Prolonged use: With long-term use, osteoporosis and hair loss may occur rarely; tolerance to heparin may develop. Periodic blood and liver function tests will be required.

Dependence rating: Low

Overdose danger rating: High

☠ OVERDOSE ACTION

Seek immediate medical advice in all cases. Take emergency action if bleeding, severe headache, or loss of consciousness occur. Heparin overdose can be reversed under medical supervision by a drug called protamine.

See Drug poisoning emergency guide (p.197).

❗ POSSIBLE SIDE EFFECTS AND WHAT TO DO

Bleeding is the most common side effect of heparin. If you experience **alopecia** or **aching bones,** discuss with your doctor in all cases. If you experience **bleeding, bruising, breathing difficulties, jaundice, vomiting blood,** or a **rash,** call your doctor now.

✋ SPECIAL PRECAUTIONS

Tell your doctor if you have: long-term liver or kidney problems; high blood pressure; any allergies; stomach ulcers. **Also discuss** if you bleed easily or if you are taking other medications.
• **Careful monitoring** is necessary during pregnancy as the drug may cause the mother to bleed excessively if taken near delivery.
• **Reduced dose** necessary for infants and children.
• **Avoid** risk of injury, since excessive bruising and bleeding may occur.
• **Discuss** with your doctor or dentist before having any surgery; heparin may need to be stopped.

↻ INTERACTIONS

The effect of heparin may be increased when it is taken with other anticoagulants such as **warfarin,** and with **clopidogrel, ticlopidine,** and **dipyridamole.** The dosage of heparin may need to be adjusted accordingly.
Do not take **ASA,** which may increase the anticoagulant effect of this drug and the risk of bleeding in the intestines or joints. Discuss with your doctor or pharmacist.

HYDROCHLOROTHIAZIDE

Product names: Apo-Hydro, DOM-Hydrochlorothiazide
Used in the following combined preparations: Atacand Plus, Avalide, Hyzaar, Inhibace Plus, Vaseretic, and others

❓ WHY IS THIS DRUG USED?

Hydrochlorothiazide is a diuretic drug, which removes excess water from the body and reduces edema (fluid retention) in people with congestive *heart failure* and kidney disorders. It is also used to treat *high blood pressure*. Taking hydrochlorothiazide may reduce potassium in the body, so it is often taken with potassium supplements.

ℹ️ INFORMATION FOR USERS

Prescription needed. Do not alter dosage without checking with your doctor.

How and when to take: Available as tablets. Take once daily, or every 2 days, early in the day.

Usual adult dosage range: 12.5–50mg daily.

Onset and duration of effect: Starts to work within 2 hours. Action lasts for 6–12 hours.

Diet advice: Use of this drug may reduce potassium in the body. Eat plenty of fresh fruit and vegetables. Discuss with your doctor the advisability of reducing your salt intake.

Storage: Keep in a closed container in a cool, dry place out of the reach of children. Protect from light.

If you miss or exceed a dose: Take missed dose as soon as you remember. If it is late in the day do not take the missed dose, or you may have to get up during the night to pass urine. Take the next scheduled dose as usual. An occasional unintentional extra dose is unlikely to be a cause for concern. If you notice any unusual symptoms, or if a large overdose has been taken, notify your doctor.

Stopping the drug: Do not stop the drug without consulting your doctor; symptoms may recur.

Prolonged use: Excessive loss of potassium and imbalances of other salts may result, especially in the elderly. Blood tests may be performed periodically to check kidney function and levels of potassium and other salts.

Dependence rating: Low

Overdose danger rating: Low

❗ POSSIBLE SIDE EFFECTS AND WHAT TO DO

Most effects are caused by excessive loss of potassium and can be dealt with by taking a potassium supplement. If you experience **lethargy, digestive disturbance,** or **temporary impotence,** discuss with your doctor if bothersome. If you experience **muscle cramps** or **dizziness,** discuss with your doctor in all cases. Stop taking the drug now and call your doctor if you develop a **rash.**

🖐️ SPECIAL PRECAUTIONS

Tell your doctor if you have: long-term liver or kidney problems; gout; diabetes; porphyria; Addison's disease; systemic lupus erythematosus; or allergy to sulpha drugs. **Also discuss if you are:** taking other medications.
- **Not usually prescribed** in pregnancy; may cause jaundice in the newborn baby. The drug passes into the breast milk while breast-feeding, but at normal doses adverse effects on the baby are unlikely. Discuss with your doctor in both cases.
- **Reduced dose necessary** for infants and children, and for those over 60.
- **Avoid** driving and hazardous work until you have learned how hydrochlorothiazide affects you because the drug may reduce mental alertness and cause dizziness.
- **Avoid** excessive intake of alcohol due to an increased likelihood of dehydration and hangovers.

🔄 INTERACTIONS

Some **non-steroidal anti-inflammatory drugs** (NSAIDs) may reduce the diuretic effect of hydrochlorothiazide, whose dosage may need to be adjusted.
　　Adverse effects of **digoxin**, including irregular heart rhythms, may be increased if excessive potassium is lost.
　　Corticosteroids further increase loss of potassium from the body when taken with hydrochlorothiazide.
　　Hydrochlorothiazide may increase **lithium** levels in the blood, leading to a risk of serious adverse effects.

IBUPROFEN

Product names: Advil, Apo-ibuprofen, Motrin IB, Novo-Profen, Nu-Ibuprofen, and many others
Used in the following combined preparations: Advil Cold and Sinus, Robax Platinum, Sudafed Sinus Advance, and many others

❓ WHY IS THIS DRUG USED?

Ibuprofen is an analgesic and a non-steroidal anti-inflammatory drug (NSAID), which reduces *pain*, stiffness, and inflammation. It is used to treat the symptoms of *osteoarthritis, rheumatoid arthritis*, and gout. Other uses of the drug include the relief of mild to moderate headache, menstrual and dental pain, pain resulting from soft tissue injuries, or the pain that may follow an operation.

ℹ️ INFORMATION FOR USERS

No prescription needed for smaller dosage forms. Call your doctor if symptoms worsen.

How and when to take: Available as tablets, chewable tablets, gel caps, liquid. Take 4–6 x daily (general pain relief); 3–4 x daily with food (arthritis).

Usual adult dosage range: *General pain relief* 600mg–1.8g daily. *Arthritis* 1.2–2.4g daily.

Onset and duration of effect: Pain relief begins in 1–2 hours. The full anti-inflammatory effect in arthritic conditions may not be felt for up to 2 weeks. Action lasts for 5–10 hours.

Diet advice: Take with food to minimize side effects.

Storage: Keep in a closed container in a cool, dry place out of the reach of children.

If you miss or exceed a dose: Take missed dose as soon as you remember. If your next dose is due within 2 hours, take a single dose now and skip the next. An occasional unintentional extra dose is unlikely to be a cause for concern. If you notice any unusual symptoms, or if a large overdose has been taken, notify your doctor.

Stopping the drug: The drug can safely be stopped if being used for short-term pain relief. If prescribed for long-term use, consult with your doctor first.

Prolonged use: There is an increased risk of bleeding from peptic ulcers and in the gastrointestinal tract with prolonged use of ibuprofen.

Dependence rating: Low

Overdose danger rating: Low

⚠️ POSSIBLE SIDE EFFECTS AND WHAT TO DO

The most common side effects are the result of gastrointestinal disturbances. If you experience **dizziness, heartburn/indigestion, nausea,** or **vomiting,** discuss with your doctor if bothersome. If you experience **swollen feet and ankles** or **ringing in the ears**, discuss with your doctor in all cases. Stop taking the drug now and call your doctor if you develop a **rash, fever, wheezing, breathlessness, black/bloodstained feces,** or **changes in vision**.

✋ SPECIAL PRECAUTIONS

Tell your doctor or pharmacist if you have: a long-term liver or kidney problem; high blood pressure, a peptic ulcer, esophagitis, or acid indigestion; asthma. **Also discuss if you are:** allergic to ASA; taking other medications.
- **Not usually prescribed** in pregnancy; may affect the unborn baby and prolong labour. The drug passes into the breast milk during breast-feeding, but at normal doses adverse effects on the baby are unlikely. Discuss with your doctor.
- **Reduced dose necessary** for infants and children, and possibly for those over 60.
- **Avoid** driving and hazardous work until you know how the drug affects you. It can cause dizziness and sleepiness. Alcohol may increase drowsiness and the risk of stomach irritation.
- **Stopping treatment** may be advised before surgery; ibuprofen may prolong bleeding.

⚙️ INTERACTIONS

Ibuprofen interacts with a wide range of drugs to increase the risk of bleeding and/or peptic ulcers. Such drugs include other **non-steroidal anti-inflammatory drugs** (NSAIDs), **ASA,** oral **anticoagulants,** and **corticosteroids.**
　The risk of seizures with **ciprofloxacin** and related antibiotics may be increased by ibuprofen.
　The beneficial effects of **antihypertensive drugs** and **diuretics** may be reduced by ibuprofen.
　Ibuprofen may increase the blood levels of **lithium, digoxin,** and **methotrexate** to an undesirable extent.

INSULIN

Product names: Humalog, Humulin, Novolin GE, and many others
Used in the following combined preparations: None

❓ WHY IS THIS DRUG USED?

Insulin is a hormone that is vital to the body's ability to use sugar. It is given by injection to treat juvenile (Type 1) *diabetes* and sometimes adult-onset (Type 2) diabetes. Insulin should be used with a carefully controlled diet. Insulin is available in a wide variety of preparations: short-, medium-, or long-acting. Combinations of types are often given. People receiving insulin should carry a warning card or tag.

ℹ️ INFORMATION FOR USERS

Prescription needed. Do not alter dosage without checking with your doctor.

How and when to take: Available as injection, infusion pump, pen injection. Short-acting insulin is usually given 15–30 minutes before meals. Some newer forms can be given directly before or after eating. The exact timing of injections and longer-acting preparations will be tailored to your individual needs.

Usual dosage range: The dose (and type) of insulin is determined according to your needs.

Onset and duration of effect: Starts to work in 15–60 minutes (short-acting); 1–2 hours (medium- and long-acting). Action lasts for 6–8 hours (short-acting); 18–26 hours (medium-acting); 28–36 hours (long-acting).

Diet advice: A low-carbohydrate diet is necessary.

Storage: Refrigerate, but once opened may be stored at room temperature for 1 month. Do not freeze. Follow the instructions on the container.

If you miss a dose: Notify your doctor.

Stopping the drug: Do not stop without consulting your doctor; confusion and coma may occur.

Prolonged use: No problems expected. Regular monitoring of levels of sugar in the blood and/or urine is required.

Dependence rating: Low

Overdose danger rating: High

☠️ OVERDOSE ACTION

Seek immediate medical advice. You may notice symptoms of low blood sugar, such as faintness, hunger, sweating, or trembling. Eat or drink something sugary. Take emergency action if seizures or loss of consciousness occur.

See Drug poisoning emergency guide (p.197).

❗ POSSIBLE SIDE EFFECTS AND WHAT TO DO

Dizziness, sweating, weakness, and confusion indicate low blood sugar. If you experience **injection-site irritation, weakness, sweating, dimpling at injection site,** or **eyesight problems,** discuss with your doctor in all cases. Call your doctor now if you develop a **rash, facial swelling,** or **shortness of breath**.

👆 SPECIAL PRECAUTIONS

Tell your doctor if you have had: a previous allergic reaction to insulin. **Also discuss if you are:** taking other medications, or your other drug treatment is changed.
• **Careful monitoring** during pregnancy required; poor control of diabetes increases the risk of birth defects.
• **Adjustment in dose** may be necessary while breast-feeding.
• **Reduced dose** necessary for infants and children.
• **Avoid** driving and hazardous work if you have warning signs of low blood sugar.
• **Avoid** alcohol as it can upset diabetic control.
• **Notify** your doctor or dentist that you are diabetic before any surgery.

🔄 INTERACTIONS

Check with your doctor or pharmacist before taking any medicines; some contain sugar and may affect control of diabetes.
    Many drugs, including some **antibiotics, monoamine oxidase inhibitors** (MAOIs), and **oral antidiabetic drugs,** increase the risk of low blood sugar.
    Corticosteroids and **diuretics** may oppose the effect of insulin.
    Beta blockers may affect insulin needs and mask signs of low blood sugar.

LACTULOSE

Product names: Apo-lactulose, PMS-lactulose, ratio-Lactulose
Used in the following combined preparations: None

❓ WHY IS THIS DRUG USED?

Lactulose is an effective laxative that softens feces by increasing the amount of water in the large intestine. It is used for the relief of *constipation* and fecal impaction. This drug is less likely than some of the other laxatives to disrupt normal bowel action. Lactulose is also used for preventing and treating brain disturbance associated with liver failure, known as hepatic encephalopathy.

ℹ️ INFORMATION FOR USERS

No prescription needed. Follow instructions on the label. Call your doctor if symptoms worsen.

How and when to take: Available as liquid. Take 2 x daily (chronic constipation); 3–4 x daily (liver failure).

Usual adult dosage range: 15–30ml daily (chronic constipation); 30–120ml daily (liver failure). May dilute drug with water or juice.

Onset and duration of effect: Starts to work in 24–48 hours. Action lasts for 6–18 hours.

Diet advice: Maintaining adequate fluid intake is important.

Storage: Keep in a closed container in a cool, dry place out of the reach of children. Do not store after diluting.

If you miss or exceed a dose: Take missed dose as soon as you remember. If your next dose is due within 3 hours, take a single dose now and skip the next. An occasional unintentional extra dose is unlikely to be a cause for concern. If you notice any unusual symptoms, or if a large overdose has been taken, notify your doctor.

Stopping the drug: In the treatment of constipation, the drug can be safely stopped as soon as you no longer need it.

Prolonged use: In children, prolonged use may contribute to the development of tooth decay.

Dependence rating: Low

Overdose danger rating: Low

❗ POSSIBLE SIDE EFFECTS AND WHAT TO DO

Side effects often disappear when your body adjusts to the medicine. Diarrhea may indicate that the dosage of lactulose is too high. If you experience **flatulence, belching, stomach cramps,** or **nausea,** discuss with your doctor if bothersome. If you develop **abdominal distension** or **diarrhea,** discuss with your doctor in all cases.

🖐 SPECIAL PRECAUTIONS

Tell your doctor or pharmacist if you have: severe abdominal pain; lactose intolerance or galactosemia. **Also discuss if you are:** taking other medications.
• **No evidence of risk** in pregnancy or breast-feeding; discuss with your doctor.
• **Reduced dose necessary** for infants and children.

🔄 INTERACTIONS

Lactulose may reduce the release of **mesalazine** at the site of action.

LATANOPROST

Product name: Xalatan
Used in the following combined preparation: Xalacom

❓ WHY IS THIS DRUG USED?

Latanoprost is used as eye drops to reduce pressure in chronic *glaucoma* and in ocular hypertension. It lowers the pressure in the eye by increasing the normal outflow of fluid inside the eye. This drug may be used alone, or in conjunction with other eye drops for glaucoma.

Latanoprost eye drops can gradually increase the amount of brown pigment in the eye, darkening the iris (because of increased amounts of melanin). It has also been reported to cause darkening, thickening, and lengthening of eyelashes.

ℹ️ INFORMATION FOR USERS

Prescription needed. Do not alter dosage without checking with your doctor.

How and when to take: Available as eye drops. Use once daily, in the evening.

Usual adult dosage range: 1 drop in the affected eye, daily.

Onset and duration of effect: Starts to work in 15–30 minutes. Action lasts for 24 hours.

Diet advice: None.

Storage: Keep the eyedrops in the outer cardboard package to protect from light. Unopened, it can be stored in a refrigerator between 2°C and 8°C, out of the reach of children. Once opened, it may be kept at room temperature up to 25°C. Discard bottle and contents after 6 weeks.

If you miss or exceed the dose: Use the next dose as normal. An occasional unintentional extra application is unlikely to cause problems. Excessive use may irritate the eye and produce adverse effects in other parts of the body; notify your doctor.

Stopping the drug: Do not stop the drug without consulting your doctor. Symptoms may recur.

Prolonged use: No known problems apart from changes to iris pigment and eyelash colour. Your doctor will monitor this as well as control of the glaucoma.

Dependence rating: Low

Overdose danger rating: Medium

⚠️ POSSIBLE SIDE EFFECTS AND WHAT TO DO

This drug can cause **darkening of the iris** and **eyelash changes.** If you experience **eye irritation** discuss with your doctor if bothersome. If you experience **eye pain, bloodshot eye, inflamed eyelids, eye/facial swelling,** or changes in **your vision,** discuss with your doctor in all cases. Stop taking the drug now and call your doctor if you develop **chest pains** or **wheezing/ breathing difficulty**.

⚠️ SPECIAL PRECAUTIONS

Tell your doctor if you are: asthmatic; wearing contact lenses; allergic to benzalkonium chloride or latanoprost; taking other medications.
• **Safety not established** in pregnancy or breast-feeding. Discuss with your doctor.
• **Not recommended** for infants and children.

🔄 INTERACTIONS

Thiomersal-containing eye drops should not be used within 5 minutes of using latanoprost (thiomersal is a preservative used in some eye drops).
   Bimatoprost should not be used with latanoprost as it may increase eye pressure.

LEVODOPA

Product names: None
Used in the following combined preparations: Apo-Levocarb, Apo-Levocarb CR, Prolopa, Sinemet, Sinemet CR, Stalevo, Teva-Levodopa carbidopa

WHY IS THIS DRUG USED?

Levodopa is a drug used to treat Parkinson's disease. Parkinson's disease is caused by an absence or shortage of a chemical messenger in the brain called dopamine. The body can transform levodopa into dopamine, which results in marked relief of the symptoms of Parkinson's disease. Levodopa causes side effects, such as nausea, dizziness, and palpitations, so it is combined with carbidopa or benserazide in a 1:4 or 1:10 ratio. Both of these combinations enhance the effects of levodopa in the brain and reduce its side effects.

INFORMATION FOR USERS

Prescription needed. Do not alter dosage without checking with your doctor.

How and when to take: Available as tablets, extended release tablets, capsules. Take 3–6 x daily with food or milk.

Usual adult dosage range: 125–500mg of levodopa initially, increased until benefits and side effects are balanced.

Onset and duration of effect: Starts to work within 1 hour (regular tablets). Action lasts for 2–12 hours.

Diet advice: None.

Storage: Keep in a closed container in a cool, dry place out of the reach of children. Protect from light.

If you miss or exceed a dose: Take missed dose as soon as you remember. If your next regular release tablet is due within 2 hours, take a single dose now and skip the next. An occasional unintentional extra dose is unlikely to cause problems. Larger overdoses may cause vomiting or drowsiness. Notify your doctor.

Stopping the drug: Do not stop taking the drug without consulting your doctor as it may lead to severe worsening of the underlying condition.

Prolonged use: Effectiveness usually declines in time; dosage may need to be increased and/or other medications added.

Dependence rating: Low

Overdose danger rating: Medium

POSSIBLE SIDE EFFECTS AND WHAT TO DO

Side effects of levodopa are related to dosage levels and may increase in severity as dosage is increased. All side effects should be discussed with your doctor, including **digestive disturbance, abnormal movement, nervousness/agitation, dark urine, dizziness, fainting, confusion,** or **vivid dreams.** Stop taking the drug now and call your doctor if you experience **palpitations.**

SPECIAL PRECAUTIONS

Tell your doctor if you have: heart problems; long-term liver or kidney problems; a lung disorder, such as asthma or bronchitis; an overactive thyroid gland; glaucoma; a peptic ulcer; diabetes; any serious mental illness. **Also discuss** if you have ever had malignant melanoma, or if you are taking other medications.
- **Unlikely to be required** in pregnancy or while breast-feeding.
- **Not normally used** in children (and rarely given to patients under 25 years).
- **Discuss** with your doctor regarding driving and hazardous work; these activities may be inadvisable due to your underlying condition, as well as the possibility of levodopa causing fainting and dizziness.

INTERACTIONS

Levodopa may interact with **monoamine oxidase inhibitors** (MAOIs) to cause a dangerous rise in blood pressure. It may also interact with **tricyclic antidepressants.**
Excessive intake of **pyridoxine** (vitamin B$_6$) may reduce the effect of levodopa, if levodopa is used on its own.
Absorption of levodopa may be reduced by **iron.**
Some **antipsychotic drugs** may reduce the effect of levodopa.
The side effects of levodopa may be increased if used with other drugs with central nervous system effects, such as **bupropion.**

LEVOFLOXACIN

Product names: Apo-Levofloxacin, CO Levofloxacin, Levaquin, Mylan-Levofloxacin, Teva-levofloxacin, and others
Used in the following combined preparations: None

❓ WHY IS THIS DRUG USED?

Levofloxacin is a quinolone antibacterial drug used for soft-tissue, respiratory, and *urinary tract infections* that have not responded to other antibiotics. The drug is usually taken as a tablet, but can be administered by intravenous infusion to people with serious systemic infections or who cannot take drugs by mouth. Levofloxacin may occasionally cause tendon inflammation and damage, especially in the elderly or in people taking corticosteroids – see below for more information.

ℹ INFORMATION FOR USERS

Prescription needed. Do not alter dosage without checking with your doctor.

How and when to take: Available as tablets, injection. Take 1 x 2 times daily for 7–14 days depending on infection (tablets). Drink plenty of fluids while on this drug.

Usual adult dosage range: 250–1,000mg daily.

Onset and duration of effect: Starts to work in 1 hour. Action lasts 12–24 hours.

Diet advice: None.

Storage: Keep in a closed container in a cool, dry place out of the reach of children.

If you miss or exceed a dose: Take missed dose as soon as you remember, then take your next dose when it is due. An occasional unintentional extra dose is unlikely to cause problems. Larger overdoses may cause mental disturbances and seizures; notify your doctor.

Stopping the drug: Take the full course. The original infection may recur if treatment is stopped too soon.

Prolonged use: Not usually prescribed for long-term use.

Dependence rating: Low

Overdose danger rating: Medium

⚠ POSSIBLE SIDE EFFECTS AND WHAT TO DO

Given by injection, levofloxacin may cause palpitations and a fall in blood pressure. Nausea and vomiting are the most common side effects of the drug taken by mouth. If you experience **nausea, vomiting, diarrhea, abdominal pain, headache, dizziness, skin rash/itching, drowsiness,** or **restlessness,** see your doctor if bothersome. Stop taking the drug now and see your doctor if you experience **painful or inflamed tendons, jaundice, confusion, hallucinations, fever** or an **allergic reaction**.

🖐 SPECIAL PRECAUTIONS

Tell your doctor if you have: kidney problems; epilepsy; glucose-6-phosphate dehydrogenase (G6PD) deficiency; porphyria; diabetes; a history of allergic reaction to a quinolone antibacterial; a personal or family history of irregular heartbeat; a history of a tendon problem with a quinolone; rheumatoid arthritis or other joint problems. **Also discuss if you are:** taking ASA or another NSAID; taking other medications.

• **Safety not established** in pregnancy or breast-feeding. Discuss with your doctor.
• **Not recommended** for infants and children.
• **Increased risk** of tendon damage for those over 60.
• **Avoid** driving and hazardous work until you have learned how levofloxacin affects you.
• **Avoid** alcohol as it may increase the sedative effects of levofloxacin.
• **Avoid** exposure to strong sunlight or artificial ultraviolet rays; photosensitization may occur.

⚙ INTERACTIONS

There is an increased risk of convulsions when **non-steroidal anti-inflammatory drugs (NSAIDs)** and **theophylline** are taken with levofloxacin.
  The effect of **anticoagulants** may be increased by levofloxacin.
  Antacids, adsorbents, sucralfate, iron, and **zinc** may reduce the absorption of levofloxacin.
  There is an increased risk of kidney damage if **cyclosporine** is taken with levofloxacin.

LEVOTHYROXINE

Product names: Eltroxin, Synthroid
Used in the following combined preparations: None

❓ WHY IS THIS DRUG USED?

Levothyroxine is the major hormone produced by the thyroid gland. A deficiency of the natural hormone causes hypothyroidism and may sometimes lead to myxedema, a condition characterized by slowing of body functions and facial puffiness. A synthetic preparation is used to replace the natural hormone when it is deficient. Levothyroxine is also used to treat or prevent the development of certain types of goiter, and is also prescribed for some forms of thyroid cancer.

ℹ️ INFORMATION FOR USERS

Prescription needed. Do not alter dosage without checking with your doctor.

How and when to take: Available as tablets. Take once daily.

Usual dosage range: *Adults* Doses of 50–100mcg daily, increased at 3–4-week intervals as required. The maximum dose is 200mcg daily. *Infants and children* Dosage depends on age and weight.

Onset and duration of effect: Starts to work within 48 hours. Full beneficial effects may not be felt for several weeks. Action lasts for 1–3 weeks.

Diet advice: None.

Storage: Keep in a closed container in a cool, dry place out of the reach of children. Protect from light.

If you miss or exceed a dose: Take missed dose as soon as you remember. If your next dose is due within 8 hours, take a single dose now and skip the next. An occasional unintentional extra dose is unlikely to cause problems. Large overdoses may cause palpitations during the next few days; notify your doctor.

Stopping the drug: Do not stop the drug without consulting your doctor; symptoms may recur.

Prolonged use: No special problems. Periodic tests of thyroid function are usually required.

Dependence rating: Low

Overdose danger rating: Medium

❗ POSSIBLE SIDE EFFECTS AND WHAT TO DO

Side effects are rare with levothyroxine and are usually the result of overdosage. If you experience **anxiety/nervousness, diarrhea, weight loss, sweating, flushing, muscle cramps,** or **insomnia,** discuss with your doctor in all cases. Call your doctor now if you experience **palpitations** or **chest pain**.

✋ SPECIAL PRECAUTIONS

Tell your doctor if you have: high blood pressure; heart problems; diabetes. **Also discuss if you are:** taking other medications.
- **Dosage adjustment** may be necessary in pregnancy.
- **Discuss** with your doctor if you are breast-feeding; the drug passes into the breast milk, but at normal doses adverse effects on the baby are unlikely.
- **Reduced dose** usually necessary for those over 60.

🔄 INTERACTIONS

Levothyroxine may increase the effect of **oral anticoagulants.**
   The doses of **antidiabetic agents** may need increasing once levothyroxine treatment is started.
   Cholestyramine and **sucralfate** may both reduce absorption of levothyroxine.
   Amiodarone may affect thyroid activity and levothyroxine dosage may need adjustment.
   Antiepileptic drugs may reduce the effect of levothyroxine.
   Calcium and iron salts may decrease absorption of levothyroxine; separate levothyroxine administration by at least 4 hours.

LOPERAMIDE

Product names: Imodium, Imodium Quick Dissolve, Loperacap, Riva-Loperamide, Sandoz Loperamide, and others
Used in the following combined preparation: Imodium Advanced multi-symptom chewable tablets

❓ WHY IS THIS DRUG USED?

Loperamide is a fast-acting antidiarrheal drug. It reduces the loss of water and salts from the bowel and slows bowel activity, resulting in the passage of firmer bowel movements at less frequent intervals.

Loperamide is widely prescribed for both sudden and recurrent bouts of *diarrhea*, but it is not generally recommended for diarrhea caused by infection because it may delay the expulsion of harmful substances from the bowel. Loperamide is often prescribed for people who have had a colostomy or an ileostomy, to reduce fluid loss from the stoma (outlet).

ℹ INFORMATION FOR USERS

Prescription not needed. Follow instructions on the label. Call your doctor if symptoms worsen.

How and when to take: Available as tablets, caplets, quick dissolve tablets, chewable tablets, liquid. *Acute diarrhea* Take a double dose (4mg) at start of treatment, then a single dose after each loose feces, up to the maximum daily dose. *Chronic diarrhea* Take 2 x daily.

Usual dosage range: *Acute diarrhea* 4mg (starting dose), then 2mg after each loose bowel movement (up to 16mg daily); usual dose 6–8mg daily. Use for up to 5 days only (3 days only for children 4–8 years), then consult your doctor. *Chronic diarrhea* 4–8mg daily (up to 16mg daily) in consultation with your doctor.

Onset and duration of effect: Starts to work within 1–2 hours. Action lasts for 6–18 hours.

Diet advice: Ensure adequate fluid, sugar, and salt intake during a diarrheal illness.

Storage: Keep in a closed container in a cool, dry place out of the reach of children.

If you miss or exceed a dose: Do not take the missed dose. Take your next dose if needed. An occasional unintentional extra dose is unlikely to be a cause for concern. Large overdoses may cause constipation, vomiting, or drowsiness, and affect breathing; notify your doctor.

Stopping the drug: Can be safely stopped as soon as you no longer need it.

Prolonged use: Although not usually taken for prolonged periods, problems are not expected during long-term use. Discuss with your doctor.

Dependence rating: Low

Overdose danger rating: Medium

❗ POSSIBLE SIDE EFFECTS AND WHAT TO DO

Side effects are rare with loperamide and often difficult to distinguish from the effects of the diarrhea it is used to treat. If you experience **bloating, abdominal pain, dry mouth, drowsiness,** or **dizziness**, discuss with your doctor if bothersome. Stop taking the drug now and call your doctor if you experience **constipation, significant abdominal distention, itching skin,** or a **rash**.

SPECIAL PRECAUTIONS

Tell your doctor or pharmacist if you have: long-term liver or kidney problems; had recent abdominal surgery; an infection or blockage in the intestine; pseudomembranous colitis, or ulcerative colitis. **Also discuss if you are:** taking other medications.
- **Safety not established** in pregnancy or breast-feeding. Discuss with your doctor.
- **Not to be given** to children under 4 years. Reduced dose necessary in older children. Children can be very sensitive to the effects of this drug.

INTERACTIONS

Opioid analgesics may cause severe constipation; avoid using them with loperamide.

LORAZEPAM

Product names: Apo-Lorazepam, Ativan, Nu-Loraz, Teva-Lorazepam, and others
Used in the following combined preparations: None

❓ WHY IS THIS DRUG USED?

Lorazepam belongs to a group of drugs known as the benzodiazepines, which help to relieve anxiety and encourage sleep. Lorazepam is used for the short-term treatment of excessive *anxiety*. In those with anxiety and *insomnia*, taking a dose at bedtime can help with sleep. The injectable form of the drug may be used as an anticonvulsant for the control of status epilepticus. Lorazepam is less likely than some of the other benzodiazepines to accumulate in the body.

ℹ️ INFORMATION FOR USERS

Prescription needed. Do not alter dosage without checking with your doctor.

How and when to take: Available as tablets, sublingual tablets, injection. Take 1–4 x daily.

Usual adult dosage range: 1–6mg daily (by mouth); varies with condition under treatment (injection) and age.

Onset and duration of effect: Starts to work in 30–60 minutes (oral tablets); 5–10 minutes (intravenous injection); less than 30 minutes (intramuscular injection, sublingual tablets). Action lasts for up to 12 hours.

Diet advice: None.

Storage: Keep in a closed container in a cool, dry place out of the reach of children. Protect from light.

If you miss or exceed a dose: If you are taking the drug once daily for insomnia, a missed dose is no cause for concern. Return to your normal dose schedule the following night, if necessary. On a daytime schedule, take the missed dose when you remember. If your next dose is due within 2 hours, take a single dose now and skip the next. An occasional unintentional extra dose is unlikely to cause problems. Larger overdoses may cause unusual drowsiness; notify your doctor.

Stopping the drug: If you have been taking the drug for less than 2 weeks, it can be safely stopped as soon as you no longer need it. If you have been taking the drug for longer, consult your doctor, who will supervise a gradual reduction in dosage. Stopping abruptly may lead to withdrawal symptoms.

Prolonged use: Regular use of this drug over several weeks can lead to a reduction in its effect as the body adapts. It may also be habit-forming when taken for extended periods, especially if large doses are taken. Its use should be reviewed regularly.

Dependence rating: High

Overdose danger rating: Medium

❗ POSSIBLE SIDE EFFECTS AND WHAT TO DO

The main side effects are related to the drug's sedative properties and normally diminish after the first few days of treatment. If you experience **daytime drowsiness,** discuss with your doctor if bothersome. If you experience **dizziness/ unsteadiness, headache, nausea,** or **vomiting,** discuss with your doctor in all cases. Stop taking the drug now and call your doctor if you experience **confusion/disorientation, rash,** or **amnesia.**

✋ SPECIAL PRECAUTIONS

Tell your doctor if you have: severe respiratory disease; sleep apnea; impaired liver or kidney function; myasthenia gravis; glaucoma; current or previous problems with alcohol or drug abuse. **Also discuss if you are:** taking other medications.
- **Safety not established** in pregnancy.
- **Discuss** with your doctor if you are breast-feeding; the drug passes into the breast milk.
- **Not recommended** for those under 18 years.
- **Reduced dose** may be necessary for those over 60 due to increased likelihood of side effects.
- **Avoid** driving and hazardous work until you have learned how the drug affects you.
- **Avoid** alcohol as it can increase the sedative effects of this drug.

⚙️ INTERACTIONS

All **sedatives,** including alcohol, are likely to increase the sedative properties of lorazepam. Such drugs include other **anti-anxiety** and **sleeping drugs, antihistamines, antidepressants, opioid analgesics, scopolamine,** and **antipsychotics.**

Benzodiazepines may enhance the adverse effects of **clozapine.**

LOSARTAN

Product name: Cozaar
Used in the following combined preparations: Hyzaar, Hyzaar DS

❓ WHY IS THIS DRUG USED?

Losartan is a member of the group of vasodilator drugs called angiotensin-II receptor blockers. Used to treat *hypertension*, the drug works by blocking the action of angiotensin-II (a naturally occurring substance that constricts blood vessels). This action causes the blood vessel walls to relax, thereby easing blood pressure. Losartan is also used in the treatment of *heart failure* when someone is intolerant to ACE inhibitors.

ℹ INFORMATION FOR USERS

Prescription needed. Do not alter dosage without checking with your doctor.

How and when to take: Available as tablets. Take once daily.

Usual adult dosage range: 25–100mg. People over 75 years, and other groups that are especially sensitive to the drug's effects, and those with liver dysfunction, may start on 25mg.

Onset and duration of effect: *Blood pressure* Starts to work in 1–2 weeks, with maximum effect in 3–6 weeks from start of treatment; *Other conditions* Within 1 hour. Action lasts for 12–24 hours.

Diet advice: None.

Storage: Keep in a closed container in a cool, dry place out of the reach of children.

If you miss or exceed a dose: Take missed dose as soon as you remember. If your next dose is due within 8 hours, take a single dose now and skip the next. An occasional unintentional extra dose is unlikely to cause problems. Large overdoses may cause dizziness and fainting; notify your doctor.

Stopping the drug: Do not stop the drug without consulting your doctor as it may lead to worsening of the underlying condition.

Prolonged use: No special problems. Periodic checks on blood potassium levels may be performed.

Dependence rating: Low

Overdose danger rating: Medium

⚠ POSSIBLE SIDE EFFECTS AND WHAT TO DO

Side effects are usually mild. If you experience **dizziness, fatigue, migraine, diarrhea,** or **taste disturbance**, discuss with your doctor if bothersome. If you experience a **rash/itching** or **jaundice,** discuss with your doctor in all cases. Stop taking the drug now and call your doctor if you develop **wheezing** or **facial swelling**.

🖐 SPECIAL PRECAUTIONS

Tell your doctor if you have: stenosis (narrowing) of the kidney arteries; liver or kidney problems; congestive heart failure; primary aldosteronism; experienced angioedema. **Also discuss if you are:** taking other medications.
- **Not prescribed** in pregnancy (may cause fetus abnormalities) or while breast-feeding.
- **Safety not established** for infants and children.
- **Reduced dose** may be necessary for those over 75 years.
- **Avoid** driving and hazardous work until you have learned how losartan affects you as the drug can cause dizziness and fatigue.
- **Avoid** alcohol; it may raise blood pressure, reducing the effectiveness of losartan, or cause blood vessels to dilate, increasing the likelihood of an excessive fall in blood pressure.

⚙ INTERACTIONS

There is a risk of a sudden fall in blood pressure when losartan is taken with **diuretics**.
Losartan increases the effect of **potassium supplements, potassium-sparing diuretics, and cyclosporine,** leading to raised levels of potassium in the blood.
Losartan may increase the levels and toxicity of **lithium**.
Certain **non-steroidal anti-inflammatory drugs** (NSAIDs) may reduce the blood-pressure lowering effect of losartan.
Antifungal drugs may increase the level of losartan.
Many **herbs** may interfere with the effectiveness of losartan. Discuss with your pharmacist or doctor.

MAGNESIUM HYDROXIDE

Product names: Milk of Magnesia Tablets (NHP), Phillips' Milk of Magnesia
Used in the following combined preparations: Almagel 200 Ls (NHP), Diovol Plus AF, Diovol caplet and Regular Liquid Dioval Ex Extra Strength Liquid (NHP), Gelusil, and others

❓ WHY IS THIS DRUG USED?

Magnesium hydroxide is a fast-acting antacid given to neutralize stomach acid and to treat *indigestion* and heartburn. It also prevents pain caused by stomach and duodenal *ulcers*, gastritis, and reflux esophagitis, although other drugs that are more effective and convenient are preferred.

It also acts as a laxative by drawing water into the intestine from the surrounding blood vessels to soften the feces and help with *constipation*. If a laxative effect is not desired, it can be taken with aluminum hydroxide, which can cause constipation, neutralizing the laxative effects.

ℹ️ INFORMATION FOR USERS

No prescription needed. Consult your pharmacist and follow instructions on the label. Call your doctor if symptoms worsen.

How and when to take: Available as tablets, chewable tablets, liquid. Take 1–4 x daily as needed with water, preferably an hour after food and at bedtime.

Usual adult dosage range: *Antacid* 2–4 tablets as needed (up to 4 x daily); 5–15ml per dose (liquid). *Laxative* 5–20ml per dose (liquid).

Onset and duration of effect: Starts to work within 15 minutes (antacid); 2–8 hours (laxative). Action lasts for 2–4 hours.

Diet advice: None.

Storage: Keep in a closed container in a cool (but not cold), dry place out of the reach of children.

If you miss or exceed a dose: Take missed dose as soon as you remember. An occasional unintentional extra dose is unlikely to be a cause for concern. If you

notice any unusual symptoms, or if a large overdose has been taken, notify your doctor.

Stopping the drug: When used as an antacid, can be safely stopped as soon as you no longer need it. When given as ulcer treatment, follow your doctor's advice.

Prolonged use: This drug should not be used for prolonged periods without consulting your doctor. If you are over 40 years of age and are experiencing long-term indigestion or heartburn, your doctor will probably refer you to a specialist. Prolonged use in people with kidney damage may cause drowsiness, dizziness, and weakness, resulting from accumulation of magnesium in the body.

Dependence rating: Low

Overdose danger rating: Low

❗ POSSIBLE SIDE EFFECTS AND WHAT TO DO

Diarrhea is the only common side effect of this drug – discuss with your doctor if bothersome. **Dizziness** and **muscle weakness** due to

absorption of excess magnesium in the body may occur in people with poor kidney function; discuss with your doctor.

✋ SPECIAL PRECAUTIONS

Tell your doctor or pharmacist if you have: a long-term kidney problem; a bowel disorder. **Also discuss if you are:** taking other medications.
- **No evidence of risk** in pregnancy or with breast-feeding; discuss the most appropriate treatment with your doctor.
- **Not recommended** for children under 1 year except on the advice of a doctor.
- **Reduced dose** necessary for older children.
- **Avoid** excessive alcohol as it irritates the stomach and may reduce the benefits of the drug.

🔄 INTERACTIONS

Magnesium hydroxide interferes with the absorption of a wide range of drugs taken by mouth, including **tetracycline antibiotics, iron supplements, diflunisal, phenytoin**, and **penicillamine**. Discuss with your pharmacist.

As with other antacids, magnesium hydroxide may allow break-up of the **enteric coating of tablets**, sometimes leading to stomach irritation.

MEMANTINE

Product names: CO Memantine, Ebixa, PMS-Memantine, ratio-Memantine, and others
Used in the following combined preparations: None

❓ WHY IS THIS DRUG USED?

Memantine is used to treat symptoms of moderate to severe Alzheimer's disease. It may be used alone or in combination with other drugs used in this condition called cholinesterase inhibitors. It works by blocking certain receptors in the brain, thereby decreasing abnormal excitement. It can help patients in performing daily activities more easily, but does not decrease the progression of Alzheimer's disease. The dose may be gradually increased.

ℹ️ INFORMATION FOR USERS

Prescription needed. Do not alter dosage without checking with your doctor.

How and when to take: Available as tablets. Usually taken once or twice daily.

Usual adult dosage range: 5–20mg daily. Doses greater than 5mg per day should be administered twice daily.

Onset of effect: Starts to work within 8 hours. Action lasts up to 24 hours.

Diet advice: None.

Storage: Keep in a closed container in a cool, dry place out of the reach of children.

If you miss or exceed a dose: Take missed dose as soon as you remember. If it is near the time of the next dose, skip the missed dose and resume your usual dosing schedule. Do not double up to catch up on a missed dose. An occasional unintentional extra dose is unlikely to cause problems, but if you notice any unusual symptoms, or if a large overdose has been taken, notify your doctor.

Stopping the drug: Do not stop the drug without consulting your doctor as it may lead to worsening of the underlying condition.

Prolonged use: May be continued for as long as there is benefit. Stopping the drug can lead to a gradual loss of the improvements. Periodic checks may be performed to test whether the drug is still providing some benefit.

Dependence rating: Low

Overdose danger rating: Medium

❗ POSSIBLE SIDE EFFECTS AND WHAT TO DO

If you experience **headache, dizziness, tiredness/sleepiness, constipation, diarrhea,** or **loss of appetite,** discuss with your doctor if bothersome. If you experience **changes in blood pressure, blurred vision, changes in walking, balance or behaviour, palpitations** or **anxiety,** discuss with your doctor in all cases. Call your doctor now if you develop **edema.**

✋ SPECIAL PRECAUTIONS

Tell your doctor if you have: asthma; seizures; kidney disease; repeated urinary tract infections. **Also discuss if you are:** a smoker; taking other medications.
- **Safety not established** in pregnancy or breast-feeding. Discuss with your doctor.
- **Safety and effectiveness not established** for infants and children.
- **Avoid** driving and hazardous work until the effect of the drug wears off and you are mentally alert.
- **Avoid** alcohol as it may increase the effect of drowsiness.

🔄 INTERACTIONS

Memantine can decrease the amount of **hydrochlorothiazide** in the blood.
  There is a potential for interaction with **amantadine, dextromethorphan (DM),** and **ketamine,** as these drugs inhibit the same receptors as memantine.
  Cimetidine, nicotine, and **quinidine** are excreted in a similar manner to memantine in the kidneys and they can affect the levels of memantine; memantine can also affect the levels of these drugs.
  Sodium bicarbonate and **acetazolamide** can lead to an accumulation of memantine in the body.

METFORMIN

Product names: Apo-Metformin, Glucophage, Glumetza, Mylan-Metformin, and others
Used in the following combined preparations: Avadamet, Janumet

❓ WHY IS THIS DRUG USED?

Metformin is an antidiabetic drug used to treat Type 2 (adult-onset) *diabetes* in which some insulin-secreting cells are still active in the pancreas. Metformin lowers blood sugar by reducing the absorption of glucose from the digestive tract into the bloodstream, by reducing the glucose production by cells in the liver and kidneys, and by increasing the sensitivity of cells to insulin so that they take up glucose more effectively from the blood. This drug may be used in conjunction with other anti-diabetic drugs or insulin.

ℹ INFORMATION FOR USERS

Prescription needed. Do not alter dosage without checking with your doctor.

How and when to take: Available as tablets, extended release tablets. Take 1–4 x daily with food.

Usual adult dosage range: 1.5–2.5g daily, with a low dose at the start of treatment.

Onset and duration of effect: Starts to work within 2 hours. It may take 2 weeks to achieve control of diabetes. Action lasts for 8–12 hours.

Diet advice: A low-fat, low-sugar diet must be maintained in order for the drug to be fully effective.

Storage: Keep in a closed container in a cool, dry place out of the reach of children.

If you miss a dose: Take missed dose as soon as you remember. If your next dose is due within 2 hours, take a single dose now and skip the next.

Stopping the drug: Consult your doctor; stopping may lead to worsening of the underlying condition.

Prolonged use: Prolonged treatment can deplete reserves of vitamin B_{12}, and this may rarely cause anemia. Regular monitoring of kidney function and sugar (glucose) levels in the blood are usually required. Vitamin B_{12} levels may also be checked annually.

Dependence rating: Low

Overdose danger rating: High

☠ OVERDOSE ACTION

Seek immediate medical advice in all cases. Take emergency action if seizures or loss of consciousness occur.

See Drug poisoning emergency guide (p.197).

❗ POSSIBLE SIDE EFFECTS AND WHAT TO DO

Nausea, vomiting, and loss of appetite are often helped by taking the drug with food. Diarrhea usually settles after a few days of continued treatment. If you experience **loss of appetite, metallic taste, nausea, vomiting,** or **diarrhea,** discuss with your doctor if bothersome. If you experience **dizziness, confusion, weakness, sweating,** or a **rash,** discuss with your doctor in all cases.

✋ SPECIAL PRECAUTIONS

Tell your doctor if you have: long-term liver or kidney problems; heart failure. **Also discuss if you are**: a heavy drinker; taking other medications.
* **Not usually prescribed** in pregnancy.
* **Safety not established** in breast-feeding.
* **Not recommended** for infants and children.
* **Reduced dose** may be necessary for those over 60 due to increased likelihood of adverse effects.
* **Avoid** driving and hazardous work if you have warning signs of low blood sugar.
* **Avoid** alcohol; it increases the risk of low blood sugar.
* **Notify** your doctor and dentist that you are diabetic before any surgery or if you are to have a contrast X-ray.

⊙ INTERACTIONS

A number of drugs reduce the effects of metformin. These include **corticosteroids, estrogens,** and diuretics. Other drugs, notably **monoamine oxidase inhibitors** (MAOIs) **and beta blockers,** increase its effects.

Metformin may increase the effect of **warfarin;** dosage may need to be adjusted accordingly.

METHOTREXATE

Product names: Apo-Methotrexate, Methotrexate, Metoject, ratio-Methotrexate Sodium, and others
Used in the following combined preparations: None

WHY IS THIS DRUG USED?

Methotrexate is an anticancer drug used in the treatment of leukemia, lymphoma, and solid cancers such as those of the breast, bladder, head, and neck. It is also used to treat severe uncontrolled psoriasis until less potent drugs can be re-introduced, and *rheumatoid arthritis*.

Methotrexate affects both healthy and cancerous cells, and its usefulness is limited by its side effects and toxicity. High doses of methotrexate are usually given with folinic acid to prevent it from destroying bone marrow cells.

INFORMATION FOR USERS

Prescription needed. Do not alter dosage without checking with your doctor.

How and when to take: Available as tablets, injection. Take as follows: *Cancer* Single dose once weekly or every 3 weeks. *Other conditions* Usually, single dose once weekly.

Usual adult dosage range: *Cancer* Dosage tailored to each individual. *Rheumatoid arthritis* 7.5–20mg weekly. *Psoriasis* 10–25mg weekly.

Onset and duration of effect: Starts to work in 30–60 minutes. Short-term effects last 10–15 hours.

Diet advice: None.

Storage: Keep in a closed container in a cool, dry place out of the reach of children. Wash your hands after handling the tablets.

If you miss or exceed a dose: Take missed dose as soon as you remember and consult your doctor. Tell your doctor if you accidentally take an extra tablet. Large overdoses damage the bone marrow and cause nausea and abdominal pain; notify your doctor immediately.

Stopping the drug: Do not stop taking the drug without consulting your doctor as it may lead to worsening of the underlying condition.

Prolonged use: Long-term treatment with methotrexate may be needed for rheumatoid arthritis. Once the condition is controlled, the drug is reduced as much as possible to the lowest effective dose. Full blood counts and kidney and liver function tests will be performed before and during treatment. Blood concentrations of methotrexate may also be measured periodically.

Dependence rating: Low

Overdose danger rating: Medium

POSSIBLE SIDE EFFECTS AND WHAT TO DO

Nausea and vomiting may occur within a few hours of taking methotrexate. If you experience **nausea, vomiting, diarrhea, dizziness, dry cough, chest pain, headache, jaundice, mood changes**, or **confusion**, discuss with your doctor in all cases. Stop taking the drug now and call your doctor if you experience **inflammation or ulcers of the mouth/gums, sore throat, fever**, or a **rash**.

SPECIAL PRECAUTIONS

Tell your doctor if you have: liver or kidney problems; porphyria; a problem with alcohol abuse; a peptic or other digestive-tract ulcer.
Also discuss if you are: taking other medications.
• **Not prescribed** in pregnancy; methotrexate may cause birth defects in the unborn baby.
• **Not advised** while breast-feeding; the drug passes into the breast milk and may affect the baby adversely.
• **Reduced dose necessary** for infants and children; used for cancer treatment only.
• **Reduced dose necessary** for those over 60.
• **Avoid** alcohol as it may increase the adverse effects of methotrexate.

INTERACTIONS

Many drugs, including **NSAIDs, diuretics, cyclosporine, phenytoin**, and **probenecid**, may increase blood levels and toxicity of methotrexate.
   Co-trimoxazole, trimethoprim, and certain **antimalarial drugs** may enhance the effects of methotrexate.

METOPROLOL

Product names: Apo-Metoprolol (Type L), Apo-Metoprolol SR, Betaloc, Lopresor, and others
Used in the following combined preparations: None

❓ WHY IS THIS DRUG USED?

Metoprolol is a member of the beta blocker group of drugs. It is used to prevent the heart from beating too quickly in conditions such as *angina*, hypertension *(high blood pressure), arrhythmias* (abnormal heart rhythms), and hyperthyroidism (overactive thyroid gland). It is also used to prevent *migraine* attacks and to protect the heart from further damage following a *heart attack*. Metoprolol is less likely to provoke breathing difficulties than some other drugs in this class, but it should be used with caution in those who have respiratory diseases such as asthma.

ℹ️ INFORMATION FOR USERS

Prescription needed. Do not alter dosage without checking with your doctor.

How and when to take: Available as tablets, SR-tablets, injection. Take 1–2 x daily (hypertension); 2–3 x daily (angina/arrhythmias); 4 x daily for 2 days, then 2 x daily (heart attack prevention); 2 x daily (migraine prevention); 4 x daily (hyperthyroidism).

Usual adult dosage range: 100–300mg daily.

Onset and duration of effect: Starts to work in 1–2 hours. Action lasts for 3–7 hours.

Diet advice: None.

Storage: Keep in a closed container in a cool, dry place out of the reach of children.

If you miss a dose: Take as soon as you remember. For the regular tablets, if your next dose is due within 2 hours, take a single dose now and skip the next.

Stopping the drug: Consult your doctor. Stopping suddenly may lead to dangerous worsening of the underlying condition.

Prolonged use: No special problems.

Dependence rating: Low

Overdose danger rating: High

☠️ OVERDOSE ACTION

Seek immediate medical advice in all cases. Take emergency action if breathing difficulties, collapse, or loss of consciousness occur.

See Drug poisoning emergency guide (p.197).

❗ POSSIBLE SIDE EFFECTS AND WHAT TO DO

Metoprolol, like other beta blockers, may be associated with nightmares and cold fingers and toes. If you experience **cold hands and feet, nightmares, drowsiness, fatigue, dizziness,** **headache, nausea, vomiting,** or **abdominal pain,** discuss with your doctor if bothersome. Call your doctor now if you experience **breathing difficulties, wheezing,** or **fainting.**

👄 SPECIAL PRECAUTIONS

Tell your doctor if you have: liver or kidney problems; asthma, bronchitis, or emphysema; heart failure; diabetes; hyperthyroidism; pheochromocytoma; psoriasis; poor circulation in the legs. **Also discuss if you are:** taking other medications.
- **Not usually prescribed** in pregnancy; may affect the baby. Discuss with your doctor.
- **Discuss** with your doctor regarding breast-feeding; the drug passes into the breast milk, but at normal doses adverse effects to the baby are unlikely.
- **Not recommended** for infants and children.
- **Reduced dose** necessary for those over 60.
- **Avoid** driving and hazardous work until you have learned how metoprolol affects you.

➕ INTERACTIONS

In general, any drug that decreases blood pressure or slows the heart rate can have additive effects when given with metoprolol. An example is **verapamil.** Discuss with your doctor.
   Taken with metoprolol, **decongestants** may increase blood pressure and heart rate.
   Taken with metoprolol, **ergotamine** increases the constriction of blood vessels in the extremities.
   Taken with metoprolol, **antidiabetic drugs** may increase the risk or mask the symptoms of low blood sugar.
   Non-steroidal anti-inflammatory drugs (NSAIDs) may oppose the blood-pressure lowering effects of metoprolol.
   Anticholinesterase inhibitors such as donepezil, may enhance the slowing of the heart rate by metoprolol.

MIRTAZAPINE

Product names: Mylan-Mirtazapine, PMS-Mirtazapine, Remeron, Remeron RD, Teva-Mirtazapine, Teva-Mirtazapine OD, and others
Used in the following combined preparations: None

❓ WHY IS THIS DRUG USED?

Mirtazapine is an antidepressant used in the treatment of mild to moderate *depression* and is as effective as other antidepressants. It can cause drowsiness and weight gain, and may also cause a decrease in blood pressure on quickly sitting or standing up. Caution should be used; stand up slowly, while supporting yourself. It is best to take mirtazapine in the evening prior to sleep.

ℹ️ INFORMATION FOR USERS

Prescription needed. Do not alter dosage without checking with your doctor.

How and when to take: Available as tablets, RD formulation (oral disintegrating tablets). Take once daily before bedtime. The RD tablet is placed on the tongue, where it disintegrates rapidly – no water is needed for these.

Usual adult dosage range: 15–45mg.

Onset and duration of effect: Starts to work within 2 weeks of starting treatment, but full antidepressant effect may not be felt for 4–6 weeks. Action lasts up to 24 hours.

Diet advice: None.

Storage: Keep in a closed container in a cool, dry place out of the reach of children.

If you miss or exceed a dose: Take missed dose as soon as you remember. Do not double up on a dose. An occasional unintentional extra dose is unlikely to be a cause for concern. Large doses may cause drowsiness, disorientation, or impaired memory; seek medical assistance right away.

Stopping the drug: Do not stop the drug without consulting your doctor. Stopping abruptly can cause withdrawal symptoms. A gradual reduction in the dose over several weeks is recommended.

Prolonged use: No problems expected.

Dependence rating: Low

Overdose danger rating: Medium

❗ POSSIBLE SIDE EFFECTS AND WHAT TO DO

Generally well tolerated. If you experience **drowsiness, dizziness, dry mouth,** or **constipation,** discuss with your doctor if bothersome. If you experience **increased appetite, weight gain, muscle weakness, or tiredness/fatigue,** discuss with your doctor in all cases.

🕒 SPECIAL PRECAUTIONS

Tell your doctor if you have: long-term liver or kidney problems; diabetes mellitus; a heart problem; a history of seizures. **Also discuss if:** you have had a TIA or stroke, or if you are taking other medications.
- **Safety not established** in pregnancy or while breast-feeding. Discuss with your doctor.
- **Not recommended** for infants and children.
- **Reduced dose** may be necessary for those over 60.
- **Avoid** driving and hazardous work until you have learned how mirtazapine affects you because the drug can cause drowsiness.
- **Avoid** alcohol as it may increase the sedative effects of this drug.

🔄 INTERACTIONS

Diazepam and other CNS depressants will have an additive effect to the sedative effects of mirtazapine.
Mirtazapine should not be used with **monoamine oxidase inhibitors** (MOAIs) or within 14 days of stopping an MAOI.
St. John's wort may increase the risk of side effects of mirtazapine.

MORPHINE

Product names: Kadian, M.O.S., M.O.S. Sulfate, MS Contin, MS IR, PMS-Morphine sulfate SR, Statex, Teva-Morphine SR, and others
Used in the following combined preparations: None

WHY IS THIS DRUG USED?

Morphine is an opioid analgesic and is used to relieve moderate to severe *pain* that can be caused by *heart attack*, injury, surgery, or chronic diseases such as cancer. It is sometimes given as premedication before surgery. Its painkilling effect wears off quickly, and it may be given in a special slow-release (long-acting) form to relieve continuous severe pain. Morphine is habit-forming, and dependence can occur. When used as prescribed for a specific pain condition, addiction rarely occurs.

INFORMATION FOR USERS

Prescription needed. Do not alter your dosage without checking with your doctor.

How and when to take: Available as tablets, extended release tablets, capsules, SR-capsules, liquid, injection, suppositories. Take every 4 hours; every 12–24 hours (SR-preparations).

Usual adult dosage range: 5–25mg per dose; however, some patients may need 75mg or more per dose. Doses vary considerably for each individual.

Onset and duration of effect: Starts to work within 1 hour; within 4 hours (SR-preparations). Action lasts for 4 hours; up to 24 hours (SR-preparations).

Diet advice: None.

Storage: Keep in a closed container in a cool, dry place out of the reach of children.

If you miss a dose: Take as soon as you remember. Return to your normal dosing schedule as soon as possible.

Stopping the drug: If the reason for taking the drug no longer exists, you may stop the drug in consultation with your doctor.

Prolonged use: The effects of this drug usually become weaker during prolonged use as the body adapts. Dependence may occur if it is taken for extended periods. Addiction is unusual in patients taking the correct dose for pain relief.

Dependence rating: High

Overdose danger rating: High

OVERDOSE ACTION

Seek immediate medical advice in all cases. Take emergency action if symptoms such as slow or irregular breathing, severe drowsiness, or loss of consciousness occur.

See Drug poisoning emergency guide (p.197).

POSSIBLE SIDE EFFECTS AND WHAT TO DO

Nausea, vomiting, and constipation are common, especially with high doses. If you experience **drowsiness, nausea, vomiting,** or **constipation,** discuss with your doctor if bothersome. If you experience **dizziness** or **confusion,** discuss with your doctor in all cases. Stop taking the drug now and call your doctor if you develop **breathing difficulties**.

SPECIAL PRECAUTIONS

Tell your doctor if you have: long-term liver or kidney problems; heart or circulatory problems; a lung disorder such as asthma or bronchitis; thyroid disease; a history of epileptic seizures; chronic heavy alcohol use; addiction problems.
Also discuss if you are: taking other medications.
- **Not prescribed in** pregnancy. The drug passes into the breast milk while breast-feeding. Discuss with your doctor.
- **Reduced dose** necessary for infants and children, and possibly for those over 60.
- **Avoid** alcohol as it may increase the sedative effects of this drug.

INTERACTIONS

Monoamine oxidase inhibitors (MAOIs) may produce a severe rise in blood pressure when taken with morphine.
The effects of **esmolol** may be increased by morphine.
Morphine increases the sedative effects of other sedating drugs including **antidepressants, antipsychotics, sleeping drugs,** and **antihistamines**.
Rifampin may decrease morphine levels.

NAPROXEN

Product names: Aleve, Anaprox, Anaprox-DS, Naprosyn SR, PMS Naproxen, and others
Used in the following combined preparations: None

❓ WHY IS THIS DRUG USED?

Naproxen is a non-steroidal anti-inflammatory drug (NSAID), and is used to reduce *pain*, stiffness, and inflammation. The drug relieves the symptoms of adult and juvenile *rheumatoid arthritis*, ankylosing spondylitis, and *osteoarthritis*, although it does not cure the underlying disease. It is also used to treat acute attacks of gout, and may sometimes be prescribed for the relief of *migraine*, menstrual cramps, and pain following orthopedic surgery, dental treatment, strains, and sprains.

ℹ INFORMATION FOR USERS

Prescription needed for some products. Do not alter dosage without checking with your doctor.

How and when to take: Available as tablets, enteric coated tablets, SR-tablets (extended release), liquid, suppositories. Take every 6–8 hours as required (general pain relief); 1–2 x daily (muscular pain and arthritis); every 8 hours (gout). Take with food.

Usual adult dosage range: *Mild to moderate pain, menstrual cramps* 500mg (starting dose), then 250mg every 6–8 hours as required. *Muscular pain and arthritis* 500–1,250mg daily. *Gout* 750mg (starting dose), then 250mg every 8 hours until attack has subsided.

Onset and duration of effect: Pain relief begins within 1 hour. Full anti-inflammatory effect may take 2 weeks. Action lasts up to 12 hours.

Diet advice: None.

Storage: Keep in a closed container in a cool, dry place out of the reach of children. Protect from light.

If you miss or exceed a dose: Take missed dose as soon as you remember. If your next dose is due within 4 hours, take a single dose now and skip the next. An occasional unintentional extra dose is unlikely to be a cause for concern. If you notice any unusual symptoms, or if a large overdose has been taken, notify your doctor.

Stopping the drug: When taken short-term, naproxen can be safely stopped as soon as you no longer need it. Otherwise, seek medical advice before stopping.

Prolonged use: Increased risk of bleeding from peptic ulcers and in the bowel when naproxen is used long term.

Dependence rating: Low

Overdose danger rating: Medium

❗ POSSIBLE SIDE EFFECTS AND WHAT TO DO

If you experience **nausea, stomach upset or heartburn, headache,** or **inability to concentrate,** discuss with your doctor if bothersome. If you develop other **gastrointestinal side effects, ringing in the ears** or **swollen feet/ankles,** discuss with your doctor in all cases. Stop taking the drug now, call your doctor and get immediate help if you experience **rash/itching, wheezing, breathlessness,** or **black/bloodstained feces.**

🖐 SPECIAL PRECAUTIONS

Tell your doctor if you have: long-term liver or kidney problems; heart problems; a bleeding disorder; high blood pressure; a history of peptic ulcers, esophagitis, or acid indigestion; asthma. **Also discuss if you are:** allergic to ASA; taking other NSAIDs, or other medications.
- **Not usually prescribed** in pregnancy. The drug passes into breast milk; discuss with your doctor.
- **Reduced dose** necessary for infants and children; prescribed only to treat juvenile arthritis.
- **Reduced dose** may be necessary for those over 60.
- **Avoid** driving and hazardous work until you have learned how naproxen affects you.
- **Avoid** excessive intake of alcohol; it may increase the risk of stomach irritation with naproxen.
- **Discuss** with your doctor or dentist before surgery; naproxen may prolong bleeding.

✳ INTERACTIONS

Naproxen interacts with a wide range of drugs to increase the risk of bleeding and/or peptic ulcers.
  Naproxen may also increase the blood levels of **lithium, methotrexate,** and **digoxin** to an undesirable extent.
  The beneficial effects of **antihypertensive drugs** and **diuretics** may be reduced by naproxen.

NICOTINE

Product names: Habitrol, Nicoderm, Nicorette, Nicorette Gum, and others
Used in the following combined preparations: None

❓ WHY IS THIS DRUG USED?

Nicotine treatment is used to aid smoking cessation for the relief of nicotine withdrawal symptoms caused by *tobacco addiction*. Nicotine comes in the form of chewing gum, lozenges, skin patches, or an inhaler. The patches should be applied every 24 hours to unbroken, dry, and non-hairy skin on the trunk or the upper arm. Replacement patches should be placed on a different area, and the same area of application avoided for several days. The chewing gum is used whenever the urge to smoke occurs; the inhaler is prescribed according to individual requirements.

ℹ️ INFORMATION FOR USERS

No prescription needed. Follow instructions on the label and consult with your pharmacist. Call your doctor if symptoms worsen.

How and when to take: Available as skin patch, chewing gum, lozenge, inhaler. Take every 24 hours, removing the patch after 16 hours (patches); when the urge to smoke is felt (gum, lozenges); 6–12 cartridges per day (inhaler).

Usual adult dosage range: Will depend on your previous smoking habits. 7–22mg per day (patches); 1 x 2mg piece to 15 x 4mg pieces per day (gum); 1 lozenge every 1.5–8 hours, max 15 per day; dose individualized (inhaler).

Onset and duration of effect: Starts to work in a few hours (patches); within minutes (gum, lozenge). Gum is chewed slowly for up to 30 minutes. Lozenge allowed to dissolve slowly over 20–30 minutes. Action lasts up to 24 hours for patches.

Diet advice: None.

Storage: Keep in a cool, dry place out of the reach of children.

If you miss or exceed a dose: Change your patch as soon as you remember, and keep the new patch on for the required amount of time before removing it. Application of several nicotine patches at the same time could result in serious overdosage. Remove the patches and seek immediate medical help. Overdosage with the gum can occur only if many pieces of gum are chewed simultaneously. Seek immediate medical help.

Stopping the drug: The dose of nicotine is normally reduced gradually.

Prolonged use: Nicotine replacement therapy should not normally be used for more than three months.

Dependence rating: Low

Overdose danger rating: Medium

❗ POSSIBLE SIDE EFFECTS AND WHAT TO DO

Any skin reaction to patches will usually disappear in a couple of days. The chewing gum may cause local irritation of the throat or nose and increased salivation. If you experience **local irritation,** **headache, dizziness, nausea, cold/flu-like symptoms, insomnia** or **indigestion,** discuss with your doctor or pharmacist if bothersome.

👆 SPECIAL PRECAUTIONS

Tell your doctor or pharmacist if you have: long-term liver or kidney problems; diabetes mellitus; thyroid disease; circulation problems; heart problems; a peptic ulcer; pheochromocytoma; any skin disorders. **Also discuss if you are:** taking other medications.
- **Do not use** nicotine in any form during pregnancy or while breast-feeding.
- **Do not administer** to infants and children.

⚙️ INTERACTIONS

Nicotine patches and chewing gum should not be used with **other nicotine-containing products,** including cigarettes.

Stopping smoking may increase the blood levels of some drugs (such as **warfarin** and **theophylline/aminophylline**). Discuss with your doctor or pharmacist.

Cimetidine may increase nicotine levels.

NITROGLYCERIN

Product names: Nitro-Dur, Nitrol, Nitrolingual Pumpspray, Transderm-Nitro, and others
Used in the following combined preparations: None

❓ WHY IS THIS DRUG USED?

Nitroglycerin is a vasodilator that is used to relieve the pain of *angina* attacks. It is available in short-acting forms (sublingual tablets and spray) and in long-acting forms (slow-release tablets and skin patches). The short-acting forms act very quickly to relieve angina. Nitroglycerin is also given by injection in hospital for anginal pain. The drug is best taken for the first time while sitting, as fainting may follow the drop in blood pressure caused by the drug.

ℹ️ INFORMATION FOR USERS

Generally prescribed by a medical practitioner. Do not alter dosage without checking with your doctor.

How and when to take: Available as sublingual tablets, injection, ointment, transdermal skin patches, sublingual metered-dose spray. Take as follows: *Prevention* once daily (patches); every 3–4 hours (ointment). *Relief* Use sublingual tablets or spray at the onset of an attack. Dose may be repeated twice in 5 minute intervals if further relief is required. If symptoms persist after 3 doses used over 15 minutes, seek immediate medical help. The relief medication (tablets or spray) can be used immediately prior to exercise.

Usual adult dosage range: *Prevention* 0.2–0.8mg/hr daily (patches); as directed (ointment). *Relief* 0.3–1mg per dose (sublingual tablets); 1–2 sprays per dose (spray).

Onset and duration of effect: Starts to work within minutes (sublingual tablets and spray); 1–3 hours (SR-tablets, patches, and ointment). Action lasts for 20–30 minutes (sublingual tablets and spray); 3–5 hours (ointment); up to 24 hours (patches).

Diet advice: None.

Storage: Keep sublingual tablets in a tightly closed glass container fitted with a foil-lined, screw-on cap in a cool, dry place out of the reach of children. Protect from light. Do not expose to heat. Discard tablets within 3 months of opening. Check label of other preparations for storage conditions.

If you miss or exceed a dose: Take missed dose as soon as you remember, or when needed. If your next dose is due within 2 hours, take a single dose now and skip the next. An occasional unintentional extra dose is unlikely to cause problems. Large overdoses may cause dizziness, vomiting, severe headache, seizures, or loss of consciousness; notify your doctor.

Stopping the drug: Do not stop taking the drug without consulting your doctor.

Prolonged use: The effects of the drug usually become slightly weaker during prolonged use as the body adapts; timing of the doses may need to be changed. To ensure continued effectiveness, the 3 daily doses are recommended to be taken 6 hours apart. Periodic checks on blood pressure are usually required.

Dependence rating: Low

Overdose danger rating: Medium

❗ POSSIBLE SIDE EFFECTS AND WHAT TO DO

The most serious side effect is **lowered blood pressure,** and this may need to be monitored periodically. If you experience **headache** or **flushing,** discuss with your doctor if severe. If you experience **dizziness,** discuss with your doctor in all cases.

✋ SPECIAL PRECAUTIONS

Tell your doctor if you have: any other heart condition; a lung condition; long-term liver or kidney problems; any blood disorders; glaucoma; thyroid disease. **Also discuss if you are:** taking other medications.
- **Safety not established** in pregnancy and breast-feeding.
- **Not usually prescribed** for infants and children.
- **Avoid** driving and hazardous work until you have learned how nitroglycerin affects you.
- **Avoid** excessive intake of alcohol as it may increase dizziness due to lowered blood pressure.

🔄 INTERACTIONS

Antihypertensive drugs increase the possibility of lowered blood pressure or fainting when taken with nitroglycerin.
The hypotensive effect of nitroglycerin is increased significantly by **sildenafil, vardenafil,** and **tadalafil.** Nitroglycerin should not be used with these drugs.

NORFLOXACIN

Product names: Apo-Norflox, Co-Norfloxacin, Novo-Floxacin, PMS-Norfloxacin, and Riva-Norfloxacin
Used in the following combined preparations: None

❓ WHY IS THIS DRUG USED?

Norfloxacin, a quinolone antibiotic, is effective against several types of bacteria that tend to be resistant to older, more commonly used antibiotics. It is particularly effective against bacteria responsible for *urinary tract infections*.

Norfloxacin is generally well tolerated, but those with a history of allergies to quinolone antibiotics are not usually given this drug.

ℹ INFORMATION FOR USERS

Prescription needed. Do not alter dosage without checking with your doctor.

How and when to take: Available as tablets. Take 2 x daily at least 1 hour before or 2 hours after meals.

Usual adult dosage range: 800mg daily for 7–10 days (acute infections); less frequent doses of 400mg daily is used if kidney function is impaired.

Onset and duration of effect: Starts to work in 1–2 days. Action lasts 12–24 hours.

Diet advice: Do not get dehydrated. Ensure that you drink fluids regularly.

Storage: Keep in a closed container in a cool, dry place out of the reach of children.

If you miss or exceed a dose: Take missed dose as soon as you remember. If your next dose is due within 4 hours, take a single dose now and skip the next. An occasional unintentional extra dose is unlikely to cause problems. If you notice any unusual symptoms, or if a large overdose has been taken, notify your doctor.

Stopping the drug: Take the full course. The original infection may recur if treatment is stopped too soon.

Prolonged use: No problems expected.

Dependence rating: Low

Overdose danger rating: Medium

❗ POSSIBLE SIDE EFFECTS AND WHAT TO DO

If you experience **nausea/vomiting, dizziness/ lightheadedness, headache, drowsiness,** or **fatigue,** discuss with your doctor if bothersome.

Discuss with your doctor in all cases if you develop a **rash/itching** or a **light sensitive rash**.

✋ SPECIAL PRECAUTIONS

Tell your doctor if you have: impaired kidney function; a history of epileptic seizures. **Also discuss if you are:** allergic to quinolone antibiotics; taking other medications.
* **Safety not established** in pregnancy or breast-feeding. Discuss with your doctor.
* **Not recommended** for infants and children.
* **Reduced dose** may be necessary for those over 60.
* **Avoid** driving and hazardous work until you have learned how the drug affects you; it can cause dizziness, drowsiness, and blurred vision.
* **Avoid** alcohol as it may increase the sedative effects of this drug.

⚙ INTERACTIONS

Norfloxacin may increase the anticoagulant action of **oral anticoagulants such as warfarin.**
Norfloxacin may increase the adverse effects of **theophylline, nilotinib, thioridazine, pimozide, quinine,** and **ziprasidone.**
Norfloxacin may increase the blood levels of **cyclosporine.**
Norfloxacin may increase the effects of **caffeine:** avoid excessive intake.
Antacids, iron, and **sucralfate** decrease the absorption of norfloxacin. Avoid taking these within 2 hours of each other.
Probenecid may increase levels of norfloxacin.

OLANZAPINE

Product names: Apo-Olanzapine, CO-Olanzapine, PMS-Olanzapine, PMS-Olanzapine ODT, Teva-Olanzapine, Teva-Olanzapine OD, Zyprexa, Zyprexa Intramuscular, Zyprexa Zydis, and others
Used in the following combined preparations: None

❓ WHY IS THIS DRUG USED?

Olanzapine is an antipsychotic drug prescribed for the treatment of schizophrenia and mania. In schizophrenia, the drug can be used to treat both positive symptoms (delusions, hallucinations, and thought disorders) and negative symptoms (blunted affect, emotional and social withdrawal). In mania, olanzapine can be used alone or in combination with other drugs. The drug stays in the body longer in women, non-smokers, and the elderly, so a lower dosage may be used.

ℹ INFORMATION FOR USERS

Prescription needed. Do not alter dosage without checking with your doctor.

How and when to take: Available as tablets, oral disintegrating tablets, and injection. Take once daily.

Usual adult dosage range: *Schizophrenia* 10mg (starting dose). *Mania* 15mg if used alone or 10mg if used in combination with other drugs (starting dose). For both conditions, the dose can be adjusted between 5mg and 20mg daily.

Onset and duration of effect: Starts to work in 4–8 hours. Action lasts 30–38 hours, but longer in women and in the elderly.

Diet advice: None.

Storage: Keep in a closed container in a cool, dry place out of the reach of children. Protect from light.

If you miss or exceed a dose: Take missed as soon as you remember. If your next dose is due within 8 hours take a single dose now and skip the next. An occasional unintentional extra dose is unlikely to cause problems. Large overdoses may cause unusual drowsiness, depressed breathing, and low blood pressure; notify your doctor.

Stopping the drug: Do not stop the drug without consulting your doctor; symptoms may recur.

Prolonged use: Prolonged use of olanzapine may, rarely, cause tardive dyskinesia, in which there are involuntary movements of the tongue and face.

Dependence rating: Low

Overdose danger rating: Medium

❗ POSSIBLE SIDE EFFECTS AND WHAT TO DO

If you experience **unusual drowsiness** or **weight gain**, discuss with your doctor if severe. If you experience **dizziness, fainting, Parkinsonism,** or **persistent sore throat**, discuss with your doctor in all cases. Call your doctor now if you develop **sudden weakness/numbness,** or **speech or vision problems**.

🚫 SPECIAL PRECAUTIONS

Tell your doctor if you have: an enlarged prostate; kidney or liver problems; diabetes; glaucoma; epilepsy. **Also discuss if you are:** taking other medications.
- **Safety not established** in pregnancy and breast-feeding. Discuss with your doctor.
- **Not recommended** for infants and children.
- **Reduced dose** necessary for those over 60, due to a higher risk of serious effects, including death, reported in those with dementia.
- **Avoid** driving and hazardous work as the drug can cause unusual drowsiness.
- **Avoid** alcohol as it increases the sedative effects of this drug.

⚙ INTERACTIONS

Sedatives that affect the central nervous system may increase the sedative effects of olanzapine.
  Olanzapine opposes the effect of **anticonvulsant drugs**.
  Carbamazepine, phenytoin, and **rifampin** decrease the effect of olanzapine.
  There is an increased risk of arrhythmias when certain **anti-arrhythmics** are used with olanzapine.
  Diltiazem, fluvoxamine, and **paroxetine** may increase the effect of olanzapine.

OSELTAMIVIR

Product name: Tamiflu
Used in the following combined preparations: None

WHY IS THIS DRUG USED?

Oseltamivir is an antiviral drug used to treat *influenza* (flu), a virus that infects and multiplies in the lungs. It helps to clear flu symptoms and may shorten the duration of the illness, and is also used to prevent influenza in those who have had close contact with the virus. Oseltamivir is not a substitute for flu vaccination, but is used to treat at-risk individuals, for example the elderly and those with long-term illnesses such as chronic heart and lung disease.

INFORMATION FOR USERS

Prescription needed. Do not alter dosage without checking with your doctor.

How and when to take: Available as capsules, suspension. Take once or twice daily.

Usual dosage range: *Treatment of influenza* 13 years of age or older, 75mg twice daily for 5 days. *Prevention* 75mg once daily for up to 14 days. For children 1–12 years of age, dose is based on the weight of the child.

Onset and duration of effect: Starts to work within 7 days. Action lasts up to 12 hours.

Diet advice: May be taken with or without food. Taking it with food may make it easier to tolerate the medication.

Storage: *Capsules* Keep in a closed container in a cool, dry place out of the reach of children. *Suspension* Store in refrigerator at 2–8°C. Suspension should be shaken well before use.

If you miss or exceed a dose: Take missed dose as soon as you remember. If it is near the time of the next dose, skip the missed dose and resume your usual dosing schedule. Do not double up to catch up on a missed dose. An occasional unintentional extra dose is unlikely to cause problems. If you notice any unusual symptoms, or if a large overdose has been taken, notify your doctor.

Stopping the drug: Do not stop the drug without consulting your doctor; symptoms may recur.

Prolonged use: This drug should only be used for 5 days for treatment or for the appropriate recommended duration for prevention. Not prescribed for long-term use.

Dependence rating: Low

Overdose danger rating: Low

POSSIBLE SIDE EFFECTS AND WHAT TO DO

Side effects are uncommon, and may sometimes be caused by the influenza virus rather than oseltamivir. If you experience **nausea, vomiting, dizziness, abdominal pain,** or **headache,** discuss with your doctor if bothersome. Call your doctor now if you develop a **rash, mood changes,** or **abnormal behaviour**.

SPECIAL PRECAUTIONS

Tell your doctor if you have: a previous allergic reaction to oseltamivir; a long-term illness; poor immunity to infections; kidney problems or kidney disease. **Also discuss if you are:** on any other medications.
• **Safety not established** in pregnancy.
• **Not to be used** by women who are breast-feeding children less than one year of age. Discuss with your doctor.
• **Not recommended** in children less than one year of age. For all children, discuss follow-up with your doctor.

INTERACTIONS

When oseltamivir is used in a patient on **warfarin,** more close monitoring of the effect of warfarin, as measured by INR, is recommended.
Oseltamivir may decrease the effect of **influenza virus vaccine**.
Probenecid may increase the level of oseltamivir; may require dose adjustment.

OXYCODONE

Product names: OxyContin, Oxy.IR, PMS Oxycodone, Supeudol
Used in the following combined preparations: Endocet, Percocet, Percocet-Demi, Ratio-Oxycodan, Rivacocet, and others

WHY IS THIS DRUG USED?

Oxycodone is an opioid analgesic and is used to relieve moderate to severe *pain*. An extended-release formulation is used when continuous pain relief is required, such as with cancer-related pain. If given continuously for severe pain, breakthrough pain medication should be made available.

Oxycodone is also available in combination with acetaminophen or ASA, which may provide additional analgesic benefit. Oxycodone should be used cautiously in those with compromised respiratory function.

INFORMATION FOR USERS

Prescription needed. Do not alter your dosage without checking with your doctor.

How and when to take: Available as tablets, extended-release tablets. Extended-release tablets should be swallowed whole and not chewed or crushed. Take every 6 hours (immediate release); every 12 hours (extended-release).

Usual adult dosage range: 5–40mg per day; however, some may need higher doses. Doses vary considerably for each individual.

Onset and duration of effect: Peak drug action at about 3 hours. Action lasts for 6 hours (immediate-release); 12 hours (extended-release).

Diet advice: None.

Storage: Keep in a closed container in a cool, dry place out of the reach of children.

If you miss a dose: Take as soon as you remember. Do not double up on your dose. Return to your normal dosing schedule as soon as possible.

Stopping the drug: If the reason for taking the drug no longer exists, you may stop the drug in consultation with your doctor. A gradual decrease in dose may minimize withdrawal effects.

Prolonged use: The effects of this drug usually become weaker during prolonged use as the body adapts. Dependence may occur if it is taken for extended periods. Addiction is unusual in patients taking the correct dose under medical supervision for pain relief.

Dependence rating: High

Overdose danger rating: High

☠ OVERDOSE ACTION

Seek immediate medical advice in all cases. Take emergency action if symptoms such as slow or irregular breathing, severe drowsiness, or loss of consciousness occur.

See Drug poisoning emergency guide (p.197).

❗ POSSIBLE SIDE EFFECTS AND WHAT TO DO

Nausea, vomiting, and constipation are common, especially with high doses. If you experience **drowsiness, nausea/vomiting,** or **constipation,** discuss with your doctor if bothersome. If you experience **dizziness** or **confusion,** discuss with your doctor in all cases. Stop taking the drug now and call your doctor if you develop **breathing difficulties**.

⬛ SPECIAL PRECAUTIONS

Tell your doctor if you have: long-term liver or kidney problems; heart or circulatory problems; a lung disorder such as asthma or bronchitis; thyroid disease; a history of epileptic fits; chronic heavy alcohol use. **Also discuss if you are:** taking other medications.
- **Not usually prescribed** in pregnancy.
- **Discuss** with your doctor if you are breast-feeding as the drug passes into the breast milk.
- **Reduced dose** necessary for children and for those over 60. Discuss use with your doctor.
- **Avoid** alcohol; it may increase sedation.

⊙ INTERACTIONS

Monoamine oxidase inhibitors (MAOIs) may produce a severe rise in blood pressure when taken with oxycodone.
Oxycodone increases the sedative effects of other sedating drugs including **antidepressants, antipsychotics, sleeping drugs,** and **antihistamines.**
Clarithromycin, itraconazole, and **ketoconazole** may increase oxycodone levels.

PANTOPRAZOLE

Product names: Apo-Pantoprazole, CO Pantoprazole, Mylan-Pantoprazole, Novo-Pantoprazole, PANTO IV, Pantoloc, and others
Used in the following combined preparations: None

❓ WHY IS THIS DRUG USED?

Pantoprazole is an anti-ulcer drug that reduces the amount of acid produced by the stomach. It is used to treat stomach and duodenal *ulcers* as well as *reflux esophagitis*, a condition in which acid from the stomach rises into the esophagus. It may also be used to prevent gastroduodenal ulceration sometimes caused by non-steroidal anti-inflammatory drugs (NSAIDs).

Pantoprazole may be given with antibiotics to eradicate the Helicobacter pylori bacteria that cause many gastric ulcers. As with other anti-ulcer drugs, it may mask signs of stomach cancer, so it is used only when the possibility of this disease has been ruled out.

ℹ️ INFORMATION FOR USERS

Prescription needed. Do not alter dosage without checking with your doctor.

How and when to take: Available as enteric-coated tablets, delayed-release tablets, injection. Tablets should be swallowed whole and not chewed or crushed. Take once daily in the morning.

Usual adult dosage range: 20–40mg daily, usually taken in the morning.

Onset and duration of effect: Starts to work in 1–3 hours. Action lasts 24 hours.

Diet advice: None, although spicy foods and alcohol may exacerbate the underlying condition.

Storage: Keep in a closed container in a cool, dry place out of the reach of children.

If you miss or exceed a dose: Take missed dose as soon as you remember. If your next dose is within 8 hours, take a single dose now and skip the next. An occasional unintentional extra dose is unlikely to be a cause for concern. If you notice any unusual symptoms, or if a large overdose has been taken, notify your doctor.

Stopping the drug: Do not stop the drug without consulting your doctor; symptoms may recur.

Prolonged use: No problems expected.

Dependence rating: Low

Overdose danger rating: Low

❗ POSSIBLE SIDE EFFECTS AND WHAT TO DO

Side effects such as diarrhea are usually mild, and often diminish with continued use of the drug. If you experience **diarrhea, nausea, vomiting, constipation, headaches,** or **dizziness,** discuss with your doctor if bothersome. Stop taking the drug now and call your doctor if you develop a **rash.**

✋ SPECIAL PRECAUTIONS

Tell your doctor if you have: liver problems; a history of allergic reaction to pantoprazole; unexplained weight loss, nausea, or dark stools.
Also discuss if you are: taking other medications.
• **Safety not established** in pregnancy or breast-feeding. Discuss with your doctor.
• **Not recommended** for infants and children.
• **Avoid** alcohol as it may aggravate your underlying condition and reduce the beneficial effects of this drug.

🔄 INTERACTIONS

By decreasing stomach acidity, pantoprazole may decrease the absorption of **ketoconazole, itraconazole, posaconazole,** and **iron salts.**
    Pantoprazole may increase the effects of **warfarin** and may require close monitoring.
    Pantoprazole may decrease the effectiveness of **atazanavir, clopidogrel, nelfinavir, erlotinib, delavirdine,** and **other drugs.**

PAROXETINE

Product names: Apo-Paroxetine, Mylan-Paroxetine, Paxil, Paxil CR, PMS-Paroxetine, Teva-Paroxetine, and others
Used in the following combined preparations: None

WHY IS THIS DRUG USED?

Paroxetine is an antidepressant drug used in the treatment of mild to moderate *depression*. It helps control the *anxiety* often accompanying depression. It is also used to treat generalized anxiety disorder, social phobia, panic disorder, and obsessive-compulsive disorders. Compared with the older tricyclic antidepressants, paroxetine and similar drugs are less likely to cause anticholinergic side effects such as dry mouth, blurred vision, and difficulty in passing urine. They are also much less dangerous if taken in overdose.

INFORMATION FOR USERS

Prescription needed. Do not alter dosage without checking with your doctor.

How and when to take: Available as tablets, extended release tablets. Take once daily, preferably in the morning.

Usual adult dosage range: 10–60mg daily.

Onset and duration of effect: The onset of therapeutic response usually occurs within 7–14 days of starting treatment, but full antidepressant effect may not be felt for 4 weeks. Action lasts up to 24 hours.

Diet advice: None.

Storage: Keep in a closed container in a cool, dry place out of the reach of children.

If you miss or exceed a dose: Take missed dose as soon as you remember. An occasional unintentional extra dose is unlikely to be a cause for concern. Large doses may cause unusual drowsiness. Notify your doctor immediately.

Stopping the drug: Do not stop the drug without consulting your doctor. Stopping abruptly can cause withdrawal symptoms.

Prolonged use: Withdrawal symptoms may occur if the drug is not stopped gradually. Such symptoms include dizziness, electric shock sensations, anxiety, nausea, and insomnia. These rarely last for more than 1–2 weeks.

Dependence rating: Low

Overdose danger rating: Medium

POSSIBLE SIDE EFFECTS AND WHAT TO DO

If you experience **nausea, sweating, drowsiness, dizziness, sexual dysfunction** (both sexes), **diarrhea,** discuss with your doctor only if severe. If you experience **nervousness, anxiety, agitation, poor appetite,** or **weight loss,** discuss with your doctor in all cases. Stop taking the drug now and call your doctor if you develop **rash, itching, hives, joint pain,** or **convulsions.**

SPECIAL PRECAUTIONS

Tell your doctor if you have: long-term liver or kidney problems; a heart problem; a history or a family history of seizures. **Also discuss if you are:** taking other medications.
- **Safety not established** in pregnancy. Discuss with your doctor.
- **Discuss** with your doctor if you are breast-feeding as the drug passes into the breast milk.
- **Not recommended** for those under 18 years.
- **Reduced dose** may be necessary for those over 60 due to increased likelihood of adverse effects.
- **Avoid** driving and hazardous work until you have learned how paroxetine affects you because the drug can cause drowsiness.
- **Avoid** alcohol as it may increase the sedative effects of this drug.

INTERACTIONS

Any drug that affects the breakdown of others in the liver may alter blood levels of paroxetine or vice versa.
Paroxetine may increase the effects of **anticoagulants**.
All **sedatives** are likely to increase the sedative effects of paroxetine.
Paroxetine may increase the toxicity of **tricyclic antidepressants**.
Paroxetine should not be taken during or within 14 days of **monoamine oxidase inhibitor** (MAOI) treatment because serious reactions may occur.

PHENYTOIN/FOSPHENYTOIN

Product names: Cerebyx (fosphenytoin), Dilantin, and others
Used in the following combined preparations: None

❓ WHY IS THIS DRUG USED?

Phenytoin decreases the likelihood of convulsions by reducing abnormal electrical discharges within the brain. It is prescribed for the treatment of epilepsy, including tonic/clonic and temporal lobe epilepsy. Fosphenytoin (Cerebryx) is a new type of phenytoin given by injection for control of seizures, if oral therapy is not temporarily possible. It is recommended that patients remain on the same brand of phenytoin.

ℹ️ INFORMATION FOR USERS

Prescription needed. Do not alter dosage without checking with your doctor.

How and when to take: Available as tablets, chewable tablets, extended release capsules, liquid, injection. Take 1–3 x daily with food or plenty of water. Once daily (extended release capsules).

Usual dosage range: *Adults* 100–500mg daily. *Children* According to age and weight.

Onset and duration of effect: Full anticonvulsant effect may not be felt for 7–10 days. Action lasts for 24 hours.

Diet advice: Folic acid and vitamin D deficiency may occasionally occur while taking this drug. Make sure you eat a balanced diet containing fresh, green vegetables.

Storage: Keep in a tightly closed container in a cool, dry place out of the reach of children.

If you miss or exceed a dose: Take missed dose as soon as you remember. An occasional, unintentional extra dose is unlikely to cause problems. If you notice excessive drowsiness, slurred speech, or confusion, notify your doctor.

Stopping the drug: Do not stop the drug without consulting your doctor; symptoms may recur.

Prolonged use: There is a slight risk of blood abnormalities, and adverse effects on skin, gums, and bones. It may also disrupt control of diabetes. Periodic blood tests may be performed to monitor levels of the drug in the body.

Dependence rating: Low

Overdose danger rating: Medium

❗ POSSIBLE SIDE EFFECTS AND WHAT TO DO

Phenytoin has a number of side effects, many of which appear only after prolonged use. If you experience **confusion, nausea, vomiting, insomnia,** or **increased body hair,** discuss with your doctor if bothersome. If you experience **dizziness, headache,** or **overgrowth of gums,** discuss with your doctor in all cases. Call your doctor now if you develop a **rash, fever, sore throat,** or **mouth ulcers.**

✋ SPECIAL PRECAUTIONS

Tell your doctor if you have: long-term liver or kidney problems; diabetes; porphyria. **Also discuss if you are:** taking other medications.
* **Discuss** with your doctor if you are pregnant; the drug may adversely affect the baby.
* **Discuss** with your doctor if you are breast-feeding; the drug passes into the breast milk.
* **Reduced dose necessary** for infants and children, and possibly for those over 60.
* **Discuss** with your doctor regarding driving and hazardous work; your underlying condition, as well as the effects of phenytoin, may make such activities inadvisable.
* **Avoid** alcohol as it will increase the sedative effects of this drug.

🔄 INTERACTIONS

Many drugs may interact with phenytoin, causing either an increase or a reduction in the phenytoin blood level. The dosage of phenytoin may need to be adjusted by your doctor.
   Blood levels of **cyclosporine** may be reduced with phenytoin.
   Phenytoin may reduce effectiveness of **oral contraceptives**.
   Antidepressants, antipsychotics, mefloquine, chloroquine, and **St John's wort** may reduce the effect of phenytoin.
   The anticoagulant effect of **warfarin** may be altered. An adjustment in its dosage may be necessary.

PRAVASTATIN

Product names: Apo-Pravastatin, Mylan-Pravastatin, Pravachol, Teva-Pravastatin, and others
Used in the following combined preparation: Pravasa

❓ WHY IS THIS DRUG USED?

Pravastatin is a lipid-lowering drug that blocks the action, in the liver, of an enzyme that is needed for the manufacture of cholesterol. As a result, blood levels of cholesterol are lowered. It is prescribed for people with *hypercholesterolemia* (high levels of cholesterol in the blood) who have not responded to other treatments, such as a special diet, and who are at risk of developing heart disease. Pravastatin is taken at night when most cholesterol is produced.

ℹ️ INFORMATION FOR USERS

Prescription needed. Do not alter dosage without checking with your doctor.

How and when to take: Available as tablets. Take once daily at night.

Usual adult dosage range: 10–40mg daily, changed after intervals of at least 4 weeks.

Onset and duration of effect: Starts to work within 2 weeks. Full beneficial effect may be felt within 4 weeks. Action lasts for 24 hours.

Diet advice: A low fat diet is usually recommended.

Storage: Keep in a closed container in a cool, dry place out of the reach of children. Protect from light.

If you miss or exceed a dose: Take missed dose as soon as you remember. If your next dose is due within 8 hours, do not take the missed dose, but take the next dose as usual. An occasional unintentional extra dose is unlikely to cause problems. Large overdoses may cause liver problems. Notify your doctor.

Stopping the drug: Do not stop taking the drug without consulting your doctor; it may lead to worsening of the underlying condition.

Prolonged use: Long-term use can affect liver function. Regular blood tests to check liver and muscle function are usually required.

Dependence rating: Low

Overdose danger rating: Medium

❗ POSSIBLE SIDE EFFECTS AND WHAT TO DO

Most side effects are mild and usually disappear with time. If you experience **headache, nausea,** or **fatigue,** discuss with your doctor if bothersome. If you experience **chest or abdominal pain, muscle pain,** or **jaundice,** discuss with your doctor in all cases. Stop taking the drug now and call your doctor if you develop a **rash, muscle weakness,** or **change in cognition**.

⚠️ SPECIAL PRECAUTIONS

Tell your doctor if you have: previous liver or kidney problems; thyroid problems; a family history of muscular disorders. **Also discuss if you are:** taking other medications; a heavy drinker; diabetic.
* **Safety not established** in pregnancy and breast-feeding. Discuss with your doctor.
* **Not recommended** for infants and children.
* **Avoid** excessive amounts of alcohol as it may increase the risk of developing liver problems.

⚙️ INTERACTIONS

Statins can increase the effect of **anticoagulants,** although this is less likely with pravastatin.
Taken with statins, **itraconazole, ketoconazole,** and possibly **other antifungal drugs** may increase the risk of muscle damage.
Orlistat increases blood levels and toxicity of pravastatin.
Taken with pravastatin, other **lipid-lowering drugs** (fibrates) may increase the risk of muscle damage.
There is an increased risk of muscle damage if pravastatin is taken with **cyclosporine** and other **immunosuppressant drugs**. They are not usually prescribed together.

PREDNISONE/PREDNISOLONE

Product names: [Prednisone] Apo-Prednisone, Pediapred, Teva-Prednisone, Winpred, and others
[Prednisolone] Pred Forte, Pred Mild, ratio-Prednisolone, and others
Used in the following combined preparations: [all with prednisolone] AK Cide Ophthalmic
Solution, Blephamide

WHY IS THIS DRUG USED?

Prednisolone is a powerful corticosteroid, and is used for a wide range of conditions, including some skin diseases, rheumatic disorders, allergic states, and certain blood disorders. Prednisolone is the active form of prednisone and is used in the form of eye drops to reduce inflammation in

conjunctivitis or iritis. Prednisone is also prescribed with fludrocortisone for pituitary or adrenal gland disorders. Other forms of corticosteroid, such as methylprednisolone, can also be injected into joints to relieve rheumatoid and other forms of *arthritis*.

INFORMATION FOR USERS

Prescription needed. Do not alter dosage without checking with your doctor.

How and when to take: Available as tablets, liquid, eye drops, ophthalmic ointment. Take 1–2 x daily or on alternate days with food (tablets); 2–4 x daily (eye drops).

Usual adult dosage range: Considerable variation. Follow your doctor's instructions.

Onset and duration of effect: Starts to work in 2–4 days. Action lasts 12–72 hours.

Diet advice: A low-sodium and high-potassium diet is recommended when the oral form of the drug is prescribed for extended periods. Follow the advice of your doctor.

Storage: Keep in a closed container in a cool, dry place out of the reach of children. Protect from light.

If you miss or exceed a dose: Take missed dose as soon as you remember. If your next dose is due within 6 hours, take a single dose now and skip the next. An occasional unintentional extra dose is unlikely to be a cause for concern. If you notice any unusual symptoms, or if a large overdose has been taken, notify your doctor.

Stopping the drug: Do not stop the drug without consulting your doctor. Abrupt cessation of long-term treatment by mouth may be dangerous.

Prolonged use: Prolonged systemic use can lead to such adverse effects as diabetes, glaucoma, cataracts, and fragile bones, and may retard growth in children. Dosages are usually tailored to minimize these effects.

Dependence rating: Low

Overdose danger rating: Low

POSSIBLE SIDE EFFECTS AND WHAT TO DO

Long-term treatment with large doses can cause fluid retention, indigestion, diabetes, hypertension, and acne. Contact your doctor if you experience **unusual weight gain**. If you experience

indigestion, acne, muscle weakness, mood changes, or **depression,** discuss with your doctor in all cases. Stop taking the drug now and call your doctor if you develop **black** or **bloodstained feces.**

SPECIAL PRECAUTIONS

Tell your doctor if you have: a history of peptic ulcer or tuberculosis; glaucoma; depression; any infection; diabetes; osteoporosis. **Also discuss if you are:** taking NSAIDs or other medications.
- **Discuss** with your doctor if you are pregnant.
- **Reduced dose** may be necessary for infants and children; only given when essential.
- **Reduced dose** may be necessary for those over 60.
- **Increased risk** of peptic ulcers when alcohol is combined with prednisone taken by mouth, especially if you are also on a NSAID; keep alcohol consumption low.
- **Avoid** exposure to chickenpox, shingles, or measles if you are on systemic treatment.

INTERACTIONS

Carbamazepine, phenytoin, and **phenobarbital** can reduce the effects of prednisolone/prednisone.
　Serious reactions can occur when **vaccinations** are given with this drug. Discuss with your doctor.
　Prednisone may affect the response to **anticoagulant drugs.**
　Prednisone may increase the adverse effects of **diuretics.**
　Prednisone may reduce the effects of **antihypertensive and antidiabetic drugs** and **insulin.**
　Cyclosporine increases the effects of prednisone.

PREGABALIN

Product name: Lyrica
Used in the following combined preparations: None

❓ WHY IS THIS DRUG USED?

Pregabalin is an anti-epileptic drug used to treat pain related to damaged nerves (neuropathic pain) in the hands, fingers, arms, feet, legs, and other areas as a result of *diabetes* (diabetic peripheral neuropathy). It is also approved for nerve pain related to rash from shingles (postherpetic neuralgia).

ℹ️ INFORMATION FOR USERS

Prescription needed. Do not alter dosage without checking with your doctor.

How and when to take: Available as capsules. Take two or three times daily, with or without food.

Adult dosage range: *Initial dose* 150mg daily; maximum of 600mg daily.

Onset and duration of effect: Starts to work in several weeks for pain relief. Action lasts for 8–12 hours.

Diet advice: None.

Storage: Keep in a closed container in a cool, dry place out of the reach of children.

If you miss or exceed a dose: If you miss a dose, take it as soon as you remember. If it is near the time of the next dose, skip the missed dose and resume your usual dosing schedule. Do not double up on a dose. An occasional unintentional extra dose is unlikely to cause problems. Large overdoses may cause serious adverse effects. Notify your doctor.

Stopping the drug: Do not stop the drug without consulting your doctor. Stopping suddenly may lead to withdrawal symptoms; a gradual decrease in dose over a period of weeks is recommended.

Prolonged use: No problems expected.

Dependence rating: Low

Overdose danger rating: Medium

❗ POSSIBLE SIDE EFFECTS AND WHAT TO DO

In general, pregabalin is well tolerated. If you experience **dizziness, tiredness, weight gain, dry mouth, constipation, difficulty concentrating, blurred vision,** or **changes in eyesight,** discuss with your doctor if bothersome. Call your doctor now if you develop **swelling of the eyes, face, or throat.**

🛑 SPECIAL PRECAUTIONS

Tell your doctor if you have: constipation or other bowel problems; previous problems with alcohol or drug abuse; a low number of platelets; heart or kidney disease; congestive heart failure. **Also discuss if you are:** on medication for diabetes; planning on becoming pregnant (either you or your partner); taking other medications.
• **Safety not established** in pregnancy or breast-feeding. Discuss with your doctor.
• **Not recommended** for infants and children.
• **Dose adjustment** may be necessary for those over 60 for changes in kidney function.
• **Avoid** driving and hazardous work until the effect of the drug wears off and you feel you are mentally alert.
• **Avoid** alcohol use as it may increase the effect of drowsiness caused by this drug.
• **Inform** your doctor or dentist if you are taking pregabalin.

⚙️ INTERACTIONS

Use of pregabalin with **central nervous system (CNS) depressants** such as benzodiazepines (e.g. lorazepam) and opioids (e.g. oxycodone) may result in additional drowsiness and tiredness.
   Alcohol may increase drowsiness caused by pregabalin.
   Methotrimeprazine may increase the CNS effects of pregabalin.
   Mefloquine may decrease the effectiveness of pregabalin.

PROPRANOLOL

Product names: Apo-Propranolol, Inderal-LA, Nu-Propranolol, PMS-Propranolol, and others
Used in the following combined preparations: None

❓ WHY IS THIS DRUG USED?

Propranolol is a beta blocker most often used to treat *hypertension, angina,* and abnormal heart rhythms (*arrhythmia*). It is also helpful in controlling the fast heart rate and other symptoms of an overactive thyroid gland, reducing the palpitations, sweating, and tremor of severe *anxiety,* and preventing *migraine* headaches. Propranolol is not prescribed to people with breathing difficulties, and should be used with caution by diabetics as it affects the body's response to low blood sugar.

ℹ INFORMATION FOR USERS

Prescription needed. Do not alter dosage without checking with your doctor.

How and when to take: Available as tablets, SR-capsules. Take 2–4 x daily; once daily (SR-capsules).

Usual adult dosage range: *Abnormal heart rhythms* 30–160mg daily. *Angina* 60–320mg daily. *Hypertension* 60–320mg daily. *Migraine prevention and anxiety* 40–160mg daily.

Onset and duration of effect: Starts to work in 1–2 hours (tablets); after 4 hours (SR-capsules). In hypertension and migraine, it may be several weeks before full benefits of this drug are felt. Action lasts 6–12 hours (tablets); 24–30 hours (SR-capsules).

Diet advice: None.

Storage: Keep in a closed container in a cool, dry place out of the reach of children. Protect from light.

If you miss a dose: Take as soon as you remember. If your next dose is due within 2 hours (tablets) or 12 hours (SR-capsules), take a single dose now and skip the next.

Stopping the drug: Do not stop the drug without consulting your doctor as it may lead to worsening of the underlying condition.

Prolonged use: No problems expected.

Dependence rating: Low

Overdose danger rating: High

☠ OVERDOSE ACTION

Seek immediate medical advice in all cases. Take emergency action if breathing difficulties, collapse, or loss of consciousness occur.

See Drug poisoning emergency guide (p.197).

❗ POSSIBLE SIDE EFFECTS AND WHAT TO DO

Minor side effects are usually temporary and diminish with long-term use. If you experience **lethargy/fatigue, cold hands and feet,** or **nausea,** discuss with your doctor if bothersome. **Fainting** may be a sign that the drug has slowed the heart beat excessively; call your doctor now. If you experience **nightmares/vivid dreams, dry eyes,** or **visual disturbances,** discuss with your doctor in all cases. Call your doctor now if you experience **breathlessness**.

✋ SPECIAL PRECAUTIONS

Tell your doctor if you have: long-term liver or kidney problems; a breathing disorder such as asthma, bronchitis, or emphysema; heart failure; diabetes; poor circulation in the legs. **Also discuss if you are:** taking other medications.
- **Discuss** with your doctor if you are pregnant or breast-feeding as the drug may affect the unborn baby and does pass into the breast milk.
- **Reduced dose** necessary for infants and children.
- **Increased risk** of side effects for those over 60.
- **Consult** with your doctor or dentist before any surgery; propranolol may need to be stopped.

🔄 INTERACTIONS

Propranolol may enhance the blood pressure lowering effect of **antihypertensive drugs**.
  Combining **diltiazem** and **verapamil** with propranolol may have adverse effects on heart function.
  Cimetidine and **hydralazine** may increase the effects of propranolol.
  Non-steroidal anti-inflammatory drugs (NSAIDs), e.g. indomethacin, may reduce the antihypertensive effect of propranolol.

PSEUDOEPHEDRINE

Product name: Drixoral ND Long Acting
Used in the following combined preparations: Actifed, Dimetapp Daytime Cold Extra Strength,
Dristan Extra Strength N.D., Dristan N.D., Sinutab Non Drowsy, and others

❓ WHY IS THIS DRUG USED?

Pseudoephedrine is a decongestant and a component of many non-prescription remedies. It reduces congestion of the nasal passages and sinuses by narrowing blood vessels in the nose. It also reduces congestion of the eustachian tube (the tube connecting the middle ear with the cavity at the back of the nose) caused by inflammation and infection of the middle ear.

At higer doses, it may cause anxiety and restlessness.

ℹ️ INFORMATION FOR USERS

No prescription needed, except when combined with a prescription drug. Follow instructions on the label. Call your doctor if symptoms worsen.

How and when to take: Available as tablets, tablets SR (as extended release), capsules, oral liquid, powder for solution. Take every 4–6 hours (tablets, liquid); every 12 hours (SR tablets).

Usual dosage range: *Adults and children 12 years and over* 60mg daily to a maximum of 240mg daily. *Children 2–11 years* Consult your pharmacist or doctor. 120mg slow-release preparations are not recommended under 12 years.

Onset and duration of effect: Starts to work in 15–30 minutes (tablets and liquid). Action lasts 4–6 hours (tablets and liquid); 8–12 hours (slow-release preparations).

Diet advice: None.

Storage: Keep in a closed container in a cool, dry place out of the reach of children. Protect from light.

If you miss a dose: Take as soon as you remember. If your next dose is due within 2 hours, take a single dose now and skip the next.

Stopping the drug: Can be safely stopped as soon as you no longer need it.

Prolonged use: Should not be taken for longer than 7 days except on the advice of your doctor. It can cause worsening of congestion after prolonged use.

Dependence rating: Low

Overdose danger rating: High

☠️ OVERDOSE ACTION

Seek immediate medical advice in all cases. Take emergency action if delirium, seizures, or loss of consciousness occur.

See Drug poisoning emergency guide (p.197).

❗ POSSIBLE SIDE EFFECTS AND WHAT TO DO

If you experience **nausea, vomiting, dizziness/lightheadedness, nervousness,** or **insomnia,** discuss with your doctor if bothersome. If you experience **tremor** or **hallucinations,** discuss with your doctor in all cases. Call your doctor now if you develop **palpitations, breathlessness,** or **headache.** Stop taking the drug now and call your doctor if you develop a **rash.**

🖐️ SPECIAL PRECAUTIONS

Tell your doctor if you have: heart problems; high blood pressure; a history of glaucoma; diabetes; an overactive thyroid; urinary difficulties; an enlarged prostate. **Also discuss if you are:** taking other medications.
• **Safety not established** in pregnancy or breast-feeding; discuss with your doctor.
• **Not recommended** for children under 2 years.
• **Reduced dose** necessary in older children, and for those over 60.
• **Avoid** driving and hazardous work until you have learned how the drug affects you.

⚙️ INTERACTIONS

Pseudoephedrine counteracts the lowered blood pressure from **antihypertensive drugs.**

Other **sympathomimetic drugs** increase the risk of adverse effects with this drug.

There is a risk of a dangerous rise in blood pressure if pseudoephedrine is taken with **monoamine oxidase inhibitors** (MAOIs).

QUETIAPINE

Product names: Apo-Quetiapine, CO-Quetiapine, Mylan-Quetiapine, Seroquel, Seroquel XR, Teva-Quetiapine, and others
Used in the following combined preparations: None

❓ WHY IS THIS DRUG USED?

Quetiapine is an atypical antipsychotic drug that is prescribed for the treatment of schizophrenia. It can be used to treat positive symptoms (thought disorders, delusions, and hallucinations) and negative symptoms (blunted affect and emotional and social withdrawal). The drug may be more effective when used for positive symptoms, however. Elderly people excrete the drug more slowly and therefore need to be prescribed much lower doses.

ℹ INFORMATION FOR USERS

Prescription needed. Do not alter dosage without checking with your doctor.

How and when to take: Available as tablets, extended release tablets. Take 2 x daily; extended release tablets taken once daily, usually in the evening.

Usual adult dosage range: *regular tablets* 50mg daily (day 1), 100mg daily (day 2), 200mg daily (day 3), 300mg daily (day 4), then changing according to response. Usual dose: 300–600mg daily.

Onset and duration of effect: Starts to work in 1 hour. Action lasts up to 12 hours.

Diet advice: None.

Storage: Keep in a closed container in a cool, dry place out of the reach of children.

If you miss or exceed a dose: Take missed dose as soon as you remember. For regular tablets, if your next dose is due within 4 hours take a single dose now and skip the next. An occasional unintentional extra dose is unlikely to cause problems. Large overdoses may cause unusual drowsiness, palpitations, and low blood pressure. Notify your doctor.

Stopping the drug: Do not stop the drug without consulting your doctor; symptoms may recur.

Prolonged use: May cause tardive dyskinesia (in which there are involuntary movements of the tongue and face).

Dependence rating: Low

Overdose danger rating: Medium

❗ POSSIBLE SIDE EFFECTS AND WHAT TO DO

If you experience **unusual drowsiness, weight gain,** or **stomach upset,** discuss with your doctor if bothersome. If you experience **parkinsonism, dizziness, fainting,** or **persistent sore throat,** discuss with your doctor in all cases. Call your doctor now if you develop **palpitations**.

✋ SPECIAL PRECAUTIONS

Tell your doctor if you have: epilepsy; Parkinson's disease; liver or kidney problems; heart problems; blood problems. **Also discuss if you are:** taking other medications.
* **Safety not established** in pregnancy or breast-feeding. Discuss with your doctor.
* **Not recommended** for infants and children.
* **Reduced dose** necessary for those over 60.
* **Avoid** driving and hazardous work and alcohol consumption due to the sedative effects of this drug.

⊘ INTERACTIONS

Quetiapine opposes the effect of **antiepileptics,** but **phenytoin** decreases the effect of quetiapine. Other liver enzyme-inducing antiepileptic drugs, such as **carbamazepine** and **barbiturates,** may have a similar effect.
   Sedatives are likely to increase the sedative properties of quetiapine.

RABEPRAZOLE

Product names: Pariet, PMS-Rabeprazole, PRO-Rabeprazole, RAN-Rabeprazole, Sandoz Rabeprazole, Teva-Rabeprazole
Used in the following combined preparations: None

WHY IS THIS DRUG USED?

Rabeprazole is an anti-ulcer drug used to treat stomach and duodenal *ulcers* as well as reflux esophagitis. In combination with antibiotics, the drug is used for ulcers caused by Helicobacter pylori infection. It reduces the amount of acid produced by the stomach, and can therefore be used to treat a rare condition called Zollinger-Ellison syndrome where the stomach produces large amounts of acid. It is also used to prevent gastroduodenal ulceration sometimes caused by non-steroidal anti-inflammatory drugs (NSAIDs) (p.12). As with other anti-ulcer drugs, it may mask signs of stomach cancer, so it is used only when the possibility of this disease has been ruled out.

INFORMATION FOR USERS

Prescription needed. Do not alter dosage without checking with your doctor.

How and when to take: Available as enteric-coated tablets, delayed-release tablets. Usually taken once daily. Tablets to be swallowed whole and not chewed or crushed.

Usual adult dosage range: 10mg–20mg. *Peptic ulcers:* 4 to 8 wks. *Reflux esophagitis:* 4 to 12 wks. *Eradication of H. pylori:* 20mg twice daily for 7 days.

Onset and duration of effect: Starts to work within 1.5 to 5 hours. Duration: 24 hours.

Diet advice: None, although spicy foods and alcohol may exacerbate the underlying condition.

Storage: Keep in a closed container in a cool, dry place out of the reach of children.

If you miss or exceed a dose: Take missed dose as soon as you remember. If your next dose is due within 8 hours, take a single dose now and skip the next. Do not double up on doses. An occasional unintentional extra dose is unlikely to cause problems. If you notice any unusual symptoms, or if a large overdose has been taken, notify your doctor.

Stopping the drug: Do not stop taking the drug without consulting your doctor; symptoms may recur.

Prolonged use: Ongoing use should be evaluated periodically.

Dependence rating: Low

Overdose danger rating: Medium

POSSIBLE SIDE EFFECTS AND WHAT TO DO

Side effects such as **headache** and **diarrhea** are usually mild, and often diminish with continued use of the drug. If you develop **dizziness**, discuss with your doctor if bothersome. If you develop a **rash** or **itchiness**, discuss with your doctor in all cases.

SPECIAL PRECAUTIONS

Tell your doctor if you have: liver problems. **Also discuss if you are:** pregnant or plan on becoming pregnant; breast-feeding; allergic to anti-ulcer medications; taking other medications.
- **Not usually prescribed** in pregnancy or while breast-feeding.
- **Not recommended** for infants and children.
- **Alcohol** avoid as it may aggravate the underlying condition and reduce the beneficial effects of this drug.

INTERACTIONS

Rabeprazole may decrease the level of **posaconazole, nelfinivir,** and **erlotinib;** do not combine.
  Rabeprazole may decrease the level of **antifungal drugs.**
  Ketoconazole may increase the level of **rabeprazole.**
  Rabeprazole may decrease the effectiveness of **clopidogrel.** Discuss with your doctor and pharmacist.
  Rabeprazole may increase the effect of **warfarin** and **digoxin;** close monitoring may be required.
  Proton pump inhibitors may also interact with other drugs. Before taking a new drug, discuss with your pharmacist.

RALOXIFENE

Product names: Apo-Raloxifene, Evista, Teva-Raloxifene
Used in the following combined preparations: None

❓ WHY IS THIS DRUG USED?

Raloxifene, a non-steroidal drug, is a selective estrogen receptor modulator (SERM), which acts like estrogen on bone. It is prescribed to prevent vertebral fractures in postmenopausal women who are at increased risk of *osteoporosis*. The drug may also be useful for preventing hip fractures. It is not prescribed to men or to women who might become pregnant. Similar to estrogens, raloxifene has an increased risk of causing a thrombosis (blood clot) in a leg vein, and for this reason treatment is usually stopped temporarily if the woman becomes immobile, until full activity is resumed.

ℹ️ INFORMATION FOR USERS

Prescription needed. Do not alter dosage without checking with your doctor.

How and when to take: Available as tablets. Take once daily.

Usual adult dosage range: 60mg daily.

Onset and duration of effect: Starts to work in 1–4 hours. Action lasts 24–48 hours.

Diet advice: Adequate daily calcium and vitamin D intake is recommended. Supplements may be needed.

Storage: Keep in a closed container in a cool, dry place out of the reach of children. Protect from light.

If you miss or exceed a dose: Take missed dose as soon as you remember. If your next dose is due within 8 hours, take a single dose now and skip the next. An occasional unintentional extra dose is unlikely to be a cause for concern. But if you notice any unusual symptoms, or if a large overdose has been taken, notify your doctor.

Stopping the drug: Do not stop the drug without consulting your doctor except under conditions specified in advance, such as immobility, which increases the risk of blood clots forming.

Prolonged use: No special problems. Raloxifene is normally used long term. Liver function tests may be performed periodically.

Dependence rating: Low

Overdose danger rating: Low

❗ POSSIBLE SIDE EFFECTS AND WHAT TO DO

If you experience **hot flushes** or **leg cramps,** discuss with your doctor if bothersome. If you experience **swollen ankles/feet, headache,** or **rash**, discuss with your doctor in all cases. Stop taking the drug now and call your doctor if you experience **leg pain/tenderness, leg swelling, leg discoloration/ulceration,** or **inflammation of the capillaries.**

SPECIAL PRECAUTIONS

Tell your doctor if you have: a history of blood clots in a vein; uterine bleeding; liver or kidney problems; a history of stroke; heart rhythm problems. **Also discuss if you are:** taking other medications.
- **Not prescribed** to men, premenopausal women, or to infants and children.

INTERACTIONS

Raloxifene may decrease the absorption of **levothyroxine**. Consider separating the doses by several hours.
   Cholestyramine reduces the absorption of raloxifene by the body.

RAMIPRIL

Product names: Altace, Apo-Ramipril, CO-Ramipril, PMS-Ramipril, Teva-Ramipril, and many others
Used in the following combined preparations: Altace HCT, Altace Plus Felodipine

❓ WHY IS THIS DRUG USED?

Ramipril belongs to a group of drugs called ACE (angiotensin converting enzyme) inhibitors. It works by dilating the blood vessels, which enables the blood to circulate more easily. It is used to treat *high blood pressure* and to reduce the strain on the heart in patients with *heart failure* after a *heart attack*. The first dose can cause the blood pressure to drop very suddenly, so a few hours bed rest afterwards may be advised.

🔹 INFORMATION FOR USERS

Prescription needed. Do not alter dosage without checking with your doctor.

How and when to take: Available as capsules. Take with water, with or without food. *High blood pressure* Usually once daily. *Heart failure after a heart attack* 2 x daily.

Usual adult dosage range: *High blood pressure* 1.25–10mg daily. *Heart failure after heart attack* 5–10mg daily.

Onset and duration of effect: Starts to work within 2 hours. Action lasts up to 24 hours.

Diet advice: A low-sodium diet may be advised to help control your blood pressure.

Storage: Keep in a closed container in a cool, dry place out of the reach of children.

If you miss or exceed a dose: Take missed dose as soon as you remember. If your next dose is due within 6 hours, take a single dose now, skip the next, then continue with your usual routine. If you exceed the dose and notice any unusual symptoms, or if a large overdose has been taken, notify your doctor.

Stopping the drug: Consult with your doctor. Treatment of hypertension and heart failure is normally lifelong; it may be necessary to substitute alternative therapy.

Prolonged use: No problems expected. If you have other medical conditions, blood counts and kidney function tests may be performed at intervals.

Dependence rating: Low

Overdose danger rating: Medium

❗ POSSIBLE SIDE EFFECTS AND WHAT TO DO

Ramipril may cause high potassium levels and may affect kidney function. If you experience **nausea, dizziness, headache, cough, dry mouth,** or **taste disturbance,** discuss with your doctor if bothersome. If you experience **jaundice,** discuss with your doctor in all cases. If you develop a **rash** or **itching,** call your doctor now. Stop taking the drug now and call your doctor if you develop **swelling of face/mouth, difficulty in breathing, chest pain,** or **unconciousness**.

🖐 SPECIAL PRECAUTIONS

Tell your doctor if you have: long-term liver or kidney problems; a history of severe allergies or heart-valve problems; peripheral vascular disease or atherosclerosis; systemic lupus erythematosus or scleroderma. **Also discuss if you are:** taking other medications.
• **Not usually prescribed** in pregnancy.
• **Discuss** with your doctor if you are breast-feeding as the drug may affect the baby.
• **Not recommended** for infants and children.
• **Reduced dose** may be necessary for those over 60.
• **Avoid** driving and hazardous work until you have learned how ramipril affects you.
• **Avoid** alcohol as it may reduce blood pressure further at first dose or dosage adjustment.
• **Notify** your doctor or dentist that you are taking ramipril before surgery.

⚙ INTERACTIONS

Non-steroidal anti-inflammatory drugs (NSAIDs) (e.g., ibuprofen) may reduce the antihypertensive effect of ramipril and increase the risk of kidney damage.
   Cyclosporine increases the risk of high potassium levels in the blood.
   Potassium supplements and **potassium-sparing diuretics** may cause excess levels of potassium in the body.
   Ramipril may cause raised blood **lithium** levels and toxicity.
   Anesthetics can increase the effects of ramipril.

RANITIDINE

Product names: Acid Reducer, Apo-Ranitidine, Mylan-Ranitidine, Novo-Ranidine, Ratio-Ranitidine, Riva-Ranitidine, Sandoz Ranitidine, Zantac, Zantac Maximum Strength Non-Prescription, and others
Used in the following combined preparations: None

❓ WHY IS THIS DRUG USED?

Ranitidine reduces the amount of stomach acid produced and is prescribed in the treatment of stomach and duodenal *ulcers*. In combination with antibiotics, the drug is used for ulcers caused by Helicobacter pylori infection. It is also used to protect against duodenal (but not stomach) ulcers in people taking NSAIDs, who may be prone to ulcers. This drug reduces the discomfort and ulceration of reflux esophagitis, and may prevent stress ulceration and gastric bleeding in severely ill patients.

As with other anti-ulcer drugs, it may mask signs of stomach cancer, so it is used only when the possibility of this disease has been ruled out.

ℹ INFORMATION FOR USERS

Prescription needed for some preparations. Do not alter dosage without checking with your doctor.

How and when to take: Available as tablets, oral liquid, injection. Take once daily at bedtime or 2–3 x daily.

Usual adult dosage range: 150–600mg daily, depending on the condition being treated. Usual dose is 150mg twice daily.

Onset and duration of effect: Starts to work within 1 hour. Action lasts up to 12 hours.

Diet advice: None.

Storage: Keep in a closed container in a cool, dry place out of the reach of children. Protect from light.

If you miss or exceed a dose: Take missed dose as soon as you remember. If your next dose is due within 3 hours, take a single dose now and skip the next. An occasional unintentional extra dose is unlikely to be a cause for concern. If you notice any unusual symptoms, or if a large overdose has been taken, notify your doctor.

Stopping the drug: Do not stop the drug without consulting your doctor; symptoms may recur.

Prolonged use: No problems expected.

Dependence rating: Low

Overdose danger rating: Low

❗ POSSIBLE SIDE EFFECTS AND WHAT TO DO

Side effects are usually related to dosage level and almost always disappear when treatment finishes. If you experience **headache, dizziness, nausea/vomiting, constipation,** or **diarrhea,** discuss with your doctor if bothersome. If you develop **jaundice** or **mental problems,** or **any other symptoms,** discuss with your doctor in all cases. Call your doctor now if you experience a **sore throat** or **fever.**

👄 SPECIAL PRECAUTIONS

Tell your doctor or pharmacist if you have: long-term liver or kidney problems; porphyria; a history of allergic reaction to ranitidine or to another H2 blocker. **Also discuss if you are:** taking other medications.
- **Safety not established** in pregnancy or breast-feeding. Discuss with your doctor.
- **Reduced dose necessary** for children 8 years and older. Safety not established for children less than 8 years.
- **Avoid** driving and hazardous work if you experience dizziness.
- **Avoid** alcohol as it may aggravate your underlying condition and reduce the beneficial effects of this drug.

🔄 INTERACTIONS

Ranitidine may reduce the absorption of **ketoconazole, itraconazole,** and **posaconazole.** Ranitidine should be taken at least 2 hours after ketoconazole.

Ranitidine may decrease the effect of **mesalamine, erlotinib, delavirdine,** and **other drugs.** Discuss with your doctor or pharmacist.

RASAGILINE

Product name: Azilect
Used in the following combined preparations: None

WHY IS THIS DRUG USED?

Rasagiline is used alone or in combination with another medication to treat Parkinson's disease. It causes an increase of dopamine in the brain, and can be used early on in the disease to control symptoms. It can be used with medications such as levodopa as it helps prolong its effect. While on this medication, it is advised that you get up slowly while supporting yourself, to minimize dizziness or lightheadedness. The maximum dose of 1mg should not be exceeded as higher doses require specific dietary restrictions.

INFORMATION FOR USERS

Prescription needed. Do not alter dosage without checking with your doctor.

How and when to take: Available as tablets. Taken usually once daily.

Adult dosage range: 0.5–1mg daily.

Onset and duration of effect: Starts to work in 1 hour. Action lasts up to 24 hours.

Diet advice: At higher doses, avoid foods rich in tyramine while on, and for 14 days after stopping, rasagiline. These include aged cheeses, salami, fava beans, red wine, soybean products. Consult your dietician.

Storage: Keep in a closed container in a cool, dry place out of the reach of children.

If you miss a dose: Take it as soon as you remember. If it is near the time of the next dose, skip the missed dose and resume your usual dosing schedule. Do not double up on a dose.

Stopping the drug: Do not stop the drug without consulting your doctor; it may lead to worsening of the underlying condition.

Prolonged use: No problems expected.

Dependence rating: Low

Overdose danger rating: High

☠ OVERDOSE ACTION

Seek immediate medical advice in all cases. Take emergency action if chest pain or loss of consciousness occurs.

See Drug poisoning emergency guide (p.197).

POSSIBLE SIDE EFFECTS AND WHAT TO DO

If you experience **constipation, diarrhea, drowsiness, mild headache, loss of appetite,** or **unsteadiness,** discuss with your doctor if bothersome. If you develop **shortness of breath** or **slow or difficult speech,** call your doctor now. Stop taking the drug now and call your doctor if you experience **severe headache, chest pain, blurred vision,** or **hallucinations.**

SPECIAL PRECAUTIONS

Tell your doctor if you have: pheochromocytoma; kidney or liver disease; a history of melanoma.
Also discuss if you are: taking herbal remedies such as St. John's wort; taking other medications.
- **Safety not established** in pregnancy or breast-feeding. Discuss with your doctor.
- **Not recommended** for infants and children.
- **Avoid** driving and hazardous work until the effect of the drug wears off and you feel you are mentally alert.
- **Avoid** alcohol use as it may increase the effect of drowsiness caused by this drug.

⚙ INTERACTIONS

Because of the wide range of possible drug interactions with rasagiline, do not take any medication, whether prescription or nonprescription, without first consulting your doctor or pharmacist.

The combination of rasagiline with **antidepressants, St. John's wort, dextromethorphan, pseudoephedrine,** or **meperidine** may cause severe and dangerous reactions. Allow at least 14 days after stopping rasagiline before taking these.

RISEDRONATE

Product names: Actonel, Teva-Risedronate
Used in the following combined preparation: Actonel Plus Calcium

❷ WHY IS THIS DRUG USED?

Risedronate is given for the prevention and treatment of *osteoporosis* in post-menopausal women and osteoporosis due to long-term use of corticosteroid drugs in men and women. Risedronate is also beneficial in individuals with Paget's disease. Calcium should be separated and given at a different time from risedronate because calcium is one of the many substances that reduces its absorption (see below).

❶ INFORMATION FOR USERS

Prescription needed. Do not alter dosage without checking with your doctor.

How and when to take: Available as tablets. May be taken daily, weekly, or monthly; dose is adjusted accordingly.

Usual adult dosage range: *Osteoporosis prevention & treatment:* The recommended regimens are daily (5mg), weekly (35mg once a week), monthly duet (75mg on two consecutive days per month, on the same calendar days each month), or monthly (1 tablet of 150mg once a month on the same calendar day each month), taken orally. *Paget's disease:* 30mg daily for 2 months; re-treatment may be considered with relapse of the condition.

Onset and duration of effect: It may take months to notice an improvement. Some effects may persist for months or years.

Diet advice: Absorption of risedronate is reduced by foods and drinks, including dairy products such as milk. The drug should be taken on an empty stomach. The diet must contain adequate calcium and vitamin D; supplements may be given.

Storage: Keep in a closed container in a cool, dry place out of the reach of children.

If you miss or exceed a dose: If you missed a *daily dose* by a few hours and you can take it on an empty stomach and remain upright for 30 minutes, take the missed dose now. If not, take the next dose at the usual time next morning. Take a missed *weekly dose* at the usual time on the next day. Do not take the weekly dose more than once a week. An occasional unintentional extra dose is unlikely to cause problems. Large overdoses may cause stomach problems including heartburn, irritation, and ulcers. Notify your doctor at once, and try to remain upright.

Stopping the drug: Do not stop taking the drug without consulting your doctor; the underlying condition may worsen.

Prolonged use: Treatment for osteoporosis may be given for several years. Initial response to therapy should be assessed after 1–2 years of use. Blood and urine tests may be carried out at intervals.

Dependence rating: Low

Overdose danger rating: Medium

❶ POSSIBLE SIDE EFFECTS AND WHAT TO DO

The most common side effect is diarrhea, which is more likely with higher doses. If you experience **diarrhea, abdominal pain, bone pain,** or **nausea,** discuss with your doctor if bothersome. If you develop **rash/itching,** or **eye pain/redness/blurred vision,** discuss with your doctor in all cases. Stop taking the drug and call your doctor now if you experience **jaw pain.**

❶ SPECIAL PRECAUTIONS

Tell your doctor if you have: an abnormality of the esophagus, stomach problems, or a history of ulcers; unusual bone pain; impaired kidney function; a history of allergic reaction to risedronate or other bisphosphonates; problems swallowing; hypocalcemia. **Also discuss if you are:** unable to stay upright for 30 minutes; taking other medications.
- **Not recommended** in pregnancy or breast-feeding, or for infants and children.
- **Avoid** alcohol as it may cause stomach irritation.

❷ INTERACTIONS

Antacids, calcium, and **dairy products** can decrease the absorption of risedronate. Take risedronate at least 30 minutes before any calcium tablets, calcium-rich foods or calcium-containing antacids.
   Risedronate could increase **warfarin's** effect. Careful monitoring is required.
   Do not take risedronate at the same time as **other medications;** take it at least 30 mins before.

ROSIGLITAZONE

Product name: Avandia
Used in the following combined preparations: Avandamet, Avandaryl

❓ WHY IS THIS DRUG USED?

Rosiglitazone is used to treat non-insulin-dependent *diabetes mellitus* (NIDDM, Type 2 diabetes). It works by reducing insulin resistance in fatty tissue, skeletal muscle, and in the liver, which leads to a reduction of blood glucose levels. This drug is not approved for use alone, unless drugs such as metformin are considered inappropriate. Rosiglitazone is not approved for use with insulin or in triple combination with other anti-diabetic drugs; it is also not to be used by individuals with heart failure.

ℹ️ INFORMATION FOR USERS

Prescription needed. Do not alter dosage without checking with your doctor.

How and when to take: Available as tablets. Take 1–2 x daily.

Usual adult dosage range: 4–8mg daily.

Onset and duration of effect: Starts to work in 60 minutes; it can take 8 weeks for full effects to appear. Action lasts 12–24 hours.

Diet advice: An individualized low fat, low sugar diet must be maintained in order for the drug to be fully effective. Follow your doctor's advice.

Storage: Keep in a closed container in a cool dry place out of the reach of children.

If you miss a dose: Take as soon as you remember. If your next dose is due within 2 hours, take a single dose now and skip the next.

Stopping the drug: Do not stop taking the drug without consulting your doctor as it may lead to worsening of the underlying condition.

Prolonged use: Periodic blood tests of liver function and hemoglobin levels will be performed. Heart performance and weight will be monitored regularly.

Dependence rating: Low

Overdose danger rating: High

☠️ OVERDOSE ACTION

Seek immediate medical advice in all cases. Take emergency action if loss of consciousness occurs.

See Drug poisoning emergency guide (p.197).

❗ POSSIBLE SIDE EFFECTS AND WHAT TO DO

Anemia and weight gain (even on a strict diabetic diet) are two of the more common side effects. If you experience **nausea, abdominal pain, indigestion,** or **flatulence,** discuss with your doctor if bothersome. If you experience **fatigue, weakness, headache, weight gain, dark urine, dizziness, pins and needles, sleepiness, night cough,** or **blurred vision,** discuss with your doctor in all cases. Call your doctor now if you experience **edema** (swelling), and get immediate help if you develop **difficulty breathing.**

✋ SPECIAL PRECAUTIONS

Tell your doctor if you have: liver problems; heart problems, especially heart failure; shortness of breath or are easily fatigued; high cholesterol; osteoporosis or a decrease in bone mineral density. **Also discuss if you are:** anemic; not using birth control; taking nitrates or other medications.
- **Safety not established** in pregnancy and while breast-feeding. Discuss with your doctor.
- **Not recommended** for infants and children.

🔄 INTERACTIONS

Many drugs may affect the anti-diabetic effects of rosiglitazone; discuss with your pharmacist or doctor.
Paclitaxel may reduce the metabolism and increase the effects of rosiglitazone.
ACE inhibitors may increase the effects of rosiglitazone.
Diazoxide reduces the effects of rosiglitazone.

ROSUVASTATIN

Product name: Crestor
Used in the following combined preparations: None

❓ WHY IS THIS DRUG USED?

Rosuvastatin is a lipid-lowering drug that works to lower the blood levels of cholesterol. The drug is prescribed for people who will benefit from the lowering of their *blood cholesterol* level and have not responded to a special diet, and are at risk of developing or have existing coronary heart disease. Rosuvastatin should be taken at the same time daily, and should be continued even when cholesterol levels are normal as the benefits seen with this class of drugs are long-term.

ℹ INFORMATION FOR USERS

Prescription needed. Do not alter dosage without checking with your doctor.

How and when to take: Available as tablets. Usually taken once daily.

Adult dosage range: 5–40mg daily.

Onset and duration of effect: 2–4 weeks to see a change in cholesterol levels. Action lasts up to 24 hours.

Diet advice: A diet low in saturated fats and cholesterol.

Storage: Keep in a closed container in a cool, dry place out of the reach of children.

If you miss or exceed a dose: Take missed dose as soon as you remember. If it is near the time of the next dose, skip the missed dose and resume your usual dosing schedule. An occasional unintentional extra dose is unlikely to cause problems. Large overdoses may cause liver problems; notify your doctor.

Stopping the drug: Do not stop the drug without consulting your doctor as it may lead to worsening of the underlying condition.

Prolonged use: Prolonged treatment can adversely affect liver function. Regular blood tests to check liver enzymes are recommended. Tests of muscle enzymes may be carried out if problems are suspected.

Dependence rating: Low

Overdose danger rating: Medium

❗ POSSIBLE SIDE EFFECTS AND WHAT TO DO

Most side effects are mild and usually disappear with time. If you experience **headache, nausea,** or **fatigue,** discuss with your doctor if bothersome. If you experience **chest or abdominal pain, muscle pain,** or **jaundice,** discuss with your doctor in all cases. Stop taking the drug now and call your doctor if you develop a **rash, muscle weakness,** or **change in cognition**.

✋ SPECIAL PRECAUTIONS

Tell your doctor if you have: liver or kidney problems; eye or vision problems; muscle weakness; a thyroid disorder; a history of alcohol abuse; porphyria; angina; high blood pressure. **Also discuss if you are:** taking other medications.
- **Not prescribed** during pregnancy; safety not established in breast-feeding. Discuss with your doctor.
- **Not recommended** for infants and children.
- **Avoid** excessive amounts of alcohol as it may increase the risk of developing liver problems.

🔄 INTERACTIONS

Antacids may decrease the amount of rosuvastatin that is absorbed. Take antacid at least 2 hours after taking rosuvastatin.
   Cyclosporine and **gemfibrozil** can both increase the level of rosuvastatin in the blood and increase the risk for adverse effects; dosage adjustment is recommended.
   Rosuvastatin may increase the effect of **warfarin**. INR should be monitored before starting rosuvastatin and periodically after.
   Lopinavir/ritonavir can increase the level of rosuvastatin and increase its adverse effects.

SALBUTAMOL

Product names: Airomir, Apo-Salvent, ratio-Salbutamol, Ventolin, Ventolin Diskus, Ventolin HFA, and others
Used in the following combined preparations: Combivent UDV, ratio-Ipra Sal UDV

❓ WHY IS THIS DRUG USED?

Salbutamol is a sympathomimetic bronchodilator that relaxes the muscle surrounding the bronchioles (airways in the lungs). This drug is used to relieve symptoms of *asthma*, chronic *bronchitis*, and *emphysema*. Although it can be taken by mouth, inhalation is considered more effective because the drug is delivered directly to the bronchioles, thus giving rapid relief, allowing smaller doses, and causing fewer side effects. Compared with some similar drugs, when inhaled, salbutamol has little stimulant effect on the heart rate and blood pressure, making it safer for people with heart problems or high blood pressure. Because salbutamol relaxes the muscles of the uterus, it may also be used to prevent premature labour.

ℹ️ INFORMATION FOR USERS

Prescription needed. Do not alter dosage without checking with your doctor.

How and when to take: Available as inhalation solution, injection, inhaler (aerosol), powder for inhalation, tablets. Take 1–2 inhalations 3–4 x daily (inhaler); 3–4 x daily (liquid).

Usual adult dosage range: 400–800mcg daily (inhaler); 6–16mg daily (by mouth).

Onset and duration of effect: Starts to work within 5–15 minutes (inhaler); within 30–60 minutes (by mouth). Action lasts up to 6 hours (inhaler); up to 8 hours (by mouth).

Diet advice: None.

Storage: Keep in a closed container in a cool, dry place out of the reach of children. Protect from light. Do not puncture or burn inhalers.

If you miss or exceed a dose: Take missed dose as soon as you remember if you need it. If your next dose is due within 2 hours, take a single dose now and skip the next. An occasional unintentional extra dose is unlikely to be a cause for concern. If you notice any unusual symptoms, or if a large overdose has been taken, notify your doctor.

Stopping the drug: Do not stop the drug without consulting your doctor; symptoms may recur.

Prolonged use: No problems expected. However, you should contact your doctor if you need to use your salbutamol inhaler more than usual or are exceeding 8 puffs in 24 hours. This may indicate that your asthma is worsening. Periodic blood tests for potassium may be needed in people on high-dose treatment with salbutamol combined with other asthma drugs.

Dependence rating: Low

Overdose danger rating: Low

❗ POSSIBLE SIDE EFFECTS AND WHAT TO DO

If you experience **anxiety, nervous tension, tremor of the hands,** or **restlessness,** contact your doctor if bothersome. If you experience **headache** or **muscle cramps,** discuss with your doctor in all cases. Stop taking the drug now and call your doctor if you develop **palpitations.**

🖐️ SPECIAL PRECAUTIONS

Tell your doctor if you have: heart problems; high blood pressure; an overactive thyroid gland; diabetes. **Also discuss if you are:** taking other medications.
- **No evidence of risk** when used to treat asthma by inhalation in pregnancy, or to treat or prevent premature labour. Discuss with your doctor.
- **Discuss** with your doctor if you are breast-feeding; the drug passes into the breast milk, but at normal doses adverse effects to the baby are unlikely.
- **Reduced dose necessary** for infants and children, and possibly for those over 60.
- **Avoid** driving and hazardous work until you have learned how salbutamol affects you.

⊘ INTERACTIONS

There is a risk of low potassium levels in the blood occurring if **theophylline** is taken with salbutamol.
    Monoamine oxidase inhibitors (MAOIs) can interact with salbutamol to produce a dangerous rise in blood pressure.
    Other **sympathomimetic drugs** may increase the effects of salbutamol, thereby also increasing the risk of adverse effects.
    Beta blockers may reduce the action of salbutamol.

SALMETEROL

Product name: Serevent Diskus
Used in the following combined preparations: Advair, Advair Diskus

❓ WHY IS THIS DRUG USED?

Salmeterol is a sympathomimetic bronchodilator used to treat conditions, such as *asthma* and bronchospasm, in which the airways become constricted. For these conditions, it is usually added to an inhaled corticosteroid. Salmeterol is also used in the management of *chronic obstructive pulmonary disease* such as bronchitis or emphysema. Its advantage over salbutamol (p.163) is that it is longer acting. It is not used for immediate relief of asthma because of its slow onset of effect. It is prescribed to prevent attacks, however, and can be helpful in preventing night-time asthma.

ℹ️ INFORMATION FOR USERS

Prescription needed. Do not alter dosage without checking with your doctor.

How and when to take: Available as inhaler (aerosol), powder for inhalation. Take 2 x daily.

Usual adult dosage range: 100mcg daily (2 inhalations twice daily).

Onset and duration of effect: Starts to work in 10–20 minutes. Action lasts for 12 hours.

Diet advice: None.

Storage: Keep in a cool, dry place out of the reach of children.

If you miss or exceed a dose: Take missed dose as soon as you remember. If your next dose is due within 4 hours, take a single dose now and skip the next. An occasional unintentional extra dose is unlikely to be a cause for concern. But if you notice any unusual symptoms, or if a large overdose has been taken, notify your doctor.

Stopping the drug: Do not stop the drug without consulting your doctor; symptoms may recur.

Prolonged use: Salmeterol is intended to be used long term. The main problem comes from using combinations of anti-asthma drugs, leading to low blood potassium levels. Periodic blood tests are usually carried out to monitor potassium levels.

Dependence rating: Low

Overdose danger rating: Low

❗ POSSIBLE SIDE EFFECTS AND WHAT TO DO

Side effects are usually mild. If you experience **tremor**, discuss with your doctor if bothersome. If you experience **palpitations** or **headache**, discuss with your doctor in all cases. Stop taking the drug now and call your doctor if you develop **sudden breathlessness**.

✋ SPECIAL PRECAUTIONS

Tell your doctor if you have: heart problems; high blood pressure; an overactive thyroid; diabetes; untreated respiratory infection; allergy to milk or lactose. **Also discuss if you are:** taking other medications.
• **No evidence of risk** in pregnancy known when used by inhalation to treat asthma. Discuss with your doctor.
• **Discuss** with your doctor if you are breast-feeding: the drug passes into the breast milk, but at normal doses adverse effects on the baby are unlikely.
• **Reduced dose necessary** for children. Not recommended for children under 4 years.
• **Avoid** driving and hazardous work until you have learned how salmeterol affects you because the drug can cause tremors.

🔄 INTERACTIONS

There is an increased risk of low blood potassium levels when high doses of salmeterol are taken with **corticosteroids, theophylline, diuretics** and other drugs.

Drugs that inhibit CP450 3A4 enzyme, such as **ketoconazole** or **clarithromycin,** should be used cautiously with salmeterol.

Any **sympathomimetic drug** when used with salmeterol may increase side effects, especially the cardiovascular effects.

SIMVASTATIN

Product names: Apo-Simvastatin, CO-Simvastatin, Mylan Simavastatin, Teva-Simvastatin, Zocor, and others
Used in the following combined preparations: None

WHY IS THIS DRUG USED?

Simvastatin is a lipid-lowering drug that lowers the blood levels of cholesterol. The drug is prescribed for people with hypercholesterolemia (*high levels of cholesterol* in the blood) who have not responded to other forms of therapy, such as a special diet, and who are at risk of developing or have existing coronary heart disease. Simvastatin should be taken at the same time daily, and should be continued even when cholestrol levels are normal as the benefits seen with this class of drugs are long-term.

INFORMATION FOR USERS

Prescription needed. Do not alter dosage without checking with your doctor.

How and when to take: Available as tablets. Take once daily in the evening.

Usual adult dosage range: 10–80mg daily.

Onset and duration of effect: Starts to work within 2 weeks; full beneficial effects may not be felt for 4–6 weeks. Action lasts up to 24 hours.

Diet advice: A low-fat diet is usually recommended.

Storage: Keep in a closed container in a cool, dry place out of the reach of children. Protect from light.

If you miss or exceed a dose: Take missed dose as soon as you remember. If your next dose is due within 8 hours, do not take the missed dose, but take the next dose on schedule. An occasional unintentional extra dose is unlikely to cause problems. Large overdoses may cause liver problems. Notify your doctor.

Stopping the drug: Do not stop taking the drug without consulting your doctor as it may lead to worsening of the underlying condition.

Prolonged use: Prolonged treatment can adversely affect liver function. Regular blood tests to check liver function are recommended. Tests of muscle function may be carried out if problems are suspected.

Dependence rating: Low

Overdose danger rating: Medium

POSSIBLE SIDE EFFECTS AND WHAT TO DO

Most side effects are mild and usually disappear with time. If you experience **headache, nausea,** or **fatigue,** discuss with your doctor if bothersome. If you experience **chest or abdominal pain, muscle weakness,** or **jaundice,** discuss with your doctor in all cases. Stop taking the drug now and call your doctor if you develop a **rash** or **change in cognition.**

SPECIAL PRECAUTIONS

Tell your doctor if you have: liver or kidney problems; eye or vision problems; muscle weakness; a family history of muscular disorders; a thyroid disorder; a history of alcohol abuse; porphyria; angina; high blood pressure. **Also discuss if you are:** taking other medications.
- **Not usually prescribed** in pregnancy; safety not established in breast-feeding. Discuss with your doctor.
- **Not recommended** for infants and children.
- **Avoid** excessive amounts of alcohol as it may increase the risk of developing liver problems with this drug.

INTERACTIONS

Simvastatin may increase the effect of **anticoagulants.** Close monitoring and dose adjustment may be required.
　　The use of other **lipid-lowering drugs** with simvastatin may increase the risk of muscle toxicity.
　　Amiodarone and **grapefruit juice** may increase blood levels of simvastatin.
　　Cyclosporine, immunosuppressants, or **antivirals,** given with simvastatin, can increase the risk of muscle toxicity; not usually prescribed together.
　　Itraconazole, ketoconazole erythromycin, or **protease inhibitors,** given with a statin, may increase the risk of muscle damage.
　　Simvastatin may decrease the effect of **clopidogrel.**

SITAGLIPTIN PHOSPHATE

Product name: Januvia
Used in the following combined preparation: Janumet

❓ WHY IS THIS DRUG USED?

Sitagliptin is used to treat non-insulin-dependent *diabetes mellitus* (NIDDM, Type 2 diabetes) when metformin cannot be used to control blood glucose levels. It can also be used in combination with metformin and other oral anti-diabetic medications. It works by inhibiting an enzyme called dipeptidyl peptidase 4 (DPP-4). The drug helps to increase the insulin level when blood sugar levels are high, such as after a meal, and also decreases the amount of sugar made by the body. This drug is not recommended to be used in those with Type 1 diabetes.

ℹ️ INFORMATION FOR USERS

Prescription needed. Do not alter dosage without checking with your doctor.

How and when to take: Available as tablets. Take 1 tablet once daily. The combination product (Janumet) is to be taken twice daily.

Usual adult dosage range: 100mg daily.

Onset and duration of effect: Starts to work within 1–4 hours; action lasts at least 24 hours.

Diet advice: A low-fat, low-sugar diet must be maintained in order for the drug to be fully effective. Follow your doctor's advice.

Storage: Keep in a closed container in a cool, dry place out of the reach of children.

If you miss or exceed a dose: Once daily regimen: If you remember a missed dose within 12 hours, take it as soon as you remember. If you do not remember until later, do not take the missed dose and do not double up the next one. Instead, go back to your regular schedule. An occasional unintentional extra dose is unlikely to cause problems. Notify your doctor and seek medical help with large overdoses.

Stopping the drug: Consult your doctor, as stopping the drug may lead to worsening of the underlying condition

Prolonged use: No problems expected.

Dependence rating: Low

Overdose danger rating: Medium

❗ POSSIBLE SIDE EFFECTS AND WHAT TO DO

If you develop a **stuffy or runny nose, sore throat, diarrhea,** or **constipation,** discuss with your doctor if bothersome. When combined with other anti-diabetic medication, low blood sugar may occur. If symptoms of low blood sugar develop such as **headache, drowsiness, weakness, dizziness, confusion,** a **fast heartbeat,** or **sweating,** call your doctor and seek medical help. If you develop **severe abdominal pain** and **nausea,** or a **rash, swelling of the face,** or **difficulty breathing,** stop taking the drug now and call your doctor.

👋 SPECIAL PRECAUTIONS

Tell your doctor if you have: pancreatitis; gall stones; high triglyceride levels; kidney or liver problems; congestive heart failure; a history of allergic reaction to sitagliptan, or if you drink alcohol regularly. **Also consult if you are:** pregnant; breast-feeding; taking other medications.
- **Safety not established** in pregnancy and breast-feeding.
- **Not recommended** for those less than 18 years of age.
- **Reduced dose** may be needed for those over 60 based on kidney function.
- **Avoid** driving and hazardous work if you have warning signs of low blood sugar.
- **Avoid** alcohol as it increases the risk of low blood sugar.

🎯 INTERACTIONS

Sitagliptin may cause hypoglycemia when administered with other drugs that lower blood glucose levels.
    Sitagliptin may increase the risk of facial swelling (angioedema) with **ACE inhibitors.**
    Somatriptin may decrease the effectiveness of sitagliptin.

SULFAMETHOXAZOLE-TRIMETHOPRIM

Product names: Apo Sulfatrim, Apo Sulfatrim DS, Protrin DS, Septra, Teva-Sulfamethoxazole Trimethoprim, Trisulfa, Trisulfa DS, and others
Used in the following combined preparations: This is a combination product.

❓ WHY IS THIS DRUG USED?

Sulfamethoxazole-trimethoprim is a mixture of two antibacterial drugs, also known as co-trimoxazole. It is prescribed for prevention and treatment of *urinary tract infections* and treatment of skin, ear, and gastrointestinal infections. It is also used to treat pneumocystis pneumonia, toxoplasmosis, and the bacterial infection nocardiasis. Although co-trimoxazole was widely prescribed in the past, its use has declined in recent years with development of resistance to it by some bacteria and the introduction of new, more effective, and safer drugs.

ℹ️ INFORMATION FOR USERS

Prescription needed. Do not alter dosage without checking with your doctor.

How and when to take: Available as tablets, tablets double strength (DS), liquid, injection. Normally taken 2 x daily, preferably with food.

Usual adult dosage range: Usually 4 tablets daily (each standard tablet is 400mg sulfamethoxazole and 80mg trimethroprim) or 2 DS daily. Higher doses may be used for the treatment of pneumocystis pneumonia, toxoplasmosis, and nocardiasis.

Onset and duration of effect: Starts to work in 1–4 hours. Action lasts for 12 hours.

Diet advice: Drink plenty of fluids, particularly in warm weather.

Storage: Keep in a closed container in a cool, dry place out of the reach of children. Protect from light.

If you miss or exceed a dose: Take missed dose as soon as you remember. If your normal dose is 80/400mg, double this; if it is more than 80/400mg, take one dose only. An occasional unintentional extra dose is unlikely to be a cause for concern. Large overdoses may cause nausea, vomiting, dizziness, and confusion; notify your doctor.

Stopping the drug: Take the full course. The original infection may recur if treatment is stopped too soon.

Prolonged use: May lead to folic acid deficiency, which can cause anemia. Folic acid supplements may be needed. Regular blood tests are recommended.

Dependence rating: Low

Overdose danger rating: Medium

❗ POSSIBLE SIDE EFFECTS AND WHAT TO DO

If you develop **diarrhea**, discuss with your doctor if bothersome. If you experience **nausea/vomiting, sore tongue, headache,** or **jaundice,** discuss with your doctor in all cases. Stop taking the drug now and call your doctor if you experience a **rash** or **itching.**

🖐️ SPECIAL PRECAUTIONS

Tell your doctor if you have: long-term liver or kidney problems; a blood disorder including anemia; glucose-6-phosphate dehydrogenase (G6PD) deficiency; porphyria. **Also discuss if you are:** allergic to sulfonamide drugs; taking other medications.
- **Not usually prescribed** in pregnancy, especially as trimethoprim may cause defects in the baby.
- **Discuss** with your doctor if breast-feeding. The drug passes into the breast milk, but at normal levels adverse effects on the baby are unlikely.
- **Not recommended** in infants under 2 months. Reduced dose necessary in older children.
- **Used only when necessary** in those over 60 due to increased likelihood of adverse effects.

⚙️ INTERACTIONS

Sulfamethoxazole-trimethoprim may increase the anticoagulant effect of **warfarin**; reduced dose of warfarin may be necessary.
  Taking **cyclosporine** with sulfamethoxazole-trimethoprim can impair kidney function.
  Sulfamethoxazole-trimethoprim may cause a build-up of **phenytoin** in the body; reduced dose of phenytoin may be necessary.
  Sulfamethoxazole-trimethoprim may increase the blood sugar lowering effect of **oral antidiabetic drugs**.
  Trimethoprim may enhance the toxic effect of **methotrexate.**
  Antibiotics may diminish the effect of **live vaccines,** like Typhoid.
  Methenamine may enhance the toxic effects of sulfonamides.
  Fluconazole and **ketoconazole** may cause a build-up of sulfamethoxazole.

TERAZOSIN

Product names: Apo-Terazosin, Hytrin, PMS-Terazosin, Teva-Terazosin, and others
Used in the following combined preparations: None

❓ WHY IS THIS DRUG USED?

Terazosin is an antihypertensive drug and is used to treat *high blood pressure* (hypertension). The drug works by relaxing the muscles in the blood vessel walls. Terazosin is also used to relieve the obstruction caused by an enlarged prostate

(benign prostatic hyperplasia, or BPH), thereby improving the flow of urine. Dizziness and fainting, especially on standing up, are common side effects at the start of treatment, so it is advisable to take the drug just before going to bed.

ℹ️ INFORMATION FOR USERS

Prescription needed. Do not alter dosage without checking with your doctor.

How and when to take: Available as tablets. Take once daily.

Usual adult dosage range: *Hypertension* 1mg at bedtime (starting dose) doubled after 7 days if necessary. Usual dosage range 1–5mg. *Benign prostatic hyperplasia* 1mg at bedtime (starting dose); may increase gradually after 1–2 weeks if necessary. Usual dosage range 5–10mg.

Onset and duration of effect: *Hypertension* Starts to work within 3 hours. *Benign prostatic hypertrophy* Improvements in symptoms can occur as early as 2 weeks after starting treatment. Full beneficial effects may not be felt for 4–6 weeks. Action lasts for 24 hours.

Diet advice: None.

Storage: Keep in a closed container in a cool dry place out of the reach of children.

If you miss or exceed a dose: Do not double up on a missed dose. Take the next dose at the usual time. An occasional unintentional extra dose is unlikely to be a cause for concern. Large overdoses may drop blood pressure and cause dizziness or fainting; notify your doctor.

Stopping the drug: Do not stop the drug without consulting your doctor as it may lead to an increase in blood pressure.

Prolonged use: No problems expected.

Dependence rating: Low

Overdose danger rating: Medium

❗ POSSIBLE SIDE EFFECTS AND WHAT TO DO

A common problem with terazosin is that it may cause dizziness or fainting when you stand up.
    If you experience **weakness, nausea, drowsiness, stuffy nose,** or **headache,** discuss

with your doctor if bothersome. If you experience **dizziness/faintness, palpitations, ankle swelling,** or **blurred vision,** discuss with your doctor in all cases.

✋ SPECIAL PRECAUTIONS

Tell your doctor if you are: taking other medications.
* **Safety not established** in pregnancy or breast-feeding. Discuss with your doctor.
* **Not recommended** for infants and children.
* **Avoid** driving and hazardous work until you have learned how terazosin affects you because the drug can cause dizziness, lightheadedness, or drowsiness.
* **Avoid** alcohol as it may increase some of the adverse effects of terazosin, such as drowsiness.
* **Discuss** with your doctor or dentist before you have any surgery; terazosin may need to be stopped.

↻ INTERACTIONS

Anesthetics, antidepressants, and **hypotensive drugs** may enhance the blood pressure-lowering effect of terazosin.
    Beta blockers may enhance the blood pressure decrease cause by terazosin. Use with caution.
    Avoid using terazosin with other alpha-1 blocking agents such as **tamsulosin** or **prazosin**.

TIOTROPIUM

Product name: Spiriva
Used in the following combined preparations: None

❓ WHY IS THIS DRUG USED?

Tiotropium, inhaled as a powder, is an anticholinergic bronchodilator that relaxes the muscles surrounding the bronchioles (airways in the lung). It is used in the maintenance treatment of reversible airway disorders, such as chronic *bronchitis*. Tiotropium is a long-acting drug, but its effects are felt after only 5 minutes or so. It is used in the maintenance treatment of airway disorders, such as *chronic obstructive pulmonary disease* (COPD) and chronic bronchitis.

ℹ INFORMATION FOR USERS

Prescription needed. Do not alter dosage without checking with your doctor.

How and when to take: Available as powder in capsules for inhalation. Take once daily, at the same time each day.

Usual adult dosage range: 18mcg daily.

Onset and duration of effect: Starts to work in 5 minutes. Action lasts 24 hours.

Diet advice: None.

Storage: Keep in a closed container in a cool, dry place out of the reach of children.

If you miss or exceed a dose: Take missed dose as soon as you remember. If your next dose is due within 8 hours, take a single dose now and skip the next. An occasional unintentional extra dose is unlikely to be a cause for concern. If you notice any unusual symptoms, or if a large overdose has been taken, notify your doctor.

Stopping the drug: Do not stop taking the drug without consulting your doctor; symptoms may recur.

Prolonged use: No known problems.

Dependence rating: Low

Overdose danger rating: Low

❗ POSSIBLE SIDE EFFECTS AND WHAT TO DO

If you get the powder in your eyes, it could trigger glaucoma; call your doctor immediately.
  If you experience **dry mouth, sore throat** or **constipation,** discuss with your doctor if bothersome. If you experience **fast heart** beat/palpitations, difficulty in passing urine, rash, or wheezing after inhalation,** discuss with your doctor in all cases. Call your doctor now if you develop **eye pain, blurred vision,** or **visual halos**.

🖐 SPECIAL PRECAUTIONS

Tell your doctor if you have: prostate problems; urinary retention; glaucoma; kidney problems.
Also discuss if you are: allergic to atropine or ipratropium; taking other medications.
• **Safety not established** in pregnancy or breast-feeding.
• **Not recommended** for children under 18 years of age.
• **Avoid** getting the powder into the eyes as it could trigger glaucoma or make existing glaucoma worse. If you develop eye or vision problems, call your doctor immediately.

⊘ INTERACTIONS

The effects and toxicity of tiotropium are likely to be increased if it is used at the same time as **atropine** and **ipratropium.**

TIZANIDINE

Product names: Apo-Tizanidine, Mylan-Tizanidine, Zanaflex
Used in the following combined preparations: None

❓ WHY IS THIS DRUG USED?

Tizanidine is a medication used to treat muscle spasms. It can be used in many conditions where spasticity or muscle tone needs to be controlled, such as multiple sclerosis or spinal cord injury. The dose should be scheduled so that the peak effect coincides with the time when relief of spasticity is most desirable. Generally, the drug is well tolerated. Side effects can be minimized by increasing the dose gradually.

ℹ️ INFORMATION FOR USERS

Prescription needed. Do not alter dosage without checking with your doctor.

How and when to take: Available as tablets. Take up to three or four times daily.

Usual adult dosage range: 4–8mg (1–2 tablets) two to four times daily; starting dose 4mg once daily. Daily maximum: 36mg.

Onset and duration of effect: Peak effect usually occurs in 1–2 hours. Action may last between 3–6 hours.

Diet advice: None.

Storage: Keep in a closed container in a cool, dry place out of the reach of children.

If you miss or exceed a dose: Take missed dose as soon as you remember. If it is near the time of the next dose, skip the missed dose and resume your usual dosing schedule. Do not double up on a dose to catch up. An occasional unintentional extra dose is unlikely to cause problems. Large overdoses may cause severe drowsiness, fainting, or trouble breathing. If overdose is suspected, notify your local poison control centre right away.

Stopping the drug: Do not stop the drug without consulting your doctor as it may lead to worsening of the underlying condition.

Prolonged use: If this medication has been taken for a prolonged time, it should not be stopped suddenly without consulting with your doctor; a gradual withdrawal is recommended. Periodic blood tests may be performed to check for liver function.

Dependence rating: Low

Overdose danger rating: Medium

❗ POSSIBLE SIDE EFFECTS AND WHAT TO DO

High doses can cause blood pressure to decrease significantly; stand up slowly when arising from a sitting or lying position to minimize dizziness. If you experience **dizziness, drowsiness, nausea, dry mouth, constipation,** or **muscle fatigue/weakness,** discuss with your doctor if bothersome. Call your doctor now if you experience **stomach pain, vomiting, yellowing of skin or eyes,** or **vision/hearing changes**.

✋ SPECIAL PRECAUTIONS

Tell your doctor if you have: fainted before or have low blood pressure; kidney problems; psychiatric illness. **Also discuss if you are:** allergic to tizanidine; taking blood pressure medications; on any other medications.
- **Safety not established** in pregnancy or breast-feeding. Discuss with your doctor.
- **Not recommended** for infants and children.
- **Reduced dose** may be necessary for those over 60.
- **Avoid** driving and hazardous work until you have learned how the drug affects you; it can cause reduced alertness and slowed reactions.
- **Avoid** alcohol as it can increase side effects of tizanidine.

🔄 INTERACTIONS

All **drugs that cause drowsiness,** such as alcohol, anti-anxiety and sleeping drugs, **antihistamines,** antidepressants, opioid analgesics, and antipsychotics, can increase the sedative properties of tizanidine.
   The effect of **antihypertensive and diuretic drugs** may be increased.
   Oral contraceptives may increase the effect of tizanidine; dose of tizanidine may need to be adjusted.
   Ciprofloxacin and **fluvoxamine** can increase the levels of tizanidine; not recommended to be used together.

TOLTERODINE

Product names: Detrol, Detrol LA
Used in the following combined preparations: None

❓ WHY IS THIS DRUG USED?

Tolterodine is an anticholinergic and antispasmodic drug used to treat urinary frequency and *incontinence* in adults. Tolterodine works by reducing contraction of the bladder, allowing it to expand and hold more urine. It also stops spasms and delays the desire to empty the bladder.

Tolterodine's usefulness is limited to some extent by its side effects, and dosage needs to be reduced in the elderly. Children are more susceptible than adults to the drug's anticholinergic effects. Tolterodine can also trigger glaucoma.

ℹ INFORMATION FOR USERS

Prescription needed. Do not alter dosage without checking with your doctor.

How taken: Available as tablets, ER capsules. Take 2 x daily, once daily for extended release.

Usual adult dosage range: 4mg daily, reduced to 2mg daily, if necessary, especially in those with kidney or liver problems, to minimize side effects.

Onset and duration of effect: Starts to work in 1 hour. Action lasts for 12 hours; 24 hours for ER capsules.

Diet advice: None.

Storage: Keep in a closed container in a cool, dry place out of the reach of children.

If you miss or exceed a dose: Take missed dose as soon as you remember. If your next dose is due within 2 hours, take a single dose now and skip the next.

An occasional unintentional extra dose is unlikely to cause problems. Large overdoses may cause visual disturbances, urinary difficulties, hallucinations, convulsions, and breathing difficulties; notify your doctor.

Stopping the drug: Do not stop taking the drug without consulting your doctor; symptoms may recur.

Prolonged use: No special problems. Effectiveness of the drug, and continuing clinical need for it, are usually reviewed after 6 months. Periodic eye tests for glaucoma may be performed.

Dependence rating: Low

Overdose danger rating: Medium

❗ POSSIBLE SIDE EFFECTS AND WHAT TO DO

If you experience **dry mouth, digestive upset, constipation, abdominal pain, headache, dry eyes, blurred vision, drowsiness,** or **nervousness,** discuss with your doctor if bothersome. If you develop **chest pain, confusion,** or **urinary difficulties,** discuss with your doctor in all cases.

✋ SPECIAL PRECAUTIONS

Tell your doctor if you have: liver or kidney problems; thyroid problems; heart problems; porphyria; hiatus hernia; prostate problems or urinary retention; ulcerative colitis; glaucoma; myasthenia gravis. **Also discuss if you are:** taking other medications.
- **Safety not established** in pregnancy or breast-feeding. Discuss with your doctor.
- **Not recommended** for infants and children.
- **Reduced dose** may be necessary for those over 60.
- **Avoid** driving and hazardous work; tolterodine may cause drowsiness, disorientation, and blurred vision.
- **Avoid** alcohol as it increases the drug's sedative effects.

🔄 INTERACTIONS

All drugs that have an anticholinergic effect will have increased side effects when taken with tolterodine.
  Bupropion, fluoxetine, paroxetine, ritonavir, lopinavir, erythromycin, clarithromycin, ketaconazole, itraconazole and **other drugs** may increase tolterodine levels.
  The effects of **domperidone** and **metoclopramide** may be decreased by tolterodine.

TOPIRAMATE

Product names: Apo-Topiramate, Dom-Topiramate, Mylan-Topiramate, PMS-Topiramate, Sandoz Topiramate, Teva-Topiramate, Topamax, and others
Used in the following combined preparations: None

❓ WHY IS THIS DRUG USED?

Topiramate is an anticonvulsant drug, usually prescribed in combination with other anticonvulsants, such as valproic acid, carbamazepine, or phenytoin, for the treatment of epilepsy. It may also be used in adults to prevent or reduce the frequency of *migraine* headaches. Topiramate may cause a number of dose-related side effects. Some individuals may experience weight loss; if this occurs, an increase in food intake or dietary supplements may be helpful.

ℹ️ INFORMATION FOR USERS

Prescription needed. Do not alter dosage without checking with your doctor.

How and when to take: Available as tablets, sprinkle capsules. Usually taken twice daily; can sprinkle capsule contents on soft food or swallow whole. Do not crush tablets; swallow whole.

Usual adult dosage range: 50mg (starting); 200–400mg daily (maintenance).

Onset and duration of effect: Starts to work approximately 4–8 days at a constant dose. Action lasts up to 24 hours.

Diet advice: None.

Storage: Keep in a closed container in a cool, dry place out of the reach of children.

If you miss or exceed a dose: If it is almost time for the next dose, take a single dose now and skip the next. Do not double up on a dose. An occasional unintentional extra dose is unlikely to be a cause for concern. Large overdoses may cause sedation, loss of muscular coordination, nausea, and vomiting. Contact your doctor immediately.

Stopping the drug: Do not stop taking the drug without consulting your doctor. A gradual reduction is necessary to reduce the risk of rebound seizures.

Prolonged use: No problems expected.

Dependence rating: Low

Overdose danger rating: Medium

❗ POSSIBLE SIDE EFFECTS AND WHAT TO DO

Generally well tolerated. If you experience **headache, dizziness,** or **drowsiness,** discuss with your doctor if bothersome. If you experience **nervousness, difficulty coordinating muscle movements/speech problems, difficulty** concentrating or with memory, tingling in fingers or toes, confusion, mood changes, vision changes, or **decreased sweating,** discuss with your doctor in all cases.

✋ SPECIAL PRECAUTIONS

Tell your doctor if you have: long-term liver or kidney problems; a heart condition. **Also discuss if you are:** taking other medications.
* **Safety not established** in pregnancy or breast-feeding. Discuss with your doctor.
* **Not recommended** in children younger than 2 years.
* **Reduced dose** recommended in children between 2 and 18 years of age, and possibly for those over 60.
* **Avoid** driving and hazardous work until you have learned how topiramate affects you because the drug can cause drowsiness.
* **Avoid** alcohol as it may increase the adverse effects of this drug.

🔄 INTERACTIONS

Phenytoin and **carbamazepine** can decrease the effectiveness of topiramate and the dose of topiramate may need to be adjusted.
   Acetazolamide, when taken with topiramate, can increase the risk of kidney stones.
   Topiramate may decrease the amount of estrogen in the bodies of women taking **oral contraceptives,** possibly decreasing their effectiveness.
   When **metformin** (used in diabetic management) is given with topiramate, blood glucose levels should be closely followed.
   CNS depressants can have additive side effects with topiramate.
   Thiazide diuretics may increase the effect of topiramate; dose adjustment of topiramate may be needed. Also, when both are used together, potassium levels need to be monitored closely.

VALSARTAN

Product name: Diovan
Used in the following combined preparation: Diovan-HCT

❷ WHY IS THIS DRUG USED?

Valsartan is a vasodilator drug that works by causing the blood vessel walls to relax, thereby easing *high blood pressure*. It can also be used after a *heart attack* to improve prognosis and in those with *heart failure*, who cannot take ACE inhibitors. Valsartan is prescribed with caution to people with stenosis (narrowing) of the arteries of the kidneys.

❸ INFORMATION FOR USERS

Prescription needed. Do not alter dosage without checking with your doctor.

How and when to take: Available as tablets. Take once daily (high blood pressure) to twice daily (heart failure).

Adult dosage range: 40–320mg daily.

Onset and duration of effect: Starts to work within 2 hours; it may take 1–2 weeks to see changes in blood pressure, with maximal effect in 3–6 weeks. Action of each tablet lasts up to 24 hours.

Diet advice: None.

Storage: Keep in a closed container in a cool, dry place out of the reach of children.

If you miss or exceed a dose: Take missed dose as soon as you remember. If you take the dose daily and your next dose is within 8 hours, take a single dose now and skip the next. An occasional unintentional extra dose is unlikely to cause problems. Large overdoses may cause dizziness and fainting. Notify your doctor.

Stopping the drug: Do not stop the drug without consulting your doctor as it may lead to worsening of the underlying condition.

Prolonged use: No special problems. Periodic checks on blood potassium levels may be performed.

Dependence rating: Low

Overdose danger rating: Medium

❶ POSSIBLE SIDE EFFECTS AND WHAT TO DO

Dizziness is a common side effect; make sure to get up slowly from a chair or bed while supporting yourself. If you experience **dizziness, fatigue, headache, diarrhea,** or **abdominal pain,** discuss with your doctor if bothersome. If you experience **chills, fever, sore throat, rash/itching,** or **jaundice,** discuss with your doctor in all cases. Stop taking the drug now and call your doctor if you develop **wheezing** or **facial swelling.**

❿ SPECIAL PRECAUTIONS

Tell your doctor if you have: kidney or liver problems. **Also discuss if you are:** at risk for dehydration; allergic to valsartan or any other medications; taking other medications.
- **Not prescribed** in pregnancy or while breast-feeding.
- **Not recommended** for infants and children.
- **Reduced dose** may be necessary for those over 60.
- **Avoid** driving and hazardous work until you have learned how valsartan affects you because the drug can cause dizziness and fatigue.
- **Avoid** alcohol as it may affect your blood pressure, reducing the effectiveness of valsartan.

❼ INTERACTIONS

There is a risk of a sudden fall in blood pressure when **diuretics** are taken with valsartan.

Valsartan increases the effect of **potassium supplements, potassium-sparing diuretics,** and **cyclosporine,** leading to raised levels of potassium in the blood.

Valsartan may increase the levels and toxicity of **lithium.**

Valsartan may increase the effect of **warfarin.** Close monitoring of INR levels are required, with possible dose adjustment.

Certain **non-steroidal anti-inflammatory drugs** (NSAIDs) may interfere with the blood-pressure lowering effect of valsartan.

VARENICLINE

Product name: Champix
Used in the following combined preparations: None

❓ WHY IS THIS DRUG USED?

Varenicline is used to treat *tobacco addiction* in adults by relieving symptoms of nicotine withdrawal and craving. Treatment usually starts one to two weeks prior to the date when you decide to stop smoking, and continues for 12 weeks. For those who have successfully stopped smoking at the end of 12 weeks, the medication may be continued for another 12-week cycle. Throughout treatment, you should continue any other quit-smoking strategies or counselling recommended by your doctor or pharmacist. Varenicline is not recommended to be used with nicotine-containing products.

ℹ️ INFORMATION FOR USERS

Prescription needed. Do not alter dosage without checking with your doctor.

How and when to take: Available as tablets. Take once to twice daily. Take after a meal, with a full glass of water.

Adult dosage range: 0.5–2mg daily.

Onset and duration of effect: Starts to work in 3–4 hours. Action lasts up to 24 hours.

Diet advice: None.

Storage: Keep in a closed container in a cool, dry place out of the reach of children.

If you miss or exceed a dose: Take missed dose as soon as you remember. If it is almost time for the next dose, skip the missed dose and continue your usual dosing schedule. Do not double up on a dose. An occasional unintentional extra dose is unlikely to cause problems. With large overdoses, notify your doctor immediately.

Stopping the drug: Do not stop the drug without consulting your doctor as it may lead to worsening of the underlying condition.

Prolonged use: Varenicline is not normally used for prolonged periods.

Dependence rating: Low

Overdose danger rating: Medium

❗ POSSIBLE SIDE EFFECTS AND WHAT TO DO

If you experience **nausea, vomiting, headache, constipation, flatulence,** or **taste changes,** discuss with your doctor if bothersome.
If you experience **abnormal dreams, sleep disturbance, dizziness/drowsiness, unusual tiredness/weakness,** or **abdominal pain,** discuss with your doctor in all cases. Call your doctor now if you develop **changes in your usual thought or behaviour, anxiety, agitation, mood swings** or **thoughts of harming yourself**. Stop taking the drug now and call your doctor if you experience an **allergic reaction** (puffy, swollen eyelids, lips, throat, or hands, shortness of breath).

👐 SPECIAL PRECAUTIONS

Tell your doctor if you have: kidney disease; a history of alcohol abuse. **Also discuss if you are:** taking nicotine replacement therapy; allergic to varenicline; taking other medications.
* **Safety not established** in pregnancy or breast-feeding. Discuss with your doctor.
* **Not recommended** for infants and children.
* **Reduced dose** may be recommended for those over 60 with compromised kidney function.
* **Avoid** driving and hazardous work until you have learned how varenicline affects you.
* **Avoid** alcohol, which may increase the risk of drowsiness, agitation, anxiety, or depressed mood side effects.

🔄 INTERACTIONS

When used with **nicotine** products, side effects such as nausea, vomiting, headache, and dizziness may be higher. Not recommended to be used with nicotine or nicotine replacement therapy.

VENLAFAXINE

Product names: Effexor XR, Mylan-Venlafaxine XR, PMS-Venlafaxine XR, Sandoz Venlafaxine XR, Teva-Venlafaxine XR, and others
Used in the following combined preparations: None

❶ WHY IS THIS DRUG USED?

Venlafaxine is an antidepressant that combines the therapeutic properties of both the tricyclic antidepressants and selective serotonin reuptake inhibitors (SSRIs), without anticholinergic adverse effects. It acts against *depression* to elevate mood, increase physical activity, and restore interest in everyday pursuits. It is also used to treat generalized anxiety disorder and panic disorder.

❶ INFORMATION FOR USERS

Prescription needed. Do not alter dosage without checking with your doctor.

How and when to take: Available as extended release capsules. Take once daily with food.

Usual dosage range: 75–150mg daily for outpatients; up to 375mg daily in severely depressed patients.

Onset and duration of effect: Full antidepressant effect may not be felt for 2–4 weeks or more. Action lasts for at least 24 hours. Following prolonged treatment, antidepressant effects may persist for up to 6 weeks.

Diet advice: None.

Storage: Keep in the original container in a cool, dry place out of the reach of children.

If you miss a dose: Do not make up for a missed dose. Just take your next regularly scheduled dose.

Stopping the drug: Consult your doctor; stopping abruptly can cause withdrawal symptoms.

Prolonged use: Withdrawal symptoms, including dizziness, electric shock sensations, anxiety, nausea, and insomnia, may occur if the drug is not stopped gradually. These rarely last for more than 1–2 weeks. If high doses of venlafaxine are prescribed, you will be monitored for high blood pressure.

Dependence rating: Low

Overdose danger rating: High

☠ OVERDOSE ACTION

Seek immediate medical advice in all cases. Take emergency action if seizures, slow or irregular pulse, or loss of consciousness occur.

See Drug poisoning emergency guide (p.197).

❶ POSSIBLE SIDE EFFECTS AND WHAT TO DO

If you experience **nausea, restlessness, insomnia, weakness, blurred vision, drowsiness,** or **dizziness,** discuss with your doctor if bothersome. If you experience **decreased appetite, high blood pressure,** or develop **sexual dysfunction,** discuss with your doctor in all cases. Stop taking the drug now and call your doctor if you develop a **rash/itching.**

❶ SPECIAL PRECAUTIONS

Tell your doctor if you have: a history of adverse reactions to any other antidepressants; long-term liver or kidney problems; a heart problem or elevated blood pressure; a history of epileptic seizures or alcohol or drug abuse. **Also discuss if you are:** taking other medications.
- **Safety not established** in pregnancy; not recommended while breast-feeding.
- **Not recommended** for children under 18 years.
- **Reduced dose** may be necessary for those over 60 due to increased likelihood of adverse effects.
- **Avoid** driving and hazardous work until you have learned how venlafaxine affects you.
- **Avoid** alcohol as it may increase the sedative effects of this drug.

❷ INTERACTIONS

Bupropion, fluoxetine, paroxetine, ritonavir, lopinavir, clarithromycin, itraconazole and **other drugs** may increase venlafaxine levels.
All drugs with a **sedative** effect may increase sedative effects of venlafaxine.
Venlafaxine may reduce the effectiveness of **antihypertensive drugs.**
Venlafaxine may interact with **MAOIs** to produce a dangerous rise in blood pressure. MAOIs should be stopped at least 14 days before starting venlafaxine.
Venlafaxine may interact with **sibutramine;** use together is not recommended.

VERAPAMIL

Product names: Apo-Verap, Apo-Verap SR, Isoptin SR, Mylan-Verapamil, Teva-Verapamil SR, and others
Used in the following combined preparation: Tarka

❓ WHY IS THIS DRUG USED?

Verapamil is used in the treatment of *hypertension*, *abnormal heart rhythms*, and *angina*. It reduces the frequency of angina attacks but does not help relieve pain while an attack is in progress. Verapamil increases the ability to tolerate physical exertion, and unlike some drugs it does not affect breathing so it can be used safely by asthmatics. Verapamil is not generally prescribed for people with low blood pressure, slow heart beat, or heart failure because it may worsen these conditions.

ℹ️ INFORMATION FOR USERS

Prescription needed. Do not alter dosage without checking with your doctor.

How and when to take: Available as tablets, SR-tablets, injection. Take 2–3x daily (tablets); 1–2x daily (SR-tablets). Injection: take as directed by doctor.

Usual adult dosage range: 120–480mg daily.

Onset and duration of effect: Starts to work in 1–2 hours (tablets); 2–3 minutes (injection). Action lasts 6–8 hours. During prolonged treatment some beneficial effects may last for up to 12 hours. SR-tablets start to work in 4–5 hours and act for 12–24 hours.

Diet advice: None.

Storage: Keep in a closed container in a cool, dry place out of the reach of children.

If you miss or exceed a dose: Take missed dose as soon as you remember. If your next dose is due within 3 hours (tablets) or 8 hours (SR-tablets), take a single dose now and skip the next. An occasional unintentional extra dose is unlikely to be a cause for concern. Large overdoses may cause dizziness. Notify your doctor.

Stopping the drug: Do not stop the drug without consulting your doctor; symptoms may recur.

Prolonged use: No problems expected.

Dependence rating: Low

Overdose danger rating: Medium

❗ POSSIBLE SIDE EFFECTS AND WHAT TO DO

Verapamil may cause gynecomastia (breast enlargement in males) and an increase in gum tissue after long-term use. If you experience **constipation, headache, nausea/vomiting,** or **flushing,** discuss with your doctor if bothersome. If you experience **ankle swelling, dizziness,** or **breast/gum enlargement,** discuss with your doctor in all cases. Call your doctor now if you develop a **rash.**

✋ SPECIAL PRECAUTIONS

Tell your doctor if you have: a long-term liver problem; heart failure; porphyria. **Also discuss if you are:** taking other medications.
- **Not usually prescribed** in pregnancy; may inhibit labour if taken during later stages of pregnancy.
- **Discuss** with your doctor if you are breast-feeding; the drug passes into the breast milk, but at normal doses adverse effects on the baby are unlikely.
- **Reduced dose necessary** for infants and children; usually given on specialist advice only.
- **Avoid** driving and hazardous work until you have learned how verapamil affects you because the drug can cause dizziness.
- **Avoid** alcohol as it may further reduce blood pressure, causing dizziness or other symptoms.
- **Consult** your doctor or dentist before surgery; verapamil may need to be stopped.

🔄 INTERACTIONS

When verapamil is taken with **beta blockers**, there is a slight risk of abnormal heart beat and heart failure.
The effects of **carbamazepine** may be enhanced by verapamil.
The blood levels of **cyclosporine** may be increased by verapamil and its dose may need to be reduced.
Blood pressure may be further lowered when **antihypertensive drugs** are taken with verapamil.
The effects of **digoxin** may be increased if it is taken with verapamil. The dosage of digoxin may need to be reduced.
Avoid **grapefruit juice**, which may increase blood levels of verapamil.
Clarithromycin, ketoconzole, and **itraconazole** can increase the effect of verapamil.
Verapamil can increase the level of **dabigatran**; not recommended to be used together.
Verapamil may increase adverse effects of **disopyramide.**

WARFARIN

Product names: Apo-Warfarin, Coumadin, Mylan-Warfarin, Teva-Warfarin, and others
Used in the following combined preparations: None

❓ WHY IS THIS DRUG USED?

Warfarin is an anticoagulant used to prevent blood clots, particularly in the leg and pelvic veins. Clots formed here may travel to the lungs, causing pulmonary embolism. The drug is also used to reduce the risk of clots forming in the heart in people with atrial fibrillation, or after insertion of artificial heart valves. These clots may travel to the brain, causing a *stroke*. Warfarin requires regular monitoring to ensure proper dosage. It is often prescribed initially with heparin, which is a faster-acting drug.

ℹ️ INFORMATION FOR USERS

Prescription needed. Do not alter dosage without checking with your doctor.

How and when to take: Available as tablets. Take once daily, at the same time each day.

Usual dosage range: 10mg for 2 days (starting dose); 2–9mg daily at the same time, as determined by blood tests (maintenance dose).

Onset and duration of effect: Starts to work within 24–48 hours, with full effect after several days. Action lasts for 2–3 days.

Diet advice: None.

Storage: Keep in a closed container in a cool, dry place out of the reach of children. Protect from light.

If you miss a dose: Take as soon as you remember. Take the following dose on your original schedule. Do not double up on your doses. Discuss any missed doses with your doctor.

Stopping the drug: Do not stop taking the drug without consulting your doctor as it may lead to worsening of the underlying condition.

Prolonged use: No special problems. Regular blood tests are performed during treatment.

Dependence rating: Low

Overdose danger rating: High

☠️ OVERDOSE ACTION

Seek immediate medical advice in all cases. Take emergency action if severe bleeding or loss of consciousness occur.

See Drug poisoning emergency guide (p.197).

❗ POSSIBLE SIDE EFFECTS AND WHAT TO DO

Bleeding is the most common side effect with warfarin. If you experience **abdominal pain, diarrhea, rash, or hair loss,** discuss with your doctor in all cases. If you develop **jaundice,** call your doctor now. Stop taking the drug now and call your doctor if you experience **bleeding, bruising, fever, dark stools/urine,** or **nausea/vomiting.**

✋ SPECIAL PRECAUTIONS

Tell your doctor if you have: long-term liver or kidney problems; high blood pressure; peptic ulcers. **Also discuss** if you bleed easily, or if you are taking other medications.
- **Not usually prescribed** in pregnancy.
- **Discuss** with your doctor if you are breast-feeding; the drug passes into the breast milk, but at normal doses adverse effects on the baby are unlikely.
- **Reduced dose necessary** for infants and children.
- **Use caution:** even minor bumps can cause bad bruises and excessive bleeding.
- **Avoid** excessive amounts of alcohol as it may increase the effects of this drug.
- **Consult** with your doctor or dentist before surgery; warfarin may need to be stopped.

🔄 INTERACTIONS

A wide variety of drugs, such as **ASA, barbiturates, oral contraceptives, cimetidine, diuretics,** certain **laxatives,** certain **antidepressants,** and certain **antibiotics** interact with warfarin, either by increasing or decreasing the anticlotting effect. Consult your doctor or pharmacist before using any other medications, including over-the-counter medicines.
   Do not change your diet significantly without discussion with your doctor.

ZOPICLONE

Product names: Apo-Zopiclone, CO Zopiclone, Imovane, Mylan-Zopiclone, ratio-Zopiclone, Rhovane, and others
Used in the following combined preparations: None

❓ WHY IS THIS DRUG USED?

Zopiclone is a hypnotic (sleeping drug) used for the short-term treatment of *insomnia*. Sleep problems can take the form of difficulty in falling asleep, frequent night-time awakenings, and/or early morning awakenings. Hypnotic drugs are given only when non-drug measures – for

example, avoidance of caffeine, regular sleep routine, etc. – have proved ineffective. Unlike sedatives such as benzodiazepines, zopiclone does not have anti-anxiety properties. Hypnotics are intended for occasional use only.

ℹ️ INFORMATION FOR USERS

Prescription needed. Do not alter dosage without checking with your doctor.

How and when to take: Available as tablets. Take once daily at bedtime when required.

Usual dosage range: 3.75–7.5mg.

Onset and duration of effect: Starts to work within 30 minutes. Action lasts 4–6 hours.

Diet advice: None.

Storage: Keep in a closed container in a cool, dry place out of the reach of children. Protect from light.

If you miss or exceed a dose: If you fall asleep without having taken a dose and wake some hours later, do not take the missed dose. An occasional,

unintentional extra dose is unlikely to cause problems. Large overdoses may cause prolonged sleep, drowsiness, lethargy, and poor muscle coordination and reflexes; notify your doctor immediately.

Stopping the drug: The drug can be safely stopped if you have been taking it continuously for less than 1 week. If you have been taking the drug for longer, consult your doctor and pharmacist.

Prolonged use: Intended for occasional use only. Continuous use of zopiclone – or any other sleeping drug – may cause dependence.

Dependence rating: Medium

Overdose danger rating: Medium

⚠️ POSSIBLE SIDE EFFECTS AND WHAT TO DO

If you experience **bitter taste, dizziness, weakness, nausea, vomiting,** or **diarrhea,** discuss with your doctor if bothersome. If you develop **daytime drowsiness** or **headache,**

discuss with your doctor in all cases. Stop taking the drug now and call your doctor if you experience **amnesia, confusion,** or a **rash.**

✋ SPECIAL PRECAUTIONS

Tell your doctor if you have: a history of alcohol or drug misuse/abuse; myasthenia gravis; a history of epileptic seizures; liver or kidney problems. **Also discuss if you are:** taking other medications.
- **Not recommended** during pregnancy or while breast-feeding, or for infants and children.
- **Reduced dose** may be necessary for those over 60.
- **Avoid** driving and hazardous work until you have learned how zopiclone affects you; it can cause drowsiness, reduced alertness, and slowed reactions.
- **Avoid** alcohol as it increases the sedative effects of this drug.

🔄 INTERACTIONS

All drugs, including **alcohol**, that have a sedative effect on the central nervous system are likely to increase the sedative effects of zopiclone. Such drugs include other **sleeping and anti-anxiety drugs, antihistamines, antidepressants, opioid analgesics**, and **antipsychotics**.
Antibiotics such as **clarithromycin** and **erythromycin** may increase the effect of zopiclone.
Other drugs metabolized by the same enzymes as zopiclone can interact with it. Discuss with your pharmacist or doctor.

COMMON VITAMINS, MINERALS, AND SUPPLEMENTS

This section gives detailed information on some of the major vitamins and minerals that are required by the body for good health – essential chemicals that the body cannot make by itself. There are also profiles of some Natural Health Products (NHP) that are commonly used by Canadians.

The following pages may be particularly useful as a guide for those who think their diet lacks sufficient amounts of a certain vitamin or mineral, and for those with disorders of the digestive tract, who may need larger amounts of certain vitamins. The table on p.37 gives the good dietary sources of each one.

HOW TO UNDERSTAND THE PROFILES

The vitamin, mineral, and supplement profiles are arranged in alphabetical order and contain information arranged under standard headings to enable you to find the information you need. The Natural Health Product (NHP) profiles follow a slightly different format.

Other names
Lists the chemical and non-chemical names by which the vitamin or mineral is also known.

Dietary and other natural sources
Tells you how the vitamin or mineral is obtained naturally.

Why take supplements?
Suggests when your doctor may recommend that you take supplements.

Symptoms of deficiency
Describes the common signs of deficiency.

Dosage range for treating deficiency
Gives a usual recommended dosage of vitamin or mineral supplements.

IRON

Other names: Ferrous fumarate, ferrous gluconate, ferrous sulfate, iron dextran, iron-polysaccharide complex, sodium ferric gluconate complex

Why is iron important?
Iron is important in the formation of red blood cells (which contain two-thirds of the body's iron) in which it plays an essential role in the transportation and delivery of oxygen to the body. It is also an important component of several enzymes and plays a role in the conversion of blood sugar to energy.

Dietary and other natural sources of iron
Meat (especially liver and other organ offal), eggs, chicken, fish, leafy green vegetables, dried fruit, enriched or wholegrain cereals, breads and pastas, nuts, and dried legumes. Iron is better absorbed from animal products than from vegetables. Foods containing vitamin C enhance iron absorption.

Normal daily requirement
0.27mg (birth–6 months); 11mg (7–12 months); 7mg (1–3 years); 10mg (4–8 years); 8mg (9–13 years); 11mg (males aged 14–18 years); 15mg (females aged 14–18 years); 8mg (males aged 19 years and over); 18mg (females 19–50 years); 8mg (females 51 years and over); 27mg (pregnant women). **Breast-feeding** 10mg (18 years and under); 9mg (19–50 years).

Why take iron supplements?
Most diets supply adequate amounts of iron. Supplements may be recommended by a doctor for young vegetarians, women with heavy menstrual periods, people with chronic blood loss due to disease (i.e. peptic ulcer), and premature babies. Pregnant women require higher amounts of iron than normal – supplements may be given throughout pregnancy and for 2 to 3 months after childbirth.

Availability: No prescription needed, except for injectable forms (iron dextran).

Symptoms of deficiency
Iron deficiency causes anemia (see p.35). Symptoms include pallor, fatigue, shortness of breath, and palpitations. Apathy, irritability, and lowered resistance to infection may also occur. Iron deficiency may also affect intellectual performance and behaviour.

Dosage range for treating deficiency (under medical supervision)
Depends on the individual and the nature and severity of the condition. *Adults* Usually 100mg of elemental iron (ferrous sulphate or gluconate) daily. *Children* According to age and weight. *Pregnant women* 30–60mg daily.

Risks and special precautions
Treatment should not be taken without a full medical consultation. Keep out of the reach of children. An overdose of iron tablets is very dangerous. Symptoms include pain in the abdomen, nausea, vomiting, abdominal bloating, dehydration, and dangerously lowered blood pressure; seek immediate medical attention (see p.197). Excessive long-term intake, especially when it is taken with large amounts of vitamin C, may cause iron to accumulate in organs, causing congestive heart failure, cirrhosis of the liver, and diabetes mellitus.

182

NIACIN

Other names: Niacinamide, nicotinamide, nicotinic acid, vitamin B₃

Why is niacin important?
Niacin plays a vital role in the activities of many enzymes, and is important in producing energy from blood sugar and in the manufacture of fats. Niacin is essential for the proper working of the nervous system, for a healthy skin and digestive system, and for the manufacture of steroid hormones.

Dietary and other natural sources of niacin
Liver, lean meat, poultry, fish, wholegrain cereals, nuts, and dried legumes.

Normal daily requirement
2mg (birth–6 months); 4mg (7–12 months); 6mg (1–3 years); 8mg (4–8 years); 12mg (9–13 years); 16mg (males aged 14 years and over); and 14mg (females aged 14 years and over). Daily requirements increase during pregnancy (18mg) and during breast-feeding (17mg).

Why take niacin supplements?
Dietary deficiency is rare. Supplements are required for those with bowel disorders in which absorption from the intestine is impaired, for people with liver disease or severe alcoholism, and for elderly people with poor diets. Large doses of niacin (up to 6g daily) may be used in the treatment of dyslipidemia (high cholesterol). Niacinamide is not used to treat this condition.

Availability: No prescription needed, except for high doses.

Symptoms of deficiency
Severe niacin deficiency causes pellagra (literally, rough skin); symptoms include sore, red, cracked skin in areas exposed to sun, friction, or pressure, inflammation of the mouth and tongue, abdominal pain and distension, nausea, diarrhea, and mental disturbances such as depression, anxiety, and dementia.

Dosage range for treating deficiency
Severe pellagra: *Adults* 300–500mg daily by mouth; *Children* 100–300mg daily. For less severe deficiency: 25–50mg daily.

Risks and special precautions
At doses of over 50mg, niacin may cause transient itching, flushing, tingling, or headache. Niacin in the form that occurs naturally in the body (nicotinamide), is free of these effects. Large doses of niacin may cause nausea and may aggravate a peptic ulcer. Side effects may be reduced by taking the drug on a full stomach. At doses of over 2g daily (which have been used to treat hyperlipidemia), there is a risk of gout, liver damage, and high blood sugar levels.

Why is the vitamin or mineral important?
Explains the role played by each vitamin or mineral in maintaining healthy body function.

Normal daily requirement
Gives you a guide to the recommended daily allowance (RDA)* of each vitamin or mineral.

Availability
Tells you whether the vitamin, mineral, or supplement is available over-the-counter or only by prescription.

Risks and special precautions
Explains the risks that may accompany excessive intake of each vitamin or mineral and other cautions.

*The Recommended Daily Allowance (RDA), determined by the Food and Nutrition Board, is the amount of the nutrient thought to be enough for about 97 percent of people. Precise doses need to be determined by your doctor.

CALCIUM

Available as: Calcium acetate, calcium carbonate, calcium chloride, calcium citrate, calcium glucoheptonate, calcium gluconate, calcium lactate, calcium phosphate

Why is calcium important?
Calcium is essential for the formation and maintenance of strong bones and healthy teeth, as well as blood clotting, transmission of nerve impulses, and muscle contraction.

Dietary and other natural sources of calcium
Milk and dairy products, sardines, dark green leafy vegetables, beans, peas and nuts.

Normal daily requirement
200–1,000mg (birth–6 months); 260–1,500mg (7–12 months), 700–2,500mg (1–3 years); 1,000–2,500mg (4–8 years); 1,300–3,000mg (9–18 years); 1,000–2,500mg (19–50 years); 1,000–2,000mg (men 51–70 years); 1,200–2,000mg (women 51–70); 1,200–2,000mg (over 70 years). *Pregnancy and breast-feeding* 1,300–3,000mg (18 years and under); 1,000–2,500mg (19–50 years)

Why take calcium supplements?
Your diet may not contain enough calcium unless you consume a sufficient amount of dairy products (a glass of milk contains approximately 300mg of calcium). Breast-feeding women are especially vulnerable to calcium deficiency. Calcium supplementation can help prevent bone loss. Current osteoporosis guidelines recommend 1,200mg of calcium daily in those older than 50 years, through diet or supplementation.

Availability: No prescription needed, except injectable forms are usually prescribed by a medical practitioner.

Symptoms of deficiency
If your diet doesn't contain enough calcium, your body will obtain what it needs from your skeleton. Long-term deficiency may lead to increased bone fragility (osteoporosis) and risk of fractures. Severe deficiency, resulting in low calcium levels in the blood, can result in cramp-like spasms in the hands, feet, and face.

Dosage range for treating deficiency
Vitamin D helps with calcium absorption and is needed for treatment of rickets and osteomalacia. Oral supplements of up to 800 IU vitamin D daily may be advised for children with rickets, and 800 IU to 1,000 IU daily may be given for osteoporosis and osteomalacia. Severe calcium deficiency is treated in hospital by intravenous injection of calcium.

Risks and special precautions
Excessive intake of calcium may reduce the amount of iron and zinc absorbed and may also cause constipation and nausea. Other risks related to high calcium intake, especially with large amounts of vitamin D, include palpitations and calcium deposits in the kidneys, leading to kidney stones and damage. Older women taking calcium supplements should discuss this with their doctor.

ECHINACEA (NHP)

Other names: *Echinacea angustifolia, Echinacea pallida, Echinacea purpurea,* Black Simpson, Comb Flower, Purple Coneflower, Red Sunflower

What is it?
Echinacea is a perennial herb which grows in the midwestern region of North America. It has pink or purple flowers with a central cone which may be purple or brown in colour. Echinacea is thought to stimulate the immune system when taken orally. Three species of echinacea are commonly used: *E. angustifolia, E. pallida,* and *E. purpurea.* Several compounds found in the plants are considered to contribute to its effect, including cichoric acid, polysaccharide, and alkamide. Different products may use different parts of the plant, with differing effectiveness.

Purported Uses
Used in the treatment of: colds, upper respiratory tract infections, urinary tract infections, cancer. Also used to: improve wound healing and to protect skin from photodamage.

Common Medicinal Use
Echinacea is available for the treatment and prevention of the common cold (p.27) and upper respiratory infections. Some studies involving the treatment of these conditions have indicated beneficial effects, including decreasing the number of colds and infections and decreasing the duration of symptoms when taken within two days of symptom onset, while other studies have shown little or no benefit. Studies that demonstrated benefits used the pressed juice and extracts of *E. purpurea.* It is still unclear how echinacea works pharmacologically and further research is needed to clarify its use in preventing and treating these conditions.

Dosage regimen
For oral administration, available as extracts, tinctures, tablets and capsules. For general immune system stimulation, the dose is usually recommended to be taken three times daily, for 10–14 days and not continuously.
• Dried herb: 1g three times daily
• Tincture (hydroalcoholic) (1:5): 2–5mL three times daily
• Liquid extract (1:1): 0.5–1mL three times daily
• Expressed juice: 6–9mL in divided doses

Risks and special precautions
Individuals who are allergic to plants in the sunflower family may experience allergic symptoms with echinacea. Rarely, it has caused asthma attacks or anaphylactic reaction in others. A case report of liver inflammation (acute hepatitis) has been documented. As echinacea stimulates the immune system, it should be used with caution in those with autoimmune conditions such as lupus or rheumatoid arthritis, and with conditions such as multiple sclerosis, diabetes and tuberculosis. There is limited information in using this product during pregnancy or breast-feeding. Echinacea should be avoided by those who are taking drugs to suppress the immune function (e.g. after an organ transplant). As there may be variability in the products available, a recommendation is to look for the licensed natural health product, which can be identified by its 8-digit Natural Product Number (NPN) designation on the label.

FOLIC ACID

Other names: Folacin, folate, pteroylglutamic acid, vitamin B9

Why is folic acid important?
Folic acid is essential for the activities of several enzymes. It is required for the manufacture of nucleic acids – the genetic material of cells – and thus for the processes of growth and reproduction. It is vital for the formation of red blood cells by the bone marrow and the development and function of the central nervous system.

Dietary and other natural sources of folic acid
Leafy green vegetables, yeast extract, liver, root vegetables, oranges, dried legumes, and egg yolks.

Normal daily requirement
0.065mg (birth–6 months); 0.08mg (7 months–1 year); 0.15mg (1–3 years); 0.20mg (4–8 years); 0.30mg (9–13 years); 0.40mg (14 years and over). *Pregnancy* Healthy women on a folate-rich diet: 0.4–1mg for at least 2–3 months before conception; 0.60mg throughout pregnancy; after childbirth, 0.5mg for 4–6 weeks while breast-feeding. Women with health risks (epilepsy, Type 1 diabetes mellitus, obesity, family history of neural tube defect) on a folate-rich diet: 5mg for 3 months before conception and for the first 10–12 weeks of pregnancy.

Why take folic acid supplements?
Supplements are recommended for women planning a pregnancy and during the first 12 weeks of pregnancy for the prevention of neural tube defects such as spina bifida. Premature or low-birth-weight infants and those fed on goat's milk may also need supplements. Doctors may recommend additional folic acid for people on hemodialysis, and those with certain blood disorders, psoriasis, certain conditions in which absorption of nutrients from the intestine is impaired, severe alcoholism, or liver disease. Supplements may be helpful if you are taking certain drugs that deplete folic acid such as anticonvulsants, antimalarial drugs, estrogen-containing contraceptives, sulfasalazine, methotrexate, and sulfonamide antibacterial drugs.

Availability: No prescription needed for strengths of less than 1,000mcg (1mg).

Symptoms of deficiency
Folic acid deficiency leads to abnormally low numbers of red blood cells (anemia). Common symptoms include fatigue, loss of appetite, nausea, diarrhea, hair loss, mouth sores, and a sore tongue. Deficiency may also cause poor growth in infants and children.

Dosage range for treating deficiency
Anemia is usually treated with 0.25–1mg of folic acid daily (some may need higher doses), sometimes combined with vitamin B12. A lower maintenance dose may be substituted once the anemia has responded.

Risks and special precautions
Excessive folic acid is not toxic. However, it may worsen the symptoms of a coexisting vitamin B12 deficiency and should never be taken to treat anemia without a full medical consultation.

GLUCOSAMINE

Other names: Glucosamine sulfate, Glucosamine hydrochloride

Why is glucosamine important?
Glucosamine is a natural component of cartilage found in human joints and is thought to be able to provide some protection from damage to the cartilage.

Dietary and other natural sources of glucosamine
There are no food sources of glucosamine. Supplements are generally derived from the outer shells of crabs, shrimp, and lobsters.

Normal daily requirement
There are no specific recommended daily allowances for glucosamine.

Why take glucosamine supplements?
Glucosamine has been studied in the treatment of osteoarthritis, especially of the knee. It is thought to provide benefit by strengthening the cartilage in the joints, and improving pain and joint movement associated with osteoarthritis. Based on a recent review, glucosamine, when used up to 3 months, does not seem to have a clear beneficial effect on pain or joint function.

Availability: No prescription needed. Available mainly as tablets or capsules, and as a sulfate salt (glucosamine sulfate), hydrochloride, or hydroiodide.

Symptoms of deficiency
No specific deficiency noted.

Dosage range for treatment of osteoarthritis
Glucosamine sulfate: take 500mg three times daily with food. *Glucosamine hydrochloride:* take up to 2,000mg a day. Beneficial effects may take up to 4 weeks to manifest.

Risks and special precautions
Upset stomach, heartburn, and diarrhea are some of its side effects. It is unclear whether there are any serious effects of excessive intake. Blood glucose may need to be monitored in those with diabetes or on medications that can affect blood glucose. Glucosamine may increase the effect of anti-inflammatory drugs and doses may need adjustment. Pregnant women or women who are breast-feeding should consult their doctor, as safety in these situations has not been established.

IRON

Other names: Ferrous fumarate, ferrous gluconate, ferrous sulfate, iron dextran, iron-polysaccharide complex, sodium ferric gluconate complex

Why is iron important?
Iron is important in the formation of red blood cells (which contain two-thirds of the body's iron) in which it plays an essential role in the transportation and delivery of oxygen to the body. It is also an important component of several enzymes and plays a role in the conversion of blood sugar to energy.

Dietary and other natural sources of iron
Meat (especially liver and other organ offal), eggs, chicken, fish, leafy green vegetables, dried fruit, enriched or wholegrain cereals, breads and pastas, nuts, and dried legumes. Iron is better absorbed from animal products than from vegetables. Foods containing vitamin C enhance iron absorption.

Normal daily requirement
0.27mg (birth–6 months); 11mg (7–12 months); 7mg (1–3 years); 10mg (4–8 years); 8mg (9–13 years); 11mg (males aged 14–18 years); 15mg (females aged 14–18 years); 8mg (males aged 19 years and over); 18mg (females 19–50 years); 8mg (females 51 years and over); 27mg (pregnant women). *Breast-feeding* 10mg (18 years and under); 9mg (19–50 years).

Why take iron supplements?
Most diets supply adequate amounts of iron. Supplements may be recommended by a doctor for young vegetarians, women with heavy menstrual periods, people with chronic blood loss due to disease (i.e. peptic ulcer), and premature babies. Pregnant women require higher amounts of iron than normal – supplements may be given throughout pregnancy and for 2 to 3 months after childbirth.

Availability: No prescription needed, except for injectable forms (iron dextran).

Symptoms of deficiency
Iron deficiency causes anemia (see p.35). Symptoms include pallor, fatigue, shortness of breath, and palpitations. Apathy, irritability, and lowered resistance to infection may also occur. Iron deficiency may also affect intellectual performance and behaviour.

Dosage range for treating deficiency (under medical supervision)
Depends on the individual and the nature and severity of the condition. *Adults* Usually 100mg of elemental iron (ferrous sulphate or gluconate) daily. *Children* According to age and weight. *Pregnant women* 30–60mg daily.

Risks and special precautions
Treatment should not be taken without a full medical consultation. Keep out of the reach of children. An overdose of iron tablets is very dangerous. Symptoms include pain in the abdomen, nausea, vomiting, abdominal bloating, dehydration, and dangerously lowered blood pressure; seek immediate medical attention (see p.197). Excessive long-term intake, especially when it is taken with large amounts of vitamin C, may cause iron to accumulate in organs, causing congestive heart failure, cirrhosis of the liver, and diabetes mellitus.

NIACIN

Other names: Niacinamide, nicotinamide, nicotinic acid, vitamin B_3

Why is niacin important?
Niacin plays a vital role in the activities of many enzymes, and is important in producing energy from blood sugar and in the manufacture of fats. Niacin is essential for the proper working of the nervous system, for a healthy skin and digestive system, and for the manufacture of steroid hormones.

Dietary and other natural sources of niacin
Liver, lean meat, poultry, fish, wholegrain cereals, nuts, and dried legumes.

Normal daily requirement
2mg (birth–6 months); 4mg (7–12 months); 6mg (1–3 years); 8mg (4–8 years); 12mg (9–13 years); 16mg (males aged 14 years and over); and 14mg (females aged 14 years and over). Daily requirements increase during pregnancy (18mg) and during breast-feeding (17mg).

Why take niacin supplements?
Dietary deficiency is rare. Supplements are required for those with bowel disorders in which absorption from the intestine is impaired, for people with liver disease or severe alcoholism, and for elderly people with poor diets. Large doses of niacin (up to 6g daily) may be used in the treatment of dyslipidemia (high cholesterol). Niacinamide is not used to treat this condition.

Availability: No prescription needed, except for high doses.

Symptoms of deficiency
Severe niacin deficiency causes pellagra (literally, rough skin); symptoms include sore, red, cracked skin in areas exposed to sun, friction, or pressure, inflammation of the mouth and tongue, abdominal pain and distension, nausea, diarrhea, and mental disturbances such as depression, anxiety, and dementia.

Dosage range for treating deficiency
Severe pellagra: *Adults* 300–500mg daily by mouth; *Children* 100–300mg daily. For less severe deficiency: 25–50mg daily.

Risks and special precautions
At doses of over 50mg, niacin may cause transient itching, flushing, tingling, or headache. Niacin in the form that occurs naturally in the body (nicotinamide), is free of these effects. Large doses of niacin may cause nausea and may aggravate a peptic ulcer. Side effects may be reduced by taking the drug on a full stomach. At doses of over 2g daily (which have been used to treat hyperlipidemia), there is a risk of gout, liver damage, and high blood sugar levels.

OMEGA-3 FATTY ACIDS (OFAs)

Other names: Omega-3 acid ethyl esters, Omega-3 oils

Why are Omega-3 fatty acids important?
There are many types of OFAs; some are found in plants and some in fish. Plant OFAs (such as flaxseed and soy bean oil) are broken down and used differently in the body from the OFAs found in fish. Fish oil fatty acids contain a combination of omega-3 ethyl esters called eicosapentaenoic (EPA) and docosahexaenoic acid (DHA). Omega-3-acids are polyunsaturated and are considered an essential fatty acid, as they cannot be made by the body. They may have many potential benefits and continue to be researched (see **Why take OFA supplements?** below).

Dietary and other natural sources of OFAs
EPA and DHA: salmon, trout, mackerel, sardines, and herring. *Plant OFAs:* flax seeds, walnuts, and canola oil.

Normal daily requirement
No specific recommended daily allowance for OFAs.

Why take OFA supplements?
Studies have suggested intake of omega-3 fatty acids can reduce the risk of some types of heart disease. However, this association is not well established. Fish oils may have a more positive benefit in those with heart problems than the plant fatty acids. Fish oils can decrease the amount of triglycerides (a type of cholesterol) in the blood, and should be used in conjunction with a healthy diet and exercise program. Omega-3 oils are also being evaluated in decreasing the risk of eye problems such as macular degeneration and in inflammatory conditions such as arthritis. Always consult with your doctor before deciding on a course of treatment.

Availability: No prescription needed. Preparations include capsules, oil, and liquid.

Symptoms of deficiency
No specific deficiency noted.

Dosage range for treatment
One study evaluating the potential benefits of omega-3 oils had participants eat 2 servings of fatty fish per week; in another study, participants took 850mg of omega-3 fatty acids daily. The Heart and Stroke Foundation recommends that eating fish twice weekly may be beneficial to heart health. Higher doses may be needed to decrease high triglycerides and for use in other conditions. Individuals on omega-3 oils may require monitoring by their health care provider.

Risks and special precautions
High doses may cause excessive bleeding in some, and there is also potential for interaction with medicines such as warfarin. There is concern about contaminants like mercury in some types of fish. Pregnant or breast-feeding women should consult their doctor, as safety in these situations has not been established.

SAW PALMETTO (NHP)

Other names: *Serenoa repens, Serenoa serrulata,* Sabal

What is it?
Saw palmetto is a shrub found along the Atlantic coast of North America. It has palm tree like leaves with white flowers and dark red to deep purple berries. The dried berries or its extract have been used for medicinal purposes.

Purported Uses
Used in the treatment of: urinary tract symptoms, prostate cancer.

Common Medicinal Use
Saw palmetto's most common use is for benign prostatic hyperplasia (BPH), the increase in size of the prostate in middle-aged and elderly men. It is thought that saw palmetto may work by blocking androgen receptors or by affecting an enzyme which affects the formation of dihydrotestosterone, both of which play a role in prostate growth.

Previous clinical trials indicate that saw palmetto may be better than placebo and similar to drugs used in BPH. However, more recent larger trials over 12 weeks have concluded that the effect of saw palmetto may help improve symptoms but are not significantly better than placebo. Symptoms which showed improvement include an increase in the amount of urine each time the bladder is emptied and a decrease in the need to urinate at night. There may be variability in the quality of products available when compared to the quality of the product used in the studies. Saw palmetto is available as dried berries or an extract.

Dosage range
Dried berries may be taken as a tea (0.5–1g) up to three times daily. The liquid liposterolic extract in capsules may be taken once to twice daily (160mg twice daily). The liquid extract (0.5–1.5mL) is taken once daily.

Risks and special precautions
Before taking saw palmetto, a proper diagnosis of BPH must be established to ensure that prostatic cancer is ruled out. Its long-term safety is unknown. Occasionally, it may cause stomach upset or a mild headache. There has been a case report of acute inflammation of the liver and pancreas. Saw palmetto may interact with hormonal therapy, including oral contraceptives. It may affect the absorption of iron. This herb should not be taken with medications used for BPH, such as finasteride. It may affect the blood's clotting ability and may interact with antiplatelets such as ASA, clopidogrel, and anticoagulants such as warfarin.

Its safety has not been established in children, and in women who are pregnant or breast-feeding. It should also not be used in women at risk of hormone-related cancers. As there may be variability in the products available, a recommendation is to look for the licensed natural health product, which can be identified by its 8-digit Natural Product Number (NPN) designation on the label.

ST. JOHN'S WORT (NHP)

Other names: *Hypericum perforatum*, Amber, Goatweed, Hypercium, Johnswort, Tipton Weed

What is it?
St. John's wort is a perennial plant with green leaves and yellow flowers. The flower tops and petals are commonly used for medicinal purposes. The extract contains many different substances. The two main chemical compounds responsible for its desired effects are hyperforin and hypericin.

Purported Uses
Used in the treatment of: depression, menopausal symptoms, premenstrual syndrome.

Common Medicinal Use
St. John's wort's most common use is in the treatment of mild depression. It may work by affecting the balance of neurotransmitters as components of St. John's wort are thought to have an affinity for various neurotransmitter receptors. In studies comparing St. John's wort to antidepressants, there is a suggestion that its effect is similar to standard drug therapy in mild to moderate depression. Most studies were carried out up to 12 weeks, and long-term studies are lacking. Also, variability in the quality of products available may vary from the quality of the extract used in the studies.

Dosage range
350–1,800mg daily, taken in divided doses. This is equivalent to a standardized extract of 0.3% hypericin and/or 2–5% hyperforin.

Risks and special precautions
St. John's wort may rarely cause photosensitivity. Other side effects include stomach irritation, dizziness, sedation, and restlessness. Its safety has not been established in children and in women who are pregnant or breast-feeding. St. John's wort may interact with many drugs by affecting their breakdown, including atorvastatin, oral contraceptives, anticonvulsants, medications used in the management of HIV, antidepressants such as SSRIs and MAOIs, triptans used for migraine management, and warfarin. Consult with your pharmacist or doctor before taking St. John's wort. As there may be variability in the products available, a recommendation is to look for the licensed natural health product, which can be identified by its 8-digit Natural Product Number (NPN) designation on the label.

VITAMIN A

Other names: Beta-carotene, retinol

Why is vitamin A important?
Vitamin A is essential for normal growth and strong bones and teeth in children. It is necessary for normal vision and healthy cell structure. It helps to keep skin healthy and protect the linings of the mouth, nose, throat, lungs, and digestive and urinary tracts against infection. Vitamin A is also necessary for fertility in both sexes. Beta-carotene is an important antioxidant (i.e., it protects the body from cell damage).

Dietary and other natural sources of vitamin A
Liver (the richest source), fish liver oils, eggs, dairy products, orange and yellow vegetables and fruits (carrots, tomatoes, apricots, and peaches), and leafy green vegetables. Vitamin A is also added to margarine.

Normal daily requirement
400mcg (birth–6 months); 500mcg (7–12 months); 300mcg (1–3 years); 400mcg (4–8 years); 600mcg (9–13 years); 900mcg (males aged 14 and over); 700mcg (females aged 14 and over); 770mcg (pregnancy); and 1,300mcg (breast-feeding).

Why take vitamin A supplements?
Most diets provide adequate amounts of vitamin A. Diets very low in fat or protein can lead to deficiency. Supplements may also be needed by people with cystic fibrosis, obstruction of the bile ducts, overactivity of the thyroid gland, and certain intestinal disorders, and by people on long-term treatment with certain lipid-lowering drugs (e.g., cholestyramine). They are recommended with other vitamins for pregnant women, children under 5 years, and nursing mothers.

Availability: Retinol and beta-carotene are available without prescription in various single- and multi-ingredient preparations. Derivatives of vitamin A (isotretinoin and tretinoin) are used in prescription-only treatments for acne and psoriasis.

Symptoms of deficiency
Night blindness (difficulty in seeing in dim light) is the earliest symptom of deficiency; others include dry, rough skin, loss of appetite, and diarrhea. Resistance to infection is decreased. Eyes may become dry and inflamed. Severe deficiency may lead to corneal ulcers.

Dosage range for treating deficiency
Oral doses of up to 30,000mcg daily in adults.

Risks and special precautions
Prolonged excessive intake (7.5–15mg daily) in adults can cause loss of appetite, diarrhea, dry or itchy skin, hair loss, fatigue, irregular menstruation, headache, weakness, and vomiting. In extreme cases, bone pain and enlargement of the liver and spleen may occur. High doses of beta-carotene may turn the skin orange but are not dangerous. Excessive intake in the early weeks of pregnancy may lead to birth defects, including damage of the central nervous system, face, eyes, ears, or palate. Pregnant women and those considering pregnancy should keep to the prescribed dose and not take extra vitamin A or eat liver products such as pâté (one serving of liver may contain 4–12 times the dose recommended for pregnancy).

VITAMIN B12

Other names: Cyanocobalamin, hydroxocobalamin

Why is vitamin B12 important?
Vitamin B12 plays a vital role in the activities of several enzymes. It is essential for the manufacture of the genetic material of cells and thus for growth and development. The formation of red blood cells by the bone marrow is particularly dependent on this vitamin. It is also involved in the utilization of folic acid and carbohydrates in the diet, and is necessary for maintaining a healthy nervous system.

Dietary and other natural sources of vitamin B12
Liver is the best dietary source of vitamin B12. Almost all animal products, as well as seaweed, are also rich in the vitamin, but vegetables are not.

Normal daily requirement
0.4mcg (birth–6 months); 0.5mcg (7–12 months); 0.9mcg (1–3 years); 1.2mcg (4–8 years); 1.8mcg (9–13 years); 2.4mcg (14 years and over); 2.8mcg (breast-feeding); and 2.6mcg (pregnancy).

Why take vitamin B12 supplements?
A balanced diet usually provides more than adequate amounts of this vitamin. Disorders that impair absorption from the digestive system, such as pernicious anemia, celiac disease, or fish tapeworm infestation, can lead to vitamin B12 deficiency – supplements are prescribed on medical advice. Supplements are also often needed for those on a strict vegetarian or vegan diet lacking in eggs or dairy products

Availability: Available without prescription in a wide variety of preparations. Cyanocobalamin is given by injection only under medical supervision.

Symptoms of deficiency
Vitamin B12 deficiency usually develops over months or years – the liver can store up to 6 years' supply. Deficiency leads to anemia. The mouth and tongue often become sore. The brain and spinal cord may also be affected, leading to numbness and tingling of the limbs, memory loss, and depression.

Dosage range for treating deficiency
Dosage varies depending on the individual's situation. **Pernicious anemia:** *Adults* injections of 0.1mg–1mg (100–1,000mcg) on alternate days for 1–2 weeks, then 0.1–0.2mg per week until blood counts are normal, then 1mg every 2–3 months. Monthly doses of up to 1,000mcg are given together with folic acid, if the deficiency is severe. *Children* 30–50mcg daily. **Dietary deficiency**: oral supplements of 50–150mcg or more daily (35–50mcg twice daily in infants). **Deficiency that results from a genetic defect preventing use of the vitamin**: 250mcg every three weeks throughout life.

Risks and special precautions
Harmful effects from high doses of vitamin B12 are rare. Allergic reactions may in rare cases occur with preparations given by injection.

VITAMIN C

Other name: Ascorbic acid

Why is vitamin C important?
Vitamin C is vital for the growth and maintenance of healthy bones, teeth, gums, ligaments, and blood vessels, and is an important component of all body organs. Vitamin C is also an important antioxidant and is used in the manufacture of certain neurotransmitters and adrenal hormones, and in the actions of several enzymes. It is required for the utilization of folic acid, the absorption of iron, and for normal immune responses to infection and wound healing.

Dietary and other natural sources of vitamin C
Most fresh fruits and vegetables, including citrus fruits, tomatoes, potatoes, and leafy green vegetables. Vitamin C is easily destroyed by cooking; some fresh, uncooked fruit and vegetables should be eaten daily.

Normal daily requirement
40mg (birth–6 months); 50mg (7–12 months); 15mg (1–3 years); 25mg (4–8 years); 45mg (9–13 years); 75mg (males aged 14–18 years); 65mg (females aged 14–18 years); 90mg (males aged over 19 years); 75mg (females aged over 19 years); 85mg (pregnancy); and 120mg (breast-feeding).

Why take vitamin C supplements?
A healthy diet generally contains sufficient quantities of vitamin C. However, it is used up more rapidly after a serious injury, major surgery, burns, and in extremes of temperature. Deficiency may occur in the elderly and chronically sick, smokers, and severe alcoholics. Supplements are recommended with other vitamins for pregnant women, children under 5 years, and nursing mothers. There is no convincing evidence that vitamin C in large doses prevents or treats colds, but it may reduce the severity of symptoms.

Availability: Available without prescription in a wide variety of single- or multi-ingredient preparations. Ascorbic acid: by injection under medical supervision.

Symptoms of deficiency
Mild deficiency may cause weakness and aches and pains. Severe deficiency results in scurvy – symptoms include inflamed, bleeding gums, nosebleeds, excessive bruising, and internal bleeding. In adults, teeth become loose. In children, there is abnormal bone and tooth development. Wounds fail to heal and become infected. Untreated scurvy may cause seizures, coma, and death. Deficiency of vitamin C often leads to anemia (abnormally low levels of red blood cells) – symptoms include pallor, fatigue, shortness of breath, and palpitations.

Dosage range for treating deficiency
For scurvy, 100–250mg of vitamin C is given daily for several weeks.

Risks and special precautions
Excess vitamin C is excreted in the urine, so risks of side effects from high dosages are low; however, it may affect excretion of some drugs – consult with your pharmacist. Doses of over 1g daily may cause diarrhea, nausea, and stomach cramps. Kidney stones may occasionally develop.

VITAMIN D

Other names: Alfacalcidol, calcitriol, cholecalciferol (vitamin D_3), doxercalciferol, ergocalciferol (vitamin D_2), paricalcitol

Why is vitamin D important?
Vitamin D (together with parathyroid hormone) helps regulate the balance of calcium and phosphate in the body. It aids in the absorption of calcium from the intestinal tract, and is essential for strong bones and teeth.

Dietary and other natural sources of vitamin D
Oily fish (sardines, herring, salmon, and tuna), liver, dairy products, and egg yolks. Also produced by skin with exposure to sunlight (ultraviolet (UV) light).

Normal daily requirement
400–1,000 IU (birth–6 months); 400–1,500 IU (7–12 months); 600–2,500 IU (1–3 years); 600–3,000 IU (4–8 years); 600–4,000 IU (9–70 years); 800–4,000 IU (over 70 years); 600–4,000 IU (pregnancy and breast-feeding).

Why take vitamin D supplements?
Vitamin D requirements are usually met by diet and normal exposure to sunlight. A poor diet and inadequate sunlight may lead to deficiency; dark-skinned people (particularly those living in smoggy urban areas), night-shift workers, and those who are home-bound or who live north of 40 degrees latitude in the winter are more at risk. UV light is also blocked by clothing and by use of sunscreens. Also, the ability of the skin to make vitamin D can decrease with age.

In areas of moderate sunshine, supplements may be given to infants. Premature infants, vegetarians, and the elderly may benefit from supplements. Supplements are usually necessary on medical advice for: preventing and treating vitamin D deficiency-related bone disorders, when absorption from the intestine is impaired; certain liver diseases; certain kidney disorders; prolonged use of certain drugs; some genetic defects; and the treatment of hypoparathyroidism. Supplements are recommended with other vitamins for pregnant women, children under 5 years, and nursing mothers, and with calcium to prevent or treat osteoporosis. The Osteoporosis Society of Canada and the Canadian Cancer Society recommend high daily intakes, with 800 IU daily for those 50 years of age and older and 1,000 IU for those with osteoporosis.

Availability: Vitamins D_2 and D_3 are available without prescription in a variety of multivitamin and mineral preparations. Injections are given only under medical supervision.

Symptoms of deficiency
Long-term deficiency leads to low blood levels of calcium and phosphate, which results in softening of the bones. In children, this causes abnormal bone development (rickets), and in adults, osteomalacia, causing backache, muscle weakness, bone pain, and fractures.

Dosage range for treating deficiency
Depending on the cause of the deficiency, dose to be determined; dscuss with your doctor.
Rickets caused by dietary deficiency: 1,000–4,000 IU daily initially, depending on the age of the child, followed by a maintenance dose of 400 IU.
Osteomalacia: 3,000–40,000 IU daily initially, followed by a daily maintenance dose of 400 IU. **Deficiency caused by impaired intestinal absorption**: Up to 10,000 IU daily.

Risks and special precautions
A daily maximum should not exceed 4,000 IU. Always discuss doses greater than 2,000 IU with your doctor. Prolonged excessive use disrupts the balance of calcium and phosphate in the body and may lead to abnormal calcium deposits in the soft tissues, blood vessel walls, and kidneys, and retarded growth in children. Excess calcium may lead to symptoms such as weakness, unusual thirst, increased urination, gastrointestinal disturbances, and depression.

GLOSSARY

The following pages contain definitions of drug-related terms whose technical meanings are not explained in detail elsewhere in the book, or for which an easily located precise explanation may be helpful. These are words that may not be familiar to the general reader,

or that have a slightly different meaning in a medical context from that in ordinary use.

The glossary is arranged in alphabetical order. Entries may include cross-references to further information located in other sections of the book, or to another glossary term.

A

Addiction
See *Dependence*.

Adverse effect or reaction
See *Side effect*.

Agonist
A term meaning to have a stimulating effect. An agonist drug (often called an activator) is one that binds to a receptor, and triggers or increases a particular activity in that cell.

Allergic reaction
An allergic reaction is one that appears not on first exposure to a drug but on a subsequent occasion. Causes and symptoms are similar to a reaction caused by other allergens. See also Allergies (p.33) and *Anaphylaxis*.

Anemia
A condition in which the concentration of the oxygen-carrying pigment of the blood, hemoglobin, is below normal. Many different disorders may cause anemia, and it may sometimes occur as a result of drug treatment. See also Anemia (p.35).

Anesthetic, general
A drug or drug combination given to produce unconsciousness before and during surgery or prior to potentially painful investigative procedures. General anesthesia is usually induced initially by injection and maintained by inhalation.

Anesthetic, local
A drug applied topically or injected to numb sensation in a small area.

Analgesia
Relief of pain, usually by drugs. See also Pain (p.38).

Anaphylaxis
A severe reaction to an allergen such as a bee sting or a drug (see Allergies, p.33). Symptoms may include rash, swelling, breathing difficulty, and collapse. See also Anaphylactic shock (p.200).

Antagonist
A term meaning to have an opposing effect. An antagonist drug (often called a blocker) binds to a receptor without stimulating cell activity and

prevents any other substance from occupying that receptor.

Antibiotic
A substance that kills particular bacteria. See also Other common infections (p.57–9)

Antibody
A protein manufactured by lymphocytes (a type of white blood cell) to neutralize an antigen (foreign protein) in the body. The formation of antibodies against an invading microorganism is part of the body's defence against infection. See also Infectious diseases (p.53–4).

Anticholinergic
A drug that blocks the action of acetylcholine. Acetylcholine, a neurotransmitter secreted by the endings of nerve cells, allows certain nerve impulses to be transmitted, including those that relax some involuntary muscles, tighten others, and affect the release of saliva. Anticholinergic drugs are used to treat urinary incontinence because they relax the bladder's squeezing muscles while tightening those of the sphincter.

Antidote
A substance used to neutralize or counteract the effects of a poison. Very few poisons have a specific antidote.

Antioxidant
A substance that delays deterioration due to free radicals (unstable oxygen atoms). Free radicals are generated by the body's normal processes and are thought to play a role in aging and disease. Vitamins A, C, and E are considered to be antioxidants.

Antiseptic
A chemical that destroys bacteria and sometimes other microorganisms. Antiseptics may be applied to the skin or other areas to prevent infection.

Antispasmodic
A drug that reduces spasm (abnormally strong or inappropriate contraction) of the digestive-tract muscles. These drugs may be used to relieve irritable bowel syndrome.

Autonomic nervous system
The involuntary nervous system that governs the actions of the muscles of the organs and glands in the body,

including such vital functions as heart beat, salivation, and digestion. See also *Sympathetic nervous system* and *Parasympathetic nervous system*.

B

Bactericidal
A term used to describe a drug that kills bacteria.

Bacteriostatic
A term used to describe a drug that stops the growth or multiplication of bacteria.

Balm
A soothing or healing preparation applied to the skin.

Blocker
See *Antagonist*.

Body salts
Also known as electrolytes, these are minerals that are present in body fluids such as blood, urine, and sweat, and within cells. These salts play an important role in regulating water balance, the acidity of the blood, conduction of nerve impulses, and muscle contraction. Examples of body salts include sodium, potassium, and calcium.

Bronchoconstrictor
A substance that causes the airways in the lungs to narrow, making breathing difficult. An attack of asthma (p.30–1) may be caused by the release of bronchoconstrictor substances such as histamine or certain prostaglandins.

Bronchodilator
A drug that widens the airways.

C

Cholinergic
A drug, also called a parasympathomimetic, that acts by stimulating the parasympathetic nervous system. See also *Autonomic nervous system* and *Parasympathetic nervous system*.

Contraindication
A factor in a person's current condition, medical history, or genetic make-up that may increase the risks of a side effect from a drug, to the extent that the drug should not

be prescribed (called an absolute contraindication), or should only be prescribed with caution (called a relative contraindication).

D

Dependence
Taking certain drugs regularly can cause physical withdrawal symptoms, such as sweating, shaking, and abdominal pain, if the drug is stopped suddenly. This response is called physical dependence and is prevented by gradually stopping the drug. Taking a drug for psychological reasons is called addiction or psychological dependence. Addiction involves intense mental ravings and physical withdrawal if a drug is unavailable or withdrawn. This term refers to compulsive use of drugs such as nicotine (in tobacco) and opioids when not used as prescribed for pain control. See also Tobacco addiction (p.45–6).

Double-blind
A test used to determine the effectiveness of a new drug compared to an existing medicine or a placebo. Neither patients nor the doctors administering the drug know who is receiving which substance. Only after the test is completed and the patients' responses are recorded is the identity of those who received the new drug revealed. See also Testing and approving new drugs (p.8).

Drip
A non-medical term for intravenous infusion.

E

Electrolyte
See *Body salts*.

Emetic
Any substance that causes a person to vomit. An emetic may work by irritating the lining of the stomach and/or by stimulating the part of the brain that controls vomiting.

Emulsion
A combination of two liquids that do not normally mix together but, on addition of a third substance (known as an emulsifying agent), can be mixed to give a complex liquid consisting of droplets of one liquid suspended in the other. An example of an emulsion is liquid paraffin.

Endorphins
A group of substances occurring naturally in the brain. Released in response to pain, they bind to specialized receptors and reduce the perception of pain. Opioid analgesics

such as morphine work by mimicking the action of endorphins.

Enteric coated
Treatment of a drug to give it a coating so that, after being taken orally by the individual, it passes safely and unaltered through the stomach and is released in the intestine. This can minimize stomach upsets caused by the drugs.

Enzyme
A protein that controls the rate of one or more chemical reactions in the body. Each type of cell in the body produces a specific range of enzymes. Cells in the liver contain enzymes; for example, cells in the digestive tract release enzymes that help digest food. Some drugs work by altering the activity of enzymes.

Excitatory
A term that means having a stimulating or enhancing effect. A chemical released from a nerve ending that causes muscle contraction is having an excitatory effect. See also *Inhibitory*.

Expectorant
A type of cough remedy that enhances the production of sputum (phlegm) and is used in the treatment of a productive (sputum-producing) cough. See also Common cold (p.27–8).

G

Generic name
The official name for a substance that is therapeutically active. The term generic is distinct from a product name, which is a term chosen by a manufacturer for its version of a product containing one or more generic drugs. For example: nitrazepam is a generic name; Mogadon is a brand name for a product that contains nitrazepam. See also How drugs are classified (p.9).

H

Half-life
A term used for the time taken to reduce the concentration of the drug in the blood by half. Knowledge of the half-life of a drug helps to determine frequency of dosage.

Hallucinogen
A drug that causes hallucinations (unreal perceptions of surroundings and objects). Common hallucinogens include the drugs of abuse LSD and cannabis. Certain prescribed drugs may in rare cases cause hallucinations.

Hormone
A chemical released directly into the bloodstream by a gland or tissue. The

body produces numerous hormones, each of which has a specific range of functions – for example, controlling the metabolism of cells, growth, and sexual development. Hormone-producing glands make up the endocrine system; the kidneys, intestine, and brain also release hormones.

I

Idiosyncrasy
Some side effects appear not to be dose related. Where such an effect happens when a drug is used and is pharmacologically unexpected, the phenomenon is called idiosyncrasy, or an idiosyncratic reaction. This happens because people are different genetically; they may lack a particular enzyme or an enzyme may be less active than usual. Because of this difference, they may react differently to a drug.

Immunization
The process of inducing immunity (resistance to infection) as a preventive measure against the spread of infectious diseases. See also Infectious diseases (p.56–7).

Indication
The term used to describe a disorder, symptom, or condition for which a drug or treatment may be prescribed. For example, indications for the use of beta blockers include angina and high blood pressure (hypertension).

Infusion pump
A machine for administering a continuous, controlled amount of a drug or other fluid through a needle inserted into a vein or under the skin.

Inhaler
A device used for administering a drug in powder or vapour form. Inhalers are used principally in the treatment of respiratory disorders such as asthma and chronic bronchitis. See also Methods of administration (p.13–4) and Different types of inhaler (p.30).

Inhibitory
A term meaning to have a blocking effect on cell activity, e.g., a chemical that prevents muscle contraction has an inhibitory effect. See also *Antagonist* and *Excitatory*.

INR
INR (International Normalized Ratio) is a standardized test to calculate the amount of time it takes for blood to clot. It is usually used to help determine dosage of warfarin, an anticoagulant drug.

Interaction
See p.12.

Intramuscular injection
Injection of a drug into a muscle, usually located in the upper arm or buttock. The drug is absorbed into the bloodstream from the muscle. See also Methods of administration (p.13–4).

Intravenous infusion
Prolonged, slow injection of fluid (often a solution of a drug) into a vein. The fluid flows at a controlled rate from a bag or bottle through a fine tube inserted into an opening in a vein, or via an infusion pump.

Intravenous injection
Direct injection of a drug into a vein, putting the drug immediately into the circulation. Because it has a rapid effect, intravenous injection is useful in an emergency. See also Methods of administration (p.13–4).

J

Jaundice
A condition in which the skin and whites of the eyes take on a yellow coloration. It can be caused by an accumulation in the blood of the yellow-brown bile pigment bilirubin. Jaundice is a sign of many disorders of the liver and may be caused as an adverse effect of some drugs.

M

Medication
Any substance prescribed to treat illness. See *Medicine*.

Medicine
A medication or drug that is taken in order to maintain, improve, or restore health.

Metabolism
The term used to describe all chemical processes in the body that involve either the formation of new substances or the breakdown of substances to release energy or detoxify foreign substances. The metabolism provides the energy that is required to keep the body functioning at rest and during exertion. This energy is produced by the metabolism from the breakdown of foods.

Miotic
A drug that constricts (narrows) the pupil. Opioid drugs such as morphine have a miotic effect. The pupil is sometimes deliberately narrowed by other miotic drugs, such as pilocarpine, in the treatment of glaucoma (p.24).

N

Narcotic
Once applied to drugs derived from the opium poppy, the word narcotic no longer has a precise medical meaning; some American sources use the term to mean any potent abused drug. Narcotic analgesic, a term largely replaced by opioid analgesic, is used to refer to opium-derived and synthetic drugs that have pain-relieving properties and other effects similar to those of morphine.

Neurotransmitter
A chemical released from a nerve ending after receiving an electrical impulse. A neurotransmitter may carry a message from the nerve to another nerve so that the electrical impulse passes on, or to a muscle to stimulate contraction, or to a gland to stimulate secretion of a particular hormone. Many drugs either mimic or block the action of neurotransmitters.

O

Opioid
A group of drugs (also called narcotic analgesics) that are given to relieve pain, treat diarrhea, and suppress coughs. See also Pain (p.38).

OTC
The abbreviation for over-the-counter. Over-the-counter drugs can be bought from a pharmacy without a prescription. See also Managing your drug treatment (p.18).

P

Parasympathetic nervous system
Part of the autonomic nervous system that is responsible for the stimulation of activities that typically occur when the body is at rest. These include salivation, digestion, urination, and reduced heart beat. See also *Autonomic nervous system* and *Sympathetic nervous system*.

Parasympathomimetic
A drug that is prescribed to stimulate the parasympathetic nervous system. These drugs (also called cholinergic drugs) are used as miotics and to stimulate bladder contraction in urinary retention. See also *Autonomic nervous system* and *Parasympathetic nervous system*.

Parkinsonism
Neurological symptoms including tremor of the hands, muscle rigidity, and slowness of movement that resemble Parkinson's disease. Parkinsonism may be caused by prolonged treatment with some antipsychotic drugs.

Patch
See *Transdermal patch*.

Pharmacist
A registered health professional who oversees the preparation, compounding, and dispensing of drugs, provides advice on the correct use of drugs, and helps detect, prevent, and manage potential interactions and other medication-related problems with your drug treatment.

Pharmacologist
A scientist concerned with the study of the actions and pharmacokinetics of drugs. Pharmacologists form one of the groups responsible for scientific research into new drugs and new uses for existing drugs.

Pharmacology
The science of the origin, appearance, chemistry, and action of drugs.

Pharmacy
A term that is used to describe the science and technology involved in the study of drugs. The term is also used to refer to the place where the practise of preparing drugs, making up prescriptions, and dispensing the drugs is carried out.

Photosensitivity
An abnormal reaction of the skin to light, often causing reddening. Photosensitivity may be caused by certain drugs.

Placebo
A "medicine," often in tablet or capsule form, that contains no medically active ingredient. Placebos are frequently used in clinical trials of new drugs (see *Double-blind*). See also Placebo response (p.11).

Poison
A substance that, in relatively small amounts, disrupts the structure and/or function of cells, causing harmful and sometimes fatal effects. Many drugs are poisonous if taken in overdose.

Prescription
A written instruction, usually from the doctor to the pharmacist, detailing the name of the drug to be dispensed, the dosage, how often it has to be taken, and other instructions as necessary. See also Prescription drugs (p.18–19).

Product name
The name chosen by a manufacturer for its particular version of a product containing a generic drug; e.g., Viagra is a product name for the generic drug sildenafil. See also *Generic name* and How drugs are classified (p.9).

Proprietary
A term now applied to a drug that is sold over-the-counter and having

its name registered to a private manufacturer, i.e., a proprietor.

Prostaglandin
A fatty (organic) acid that acts in a similar way to a hormone. Prostaglandins occur in many different tissues and have various effects, including causing inflammation in damaged tissue, lowering blood pressure, and stimulating contractions in labour.

R

Receptor
A specific site on the surface of a cell with a characteristic chemical and physical structure. Natural body chemicals such as neurotransmitters bind to cell receptors to initiate a response in the cell. Many drugs also have an effect on cells by binding to a receptor in the same way. They may promote cell activity or may block it. See also *Agonist* and *Antagonist*.

Replication
The duplication of genetic material (DNA or RNA) in a cell as part of the process of cell division that enables a tissue to grow or a virus to multiply.

S

Sedative
A drug that dampens the activity of the central nervous system. Sleeping drugs and anti-anxiety drugs have a sedative effect, and many other drugs, including antihistamines, can produce sedation as a side effect.

Side effect
This is a term that refers to any unwanted effects of a drug. Most of these unwanted effects are dose-related, increasing as the dose is increased. Other unwanted side effects appear not to be dose-related, such as an idiosyncratic or an allergic reaction. See also Side effects (p.11).

Subcutaneous injection
A method of giving a drug by which the drug is injected just under the skin. It is then slowly absorbed over a few hours into surrounding blood vessels. Insulin is given in this way. See also Methods of administration (p.13–4).

Sublingual
A term meaning under the tongue. Some drugs are administered sublingually in tablet or spray form. The drug is rapidly absorbed through the lining of the mouth. See also Methods of administration (p.13–4).

Suppository
A bullet-shaped pellet usually containing a drug for insertion into

the rectum or vagina. See also Methods of administration (p.13–4).

Sympatholytic
A term that means blocking the effect of the sympathetic nervous system. Sympatholytic drugs work either by reducing the release of the stimulatory neurotransmitter norepinephrine (noradrenaline) from nerve endings, or by occupying the receptors to which the neurotransmitters epinephrine (adrenaline) and noradrenaline normally bind, thereby preventing their normal actions. Beta blockers are examples of sympatholytic drugs. See also *Autonomic nervous system* and *Sympathetic nervous system*.

Sympathetic nervous system
Part of the autonomic nervous system that is responsible for the stimulation of activities that typically occur when the body is under stress. These include dilation of pupils, increased heart rate, and the dilation of bronchioles in the lungs. See also *Autonomic nervous system* and *Parasympathetic nervous system*.

Sympathomimetic
Having the same effect as stimulation of the sympathetic nervous system to cause, for example, an increase in the heart rate and widening of the airways. A drug having a sympathomimetic action may work either by causing the release of the stimulatory neurotransmitter noradrenaline from the nerve endings or by mimicking neurotransmitter action. The sympathomimetic drugs include certain bronchodilators and decongestants. See also *Autonomic nervous system* and *Sympathetic nervous system*.

Systemic
Having a generalized effect, causing physical or chemical changes in tissues throughout the body. For a drug to have a systemic effect it must be absorbed into the bloodstream, usually via the digestive tract, by injection or by rectal suppository.

T

Tardive dyskinesia
Abnormal, uncontrolled movements, mainly of the face, tongue, mouth, and neck, that may be caused by prolonged treatment with antipsychotic drugs. This condition is distinct from parkinsonism, which may also be caused by such drugs.

Tolerance
The need to take a higher dosage of a specific drug to maintain the same physical or mental effect. Tolerance can occur during prolonged treatment with opioid analgesics and benzodiazepines.

Topical
The term used to describe the application of a drug to the site where it is intended that it should have its effect. Disorders of the skin, eye, outer ear, nasal passages, anus, and vagina are often treated with drugs applied topically.

Toxic reaction
Unpleasant and possibly dangerous symptoms caused by a drug, the result of an overdose. See also The effects of drugs (p.11).

Toxin
A poisonous substance such as a harmful chemical released by bacteria.

Transdermal patch
An adhesive patch that is impregnated with the drug and placed on the skin. The drug is slowly absorbed through the skin into the underlying blood vessels. Drugs administered in this way include nicotine and travel sickness remedies. See also Methods of administration (p.13–4).

V

Vaccine
A substance administered to induce active immunity against a specific infectious disease (see Infectious diseases, p.56–7).

Vasoconstrictor
A drug that narrows blood vessels, often prescribed to reduce nasal congestion. These drugs are also frequently given with injected local anesthetics (see also *Anesthetic, local*). Ephedrine is a commonly prescribed vasoconstrictor.

Vasodilator
A drug that widens blood vessels.

W

Wafer
A thin wafer that is impregnated with a drug and placed on the tongue. The wafer slowly dissolves and the drug is absorbed through the lining of the mouth into the surrounding blood vessels.

Withdrawal symptom
Any symptom caused by abrupt stopping of a drug. These symptoms occur as a result of physical dependence on a drug. Drugs that may cause withdrawal symptoms after prolonged use include opioids, benzodiazepines, and nicotine. Symptoms vary according to each drug, but can include sweating, shaking, anxiety, and nausea.

INDEX

Entries that contain a page reference followed by letter 'g' indicate that the entry is defined in the Glossary on the page specified (pp.187–190).

Page numbers of main entries for drugs and ailment profiles are italicized.

DRUG POISONING EMERGENCY GUIDE

Although many of the first-aid techniques described here can be used in a number of different types of emergency, these instructions apply specifically to a known or suspected drug overdose or poisoning. This section is not meant to replace taking a first aid course. If possible, take a course to receive proper training in first aid techniques.

Emergency action is necessary in any of the following circumstances:
• If a person has taken an overdose of any of the high-danger drugs listed in the box on p.200.
• If a person has taken an overdose of a less dangerous drug, but has one or more of the danger symptoms listed (right).
• If a person has taken, or is suspected of having taken, an overdose of an unknown drug.
• If an infant or child has swallowed, or is suspected of having swallowed, any medications or any drug of abuse.

What to do
If you are faced with a drug poisoning emergency, it is important to carry out first aid and arrange immediate medical help in the correct order. The Priority Action Decision Chart (below) will help you to assess the situation and to determine your priorities. The following information should help you to remain calm in an emergency if you ever need to deal with a case of drug poisoning.

Danger symptoms

Take emergency action if the person has one or more of the following symptoms:
• Drowsiness or unconsciousness
• Shallow, irregular, or stopped breathing
• Vomiting
• Seizures

PRIORITY ACTION DECISION CHART

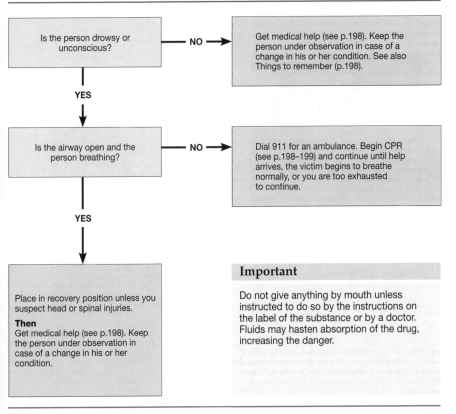

Is the person drowsy or unconscious?

NO → Get medical help (see p.198). Keep the person under observation in case of a change in his or her condition. See also Things to remember (p.198).

YES

Is the airway open and the person breathing?

NO → Dial 911 for an ambulance. Begin CPR (see p.198–199) and continue until help arrives, the victim begins to breathe normally, or you are too exhausted to continue.

YES

Place in recovery position unless you suspect head or spinal injuries.

Then
Get medical help (see p.198). Keep the person under observation in case of a change in his or her condition.

Important

Do not give anything by mouth unless instructed to do so by the instructions on the label of the substance or by a doctor. Fluids may hasten absorption of the drug, increasing the danger.

GETTING MEDICAL HELP

In an emergency, a calm person who is competent in first aid should stay with the victim, while others summon help. However, if you have to deal with a drug poisoning emergency on your own, use first aid (see the Priority Action Decision Chart, p.197) before getting help.

Calling 911 may be the quickest method of transport to hospital. Then call your local poison control centre, your doctor, or a hospital emergency department for advice. If possible, tell them what drug has been taken and how much, and the age of the victim. Follow the doctor's or hospital's instructions precisely.

THINGS TO REMEMBER

Effective treatment of drug poisoning depends on the doctor making a rapid assessment of the type and amount of drug taken. After you have carried out first aid, look for empty or opened medicine (or other)

containers. Keep any of the drug that is left, together with its container (or syringe), and give these to the nurse or doctor. Save any vomit for analysis by the hospital.

ESSENTIAL FIRST AID

CARDIOPULMONARY RESUSCITATION (CPR)

When there is no rise and fall of the chest and you can feel no movement of exhaled air, open the airway and immediately start cardiopulmonary resuscitation. This technique is used to continue breathing and output of blood from a stopped heart. It does not usually restart a heart that has stopped.

If you are untrained in CPR or unsure of your skills, provide chest compressions only and await advice from the EMS.

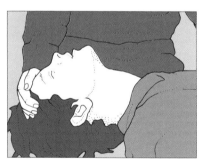

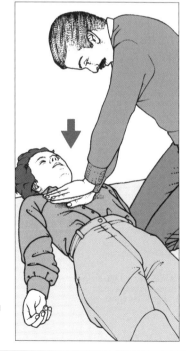

1 Lay the victim on his or her back on a firm surface. Place one hand on the victim's forehead and gently tilt the head back to open the airway. Wipe any vomit from around the mouth and clear the mouth of any obvious obstruction that might block the airway. Check quickly for normal breathing for no more than 5 seconds. If victim is not breathing, start CPR immediately.

2 Begin chest compressions. Place the heels of both hands one on top of the other on the centre of the breastbone, and press straight down to depress the chest by 4–5cm (1½–2in). Give 30 chest compressions at a rate of 100 compressions per minute.

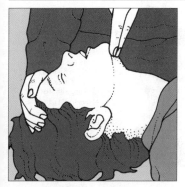

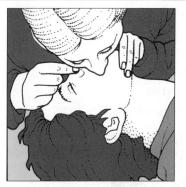

3 Return to the victim's head and check that the airway is still open by placing one hand on the forehead and two fingers under the point of the victim's chin and lifting his or her jaw.

4 Pinch the victim's nostrils closed with the hand that is placed on the forehead. Take a deep breath, seal your mouth over that of the victim, and blow steadily into the victim's mouth. The chest should rise. Repeat to give two rescue breaths.

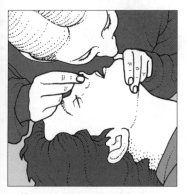

DEALING WITH A SEIZURE

Certain types of drug poisoning may provoke seizures. These may occur whether the person is conscious or not. The victim usually falls to the ground twitching or making uncontrolled movements of the limbs and body.

If you witness a seizure, remember the following points:

- Do not try to hold the person down.
- Loosen clothing around neck if possible.
- Do not attempt to put anything into the person's mouth.
- Try to ensure that the person does not suffer injury by keeping him or her away from dangerous objects or furniture.
- Once the seizure is over, place the person in the recovery position (below).

5 After each breath, turn to watch the chest falling while you listen for the sound of air leaving the victim's mouth. Continue the cycle of 30 chest compressions followed by two rescue breaths until emergency help arrives, the victim begins to breathe normally, or you are too exhausted to continue.

THE RECOVERY POSITION

The recovery position is the safest for an unconscious or drowsy person as long as you do not suspect head or spinal injuries. It allows the person to breathe easily and helps to prevent choking if vomiting occurs. A drug poisoning victim should be placed in the recovery position if more urgent first aid, such as CPR, is not needed. Place the victim on his or her side with one leg bent. Tilt the head back to keep the airway open, and support it in this position by placing the victim's hand under the cheek. Cover him or her with a blanket.

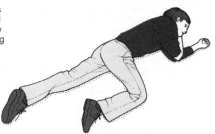

DEALING WITH ANAPHYLACTIC SHOCK

Anaphylactic shock can occur as the result of a severe allergic reaction to a drug (such as penicillin). Blood pressure drops dramatically and the airways may become narrowed. The reaction usually occurs within minutes of taking the drug.
The main symptoms are:
• Breathing difficulty
• Pallor
• Blotchy red rash
• Anxiety
• Swelling of tongue or throat

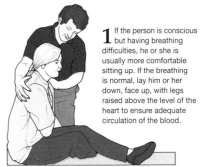

1 If the person is conscious but having breathing difficulties, he or she is usually more comfortable sitting up. If the breathing is normal, lay him or her down, face up, with legs raised above the level of the heart to ensure adequate circulation of the blood.

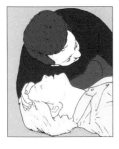

2 If the person becomes unconscious, ensure that he or she is breathing. If breathing has stopped, immediate CPR should be carried out as described on p.198–199.

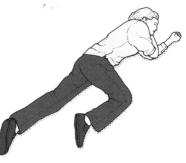

3 Call 911. While waiting, cover the person with a blanket or other article of clothing. If you have to leave the person, place him or her in the recovery position (see p.199). Do not attempt to administer anything by mouth.

High-danger drugs

The following is a list of drugs given a high overdose rating in the drug profiles. There are many other drugs not included in the profiles that also have a high overdose rating – some of them are listed here as well. If you suspect that someone has taken an overdose of any of these drugs, seek immediate medical attention.

Acetaminophen	Metformin
ASA	Metoprolol
Bupropion	Morphine
Codeine	Oxycodone
Fentanyl	Propranolol
Glyburide	Pseudoephedrine
Heparin	Quinidine
Hydrocodone	Rosiglitazone
Hydromorphone	Venlafaxine
Insulin	Warfarin
Lithium	

DEALING WITH VOMITING

Vomiting can occur as an adverse effect of some drugs and as a result of drug overdose.
 Do not attempt to provoke vomiting by pushing fingers down the victim's throat. When vomiting does occur, remember the following:
• Vomiting can be a sign of poisoning.
• Vomiting due to drugs is usually a result of an overdose rather than a side effect. Check in the relevant drug profile whether vomiting is a possible adverse effect of the suspected drug. If vomiting appears to be due to an overdose, get medical help urgently.
• Even if vomiting has stopped, keep the person under observation in case he or she loses consciousness or has a seizure.

• If the person is drowsy and is vomiting, place him or her in the recovery position (p.199).

1 Ensure that the victim leans well forward to avoid either choking or inhaling vomit. If the victim appears to be choking, encourage coughing.

2 Keep the vomit for later analysis (see Things to remember, p.198).

3 Give water to rinse the mouth. This water should be spat out; it should not be swallowed.